Categ
in
Social Psychology

Categorization
in
Social Psychology

Craig McGarty

SAGE Publications
London • Thousand Oaks • New Delhi

First published 1999

 SAGE Publications Ltd
6 Bonhill Street
London EC2A 4PU

SAGE Publications Inc
2455 Teller Road
Thousand Oaks, California 91320

SAGE Publications India Pvt Ltd
32, M-Block Market
Greater Kailash – I
New Delhi 110 048

British Library Cataloguing in Publication data

A catalogue record for this book is
available from the British Library

ISBN 0 7619 5953 X
ISBN 0 7619 5954 8 pb

Library of Congress catalog card number record available

Typeset by M Rules
Printed in Great Britain by Biddles Ltd, Guildford, Surrey

Contents

Preface

I have been planning a book about categorization for most of the last decade. However, the actual serious end of the writing started in 1997. This late start was probably fortunate given that developments in the field, and some changes in my own thinking, would have put earlier drafts out of date.

I have long been a big fan of short books. For this reason I feel I need to explain why the reader is now confronted with a tome of this length. The book is 50 per cent longer than the one I had intended to write, but contains approximately two-thirds of the material that I had intended to review. The explosion of interest in the topic of categorization has meant that I have not been able to review many topics as thoroughly as I would have liked.

Instead what I have tried to do is lay a path for the reader who wants an overview of the relevance of categorization for social psychology, from what can be termed an intergroup approach. Indeed if I had included a subtitle such as 'an intergroup perspective' this would not misrepresent the finished work.

I have reduced the scope of the work in two other ways. The first is that I have decided to restrict the pool from which I have sampled representative work to that by researchers (chiefly in social and cognitive psychology) who define the area of their work to be categorization. If I had instead sampled from research that could be said to be 'about categorization' or to 'involve categorization' I think my task would have been unmanageably large.

The second restriction that I have placed on the work is that I have largely made it a book of ideas rather than of empirical results. When I do deal with empirical results in some detail it is normally because I am attempting to make a particular point (often one quite different from the major focus of the original paper) or to show a representative example of research. My justification for this strategy is that our science has many avenues for the publication of empirical results: it has many journals that publish empirical research almost exclusively and some journals that mainly publish summaries of empirical results, and where edited book chapters are commissioned they often rely heavily on summaries of empirical results.

For reasons relating to lack of space and the inclination of authors and editors, empirically based papers often do not include much explanation of the ideas that provide the basis for the research. Furthermore, the interpretations of those results (even by the original authors) frequently change over time. The best place for providing a commentary about these changes in interpretations is in a monograph such as this one, and that is why I have devoted so much space to commentary here.

Many readers will note that my discussion of some widely accepted views in social psychology is, at times, vigorous. This stems not from any lack of respect for other workers in the field, but from my view of the duty that the author owes to the reader. No commentator on the literature can *guarantee* that s/he has adequately covered all relevant details. However, the reader should expect the author to present his or her views on the material that is covered in the clearest possible terms. I have tried to express my own views at this time as accurately as I can reflect them. If I had deeper or more serious reservations about the work of other researchers then I would have included those too.

My strategy for developing the content of this book has actually been rather simple. I have assumed that, apart from a few foundational assumptions that I present in Chapter 1, most of the key social psychological ideas about categorization are potentially deficient in important or interesting ways. Readers of Part II of the book will note that my own work, and that of colleagues with whom I have worked closely at various times, does not emerge unscathed from this critical process. Nevertheless, because I have cast a critical eye across the field it is easy to get caught up in the points of difference. I believe that the big picture shows that the study of categorization in social and cognitive psychology has made remarkable progress, that progress continues to be steady, and that much excellent work has already been done from many different approaches.

Part I of this book is the part that will be more suitable for advanced undergraduate students and graduate student courses. If the book is to be used for this purpose I strongly recommend that the text be supplemented by selected articles and chapters (some suggestions are included below). Readers will find a glossary of key terms embedded in the text for Part I. Although this form of glossary might be expected in a book aimed at a less advanced audience, I have decided that it is nevertheless very useful as a way of avoiding definitional imprecision and as a guide for navigating through the material.

Part II is my attempt to state and resolve a set of related problems in the field. To do that I open up some other larger and deeper problems. To make much progress it seems to me to be necessary to provide serviceable answers to those problems, and I also attempt that here. Chapters 9, 10 and 11 therefore may be of interest to those readers who might not otherwise be attracted to a book on the categorization process in social psychology. Given that reviews inevitably become out of date, Part II also provides a strong justification for the lasting value of a book of this type. In one sense a clear statement of answers to scientific problems never becomes out of date. Aspects may be accepted or rejected, perhaps in time the entire enterprise may be rejected, but it nevertheless stands as an alternative, providing at the very worst a guide as to what has been tried in the past and found to be unsatisfactory. This then is what I have tried to do in Part II: to provide as clear as possible a statement of my ideas (at least where those ideas are themselves reasonably clear) and the reasons for them so that you can accept or reject them as you see fit.

I accept that this is not as conventional or orthodox a practice in social psychology as it should be (except perhaps in anonymous journal reviews where much of the field's best and worst work is actually done). Much of the public discourse of social psychology today seems to me to follow the catch-cry 'Can't we all be right?' My answer is 'No, we can't' and I explain why in Chapter 9 (though this picture is qualified somewhat in Chapter 11).

My commitment to a conflictual approach to science owes much to my work with John Turner and I owe an enormous debt of gratitude to him and to other colleagues at the Australian National University including especially Alex Haslam and Penny Oakes. I trust that regardless of whether they find themselves agreeing or disagreeing with the details of my arguments they will recognize the approach.

Without in any way detracting from his great intellectual contribution to so many of my ideas here I must also single out Alex Haslam's influence in a different vein. The extent to which I have been able to manage a project of this size on my own reflects the beneficial influences of having previously worked with Alex on two books and a study guide.

Although much of the work that has provided the inspiration for this book has been collaborative in the most positive sense, the version of the views stated here is my own (with the exception of Chapter 9 which involves a collaboration with Diana Grace). The dangers in generalizing my current views to the numerous colleagues involved in that joint work more or less increase the further one goes into the book.

I would like to thank Mark Nolan, Alex Haslam, Wendy van Rijswijk, Mike Smithson and Michael Cook for commenting on sections of the manuscript or certain ideas contained herein. I would point out that in each case these people commented on an early draft: I had plenty of time and opportunity (if not motive) to introduce new errors of my own after they had looked at it!

I would like to thank those colleagues, students and friends at ANU and elsewhere who have helped me clarify my thinking about categorization over the years. Most of these individuals are referred to in the pages within, but I would like to thank Lyndon Brooks, Brenda Morrison, Peter McMahon and Mark Scarborough here and to thank Sam Penny for starting me off on categorization. Thanks also to Ziyad Marar and Naomi Meredith at Sage for their help and encouragement and to Brian Goodale for copy-editing and Seth Edwards for managing production.

Finally, I would like to thank my partner, Fiona Lynn, for her support throughout the writing of this book – even though this was somewhat tempered by her suggestion that I didn't appear to be a sufficiently 'tortured author'!

Using Part I for teaching purposes

Instructors of advanced undergraduate or graduate students may wish to consider some of the following papers as a minimum set of supplementary materials. I have selected the papers on the criteria that they strike a balance of theoretical innovation and empirical developments and that they have appeared in a wide range of readily available journals. For each section I have nominated two papers differing in approach or in a span of years to highlight developments in the field. In most cases I have selected the papers from social rather than cognitive psychology. In no case are the two papers addressing identical questions, but they provide good examples of research for instructors who will need to leaven theoretically focused seminars or lectures with empirical details.

Chapter 2

Section A: *The functions of categorization*
Anderson, J. R. & Fincham, J. M. (1996). Categorization and sensitivity to correlation. *Journal of Experimental Psychology: Learning, Memory, and Cognition, 22*, 259–277.
Bruner, J. S. (1957). On perceptual readiness. *Psychological Review, 64*, 123–152.

Section B: *Category structure and representation*
Medin, D. L. & Schaffer, M. M. (1978). Context theory of classification learning. *Psychological Review, 85*, 207–238.
Smith, E. R. & Zárate, M. A. (1992). Exemplar-based model of social judgment. *Psychological Review, 99*, 3–21.

Chapter 3

Section A: *Similarity-based approaches to category learning*
Gluck, M. A. & Bower, G. H. (1988). From conditioning to category learning: an adaptive network model. *Journal of Experimental Psychology: General, 117*, 227–247.
Nosofsky, R. M., Palmeri, T. J., & McKinley, S. C. (1994). Rule-plus-exception model of classification learning. *Psychological Review, 101*, 53–79.

Section B: *Theory-based approaches to category learning and use*
Murphy, G. L. & Medin, D. L. (1985). The role of theories in conceptual coherence. *Psychological Review, 92*, 289–316.
Medin, D. L., Lynch, E. B., Coley, J. D., & Atran, S. (1997). Categorization and reasoning among tree experts: do all roads lead to Rome? *Cognitive Psychology, 32*, 49–96.

Section C: *Categorization effects*
Krueger, J. & Clement, R. W. (1994). Memory-based judgments about multiple categories: a revision and extension of Tajfel's accentuation theory. *Journal of Personality and Social Psychology, 67*, 35–47.

Tajfel, H. & Wilkes, A. L. (1963). Classification and quantitative judgement. *British Journal of Psychology*, *54*, 101–114.

Chapter 4

Section A: Categorization as biased stimulus processing
McMullen, M. N., Fazio, R. H., & Gavanski, I. (1997). Motivation, attention and judgment: a natural sample spaces account. *Social Cognition*, *15*, 77–90.
Taylor, S. E., Fiske, S. T., Etcoff, N. L., & Ruderman, R. L. (1978). Categorical and contextual bases of person memory and stereotyping. *Journal of Personality and Social Psychology*, *36*, 778–793.

Section B: Categorization as the activation of stored knowledge
Higgins, E. T., Bargh, J. A., & Lombardi, W. L. (1985). Nature of priming effects on categorization. *Journal of Experimental Psychology: Learning, Memory, and Cognition*, *11*, 59–69.
Moskowitz, G. B. & Roman, R. J. (1992). Spontaneous trait inferences as self-generated primes: implications for conscious social judgement. *Journal of Personality and Social Psychology*, *62*, 728–738.

Section C: Affective, evaluative and motivational influences on categorization
Forgas, J. P. (1994). The role of emotion in social judgments: an introductory review and an Affect Infusion Model (AIM). *European Journal of Social Psychology*, *24*, 1–24.
Isen, A. M. (1987). Positive affect, cognitive processes, and social behavior. *Advances in Experimental Social Psychology*, *20*, 203–253.

Chapter 5

Section A: The social categorization tradition
Gaertner, S. L., Mann, J., Murrell, A., & Dovidio, J. F. (1989). Reducing intergroup bias: the benefits of recategorization. *Journal of Personality and Social Psychology*, *59*, 692–704.
Mummendey, A. & Schreiber, H.J. (1983). Better or just different? Positive social identity by discrimination against, or by differentiation from out-groups. *European Journal of Social Psychology*, *13*, 389–397.

Section B: Self-categorization and categorization
Oakes, P. J., Turner, J. C., & Haslam, S. A. (1991). Perceiving people as group members: the role of fit in the salience of social categorizations. *British Journal of Social Psychology*, *30*, 125–144.
Haslam, S. A., Oakes, P. J., Turner, J. C., & McGarty, C. (1995). Social categorization and group homogeneity: changes in the perceived applicability of stereotype content as a function of comparative context and trait favourableness. *British Journal of Social Psychology*, *34*, 139–160.

PART I

COGNITIVE AND SOCIAL PSYCHOLOGICAL APPROACHES TO CATEGORIZATION

---

1   Some Starting Assumptions: Perceivers' Perspectives and Social Consensus

A. Stating the problem

Categorization is the process of understanding what some thing is by knowing what other things it is equivalent to and what other things it is different from. It is widely studied in both cognitive psychology and social psychology and in other areas such as linguistics and philosophy. Indeed, it has such a rich and detailed usage in each one of these fields that researchers are often surprised when they discover rich veins of related work in another discipline.

The relevant research can be broken into two broad classes. There is research that is said to be about 'categorization' by the people who do that research. There is also research that *could* be said to be 'about categorization' or to 'really involve categorization' but the term is rarely or never used in discussions of such work. In this book I am only really addressing the first body of research in any detail, and even then I am largely restricting coverage to those aspects of research on cognitive and social psychology (and often their conjunction which can be referred to as **social cognition**) that I consider to be most relevant to particular (albeit sizeable) questions in social psychology. Even when we restrict discussion in this way we are left with an enormous body of research to deal with.

What I am attempting to do in the book is to (a) explain some of the important ideas in categorization research in cognitive and social psychology, (b) identify the important perspectives on these ideas in social psychology, (c) outline the major unresolved questions in social psychological treatments of categorization in a way that highlights the differences between these perspectives, and (d) suggest some answers to these questions.

The first two of these goals are difficult to achieve in their own right owing to the scope and diversity of categorization research. Many different researchers make related arguments using different terms or make conflicting arguments using the same terms. To address this difficulty I have developed a framework for describing approaches to categorization that allows us to consider them using common terms. I explain this framework later in this section.

To achieve the final two goals, however, I argue that we need a social psychological integration of the categorization process. In fact, several versions of such integrations have already been developed to varying degrees. The integration developed here is based on an articulation and further development of a particular approach which rests on four claims.

First, people categorize people including themselves. Secondly, different people commonly categorize the same things in the same way. Thirdly, people often categorize themselves in the same way as do other people. Fourthly, people often categorize things in the same ways as do the other people whom *they categorize themselves to be similar to*.

These are complex claims but they can be considered in terms of an example that will be familiar to many people in their everyday lives. Imagine you are going to watch a football match at a stadium between a team you support and a traditional rival. In order to understand the game you would, at the very least, need to categorize the players as belonging to different teams. To avoid being arrested you would need to categorize yourself as a spectator and not as a player. These categorizations are relatively obvious and may require little if any conscious thought on your part. More interestingly, however, you may come to categorize yourself as a supporter of one of the teams.

If you are like most supporters, as incidents occur on the field you will come to classify decisions by the referee or umpire as fair or unfair (and hence to be met with silence or derision) and segments of play as worthy of comment, applause or silence. You may well notice that many of your classifications seem to be shared by other people who support the same team as you.

However, you could also hardly fail to notice that the classifications that you share with other supporters of your team seem to be keenly contested by the opposition supporters. They seem to classify fair decisions as worthy of derision and often greet examples of the most scintillating play with stony silence. However, rather than being puzzled by this disagreement we actually expect this perverse behaviour from the opposition.

Let us now consider the claims I have made in terms of this example. If we accept that deciding what something is involves a process of categorization it should come as no surprise that the first claim, that people categorize themselves, is true. The alternative would be that people use some other, as yet undiscovered, process to know about themselves. However, it is obviously true that people see themselves as belonging to groups and organizations as the football supporters do.

The second claim, of common or shared categorization, also seems true given the vast evidence of consensus (and dissensus) in categorization behaviour. Supporters of different teams categorize behavioural episodes in different ways; they might also categorize clothing which bears the colours of particular teams as being appropriate or inappropriate to wear. Language provides us with terms with which to express our common categorization behaviour. We would become keenly aware of those occasions when we disagree with the categorization of something with those around us.

The third claim simply points to the existence of shared **social identity**. Not only do people see themselves as group members but, to a greater or lesser degree, other people see themselves as sharing or not sharing our group memberships. That is, the other people in the crowd can potentially see themselves as being the same as us or different from us.

While none of the first three claims has necessarily been uncontroversial in the history of social psychology, the fourth claim is the most controversial. Nevertheless, if we accept that people categorize themselves, and that they can share categories of things and persons with other people, then it follows that one excellent basis for deciding who we are similar to and different from should be the way *those people* categorize. We can determine the allegiances of supporters in the crowd behind us not by turning around to check whether they are wearing clothes of a particular colour, but by listening to the way they categorize (i.e., finding out what things they classify as good and bad or fair and unfair).

To take a more striking example in relation to the fourth claim, consider the fact that pro-life and pro-choice advocates disagree about the classification of a foetus as a child and the implications of that classification. The belief that foetuses are children drives the pro-life claim that abortion is infanticide. The pro-choice response is that that classification is far less important than the right of a woman to control her own body. Clearly, this differentiation between social groups is sharply defined by the categorization, and this provides the basis for both collective and individual action on this issue (see Chapter 9).

Exploring the merits of these claims is a large problem. How can we explain the ways people come to think the same things at the same time despite the well-established facts that (a) the contents of different people's minds cannot be *directly* communicated, and (b) there is a seemingly infinite number of different thoughts that any individual can have about any one of an infinite number of different things?

Taking the second point first, it is obvious that even the most mundane thing is open to widely different interpretations, but nevertheless we can act towards that thing in very similar ways. For most of us, wooden benches in a football stadium would be interpreted as places to sit and not as, say, sources of firewood. However, if circumstances in our own cities were to deteriorate in the way that they did in Sarajevo during the early 1990s our perceptions of those benches would change in similar ways. Still other transformations in perceptions would occur if a bench were included in an exhibition of modern art.

The idea of the transformation of perception due to changing needs and values is an old one in psychology, but it seemingly makes the task of explaining consensual behaviour more difficult. Given that, as we will see, we can eliminate coincidence and common experience as the sole general explanations of coordinated mental activity, social psychologists and others have instead posited a range of different constraining mechanisms that would enable social consensus to occur. Above all, two suggestions stand out in the history of social psychology: language and group memberships. That is, it is argued that different people act and think in the same way because they share a common language or because they share group memberships (and for two recent statements of these separate but not unrelated views, see Semin, 1997; Turner and Oakes, 1997).

We will consider some more issues that are relevant in relation to these claims in the later sections of this chapter. What I will do in the remainder of this section is to present a descriptive fram
ework that will be helpful for discussing many different models of categorization.

The descriptive framework that I propose in this book for discussing models of categorization is intended to be applied both to hypothesized relations between cognitive processes and to relations between cognitive processes and the social context. This descriptive framework is based on three components: the **perceived equivalence** of entities, **background knowledge** and **category formation/use**. These components are all psychological constructs or processes that are postulated to exist within the mind at some point in time. In order to use these terms we need assume neither that the hypothesized entity is consciously experienced by the perceiver nor that it has a long-lasting, continuing existence.

What are these components then? Perceived equivalence and category use are included in the definition of categorization that I provided at the start of the chapter. Perceived equivalence is the sense that some objects are equivalent or similar and are different or separable from other objects. Category use refers to the application of some category to a set of objects. Background knowledge refers to the ideas, beliefs, expectations and other cognitions that are currently relevant to the set of objects being considered.

These components and some of the constraints between them have been explicitly studied by both social (Berndsen et al., 1998; Turner et al., 1987; 1994) and cognitive psychologists (Medin et al., 1993; Murphy and Medin, 1985), and it is from this latter cognitive approach (especially Medin and Thau, 1992) that the idea of constraints is derived. My argument is that many different approaches to categorization can be defined in **constraint relations** terms.

Constraint relations are hypothetical causal relationships between components. The existence or strength of one component is held to increase the likelihood of occurrence or strength of the other linked component.

Constraints on category use can be understood in the following way. The recognition that two things are similar in some way (i.e., perceiving equivalence) might increase the likelihood that the stimuli will be recognized to share a category membership, or a new category membership could be identified.

To take an example of this process: the identification of many, many indistinguishable small green plants covering the ground may heighten the degree to which we understand the objects all to belong to the category *grass*. Similarly, the activation of background knowledge (e.g., knowledge of the way we have categorized in the past) may increase the likelihood that a particular categorization is used in the current situation. Thus, knowing that we have categorized small, green ground-covering plants as grass in the past may predispose us to do this in our current circumstances.

Perceived equivalence can be constrained by being increased or decreased by the other components. Our background knowledge can lead us to see things to be more or less similar to each other. You or I might see 'grass' where a lawn expert sees an array of different species and some weeds that are not properly considered to be grasses.

Background knowledge can be constrained in several different ways. A store of knowledge can be changed by being supplemented or by having its elements modified in some way. It can also be modified in the sense that certain elements or aspects become more highly activated or psychologically prominent.

Logically speaking, six constraint relations could apply between the above three components, but, as we will see, few perspectives really address all six possible constraints. The range of possible relations is shown in Figure 1.1.

My central argument is that these constraint relations can be used to define a theoretical model of categorization (i.e., a model of theories of categorization) that can be used to delineate different approaches to the categorization of non-social and social objects. In general, I consider a theorist to be discussing categorization when they discuss one or more of the constraint relations that I have detailed above (though this is most clear when category use is involved). However, the constraint relations formulation is not a theory of categorization in and of itself. Nor is it a closed system in that additional external constraints involving, for example, motivational constructs can be added readily.

Note that the same theorist might invoke different constraint relations at different times. Thus, one commonly accepted causal sequence would be that background knowledge and perceived equivalence could jointly con-

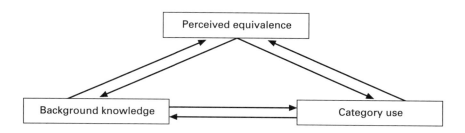

FIGURE 1.1   *The constraint relations formulation*

strain category use at time 1, but that the known use of that category could become part of the store of background knowledge at time 2. Thus, we could conclude that the ground covering is grass on the basis of prior knowledge and perceived equivalences and come to retain that recognition for future reference as part of background knowledge. When I need to depict multiple continuing constraint relations I adopt the practice of splitting the boxes to point out different aspects of the components, as in the example in Figure 1.2.

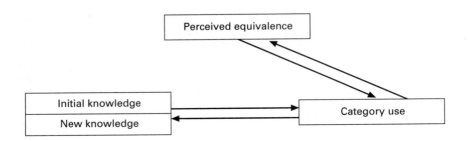

FIGURE 1.2   *Example of multiple constraint relations between subdivided components*

My strategy in the early sections of this book is to apply this constraint relations formulation to a range of issues in the study of categorization to better explicate the categorization process. I then go on to articulate a social psychological integration based on the claims that I made earlier in this section. In doing this my analysis will be guided by a number of assumptions. In the remainder of this chapter I will seek to make some of the more important of those assumptions as explicit as possible. As you will see in the chapters that follow, many other assumptions that are customary in the field will be rejected as we proceed.

To close this section though I should clarify some terminology. Throughout this discussion the terms **concept** and *category* will be used interchangeably to refer to mental representations. This has been common in the area though many cognitive psychologists prefer to reserve the term *category* to refer to things (objects, events, thoughts etc.) that exist, and *concept* to refer to mental representations of these. In practice though these writers still use the term 'category' to refer to mental constructs and I have done as these authors do rather than as they say. I will reserve the term *class* to refer to types of thing in the world.

background knowledge The store of knowledge about stimuli available to the perceiver. A subset of this knowledge may be activated at any time.

categorization The process whereby people come to understand a thing by perceiving it to be similar to some thing and different from other things. This process is treated here as a sense-making or explanatory process.

category formation/use The explicit or implicit (see later in this chapter) recognition that some stimuli share a category membership.

concept Although the idea has a long history in psychology, modern usage holds it to be a mental representation of some class of things.

constraint relations Causal links between psychological processes. The links can be positive or negative so that the link can serve to increase or decrease the dependent process.

perceived equivalence The explicit or implicit (see later in this chapter) recognition that some stimuli are alike in some way. Normally this is established in comparison with other actual or possible stimuli.

social cognition Both (a) the perception and mental processing of social phenomena and (b) the effects of social factors on perception and mental processing. The term is also used for (c) the area of social psychology that addresses these issues. Currently, the dominant approach to social psychology tends to focus on usages (a) and (c).

social identity In Tajfel and Turner's (1979) social identity theory it is that part of the self-concept that is to do with a person's membership of groups. In Turner et al.'s (1987) self-categorization theory it is a person's identity as a member of a specific group.

B. The mind is an interpretive perspective-based system

My first assumption is implied strongly in the previous section but it is well worth restating. I assume that a psychologically useful model of the mind's operation must take account of the interpretive functions of thinking, and must acknowledge that thinking occurs with respect to a perspective or vantage point.

In terms of the constraint relations model this point relates to the twin constraints between knowledge and category use. Knowledge, in the broadest sense, helps determine which perspective people will take, but the way we categorize something can also define one's perspective for future interactions. The pro-life advocate may come to categorize a foetus as a child because of a lifetime's exposure to religious, social and scientific norms (knowledge constraining category use), but once formed that categorization can serve to shape future experiences and behaviour (category use constraining knowledge). For example, it is meaningless to state that 'Abortion is murder' without first categorizing the foetus as a child. To take a different example, the claim made by certain animal liberation advocates that 'Milk is rape and meat is murder' rests on the classification of animals that other people customarily treat as natural objects as beings with rights to liberty and security which are equivalent to those of human beings.

The position I develop derives from what Turner et al., (1994; see also Turner and Oakes, 1997) refer to as **cognitive choice**. This refers to the selective representation of phenomena from the current vantage point of the perceiver. As we will see in the chapters to come, the mechanism that allows this is the *self*. In other words, the self enables the social determination of cognition by allowing the cognitive internalization of society and particular forces, groups and trends within society. This is a very complex point and we will return to it several times, but the groundwork for these ideas was laid by Asch (1952). He argued that the master problem of psychology rested on the *unique* capacity of the person and society to *contain each other*. That is, individuals are part of society but, in a special sense, society is also contained within the individual mind because we are able to conceive of society. The need to agree with relevant other people, despite many different conceptions of that same society, implies that the shape of our thinking is constrained by our presence in society. Importantly for the issue of perspective, 'society' is not uniformly distributed or stored within its members; rather particular norms, values and beliefs are endorsed by some members and contested or disputed by others.

To take an example, some aspects of the collective behaviour of supporters of rival sporting teams can be understood in terms of the shared norms of the entire crowd about appropriate conduct and the rules of the game. However, the definition of appropriate conduct is often contested by different groups as well. Exactly the same umpiring decision can be met with spontaneous delight or spontaneous derision depending upon which team is favoured by the decision. It is obvious to even the most casual observer that contesting views of the same reality are being displayed, even though there are also many aspects of common interpretation.

Irrespective of which metaphor of the mind's operation is used (popular current examples include **computational** or **propositional** metaphors), it will be of limited use unless it helps to explain how minds make sense of the world from a particular perspective. The theoretical task then is to explain the process and the experience of interpretation from a particular point of view and, as we will see, at a particular point in time.

The alternatives are worth considering briefly. A computationalist account of mind might treat interpretation, self, agency, intention and perspective as epiphenomena. That is, the mind could be seen as a system of connections which follow processing laws implied by the neural architecture – a proposition which is not disputed here. However, a common extension of the computationalist metaphor, which was shared by radical behaviourists, was that because higher-order mental phenomena are based on more primitive neurological events, there is no necessary role for the existence of those higher-level phenomena in the science of psychology.

The debate about this **reductionist** thesis is both vigorous and continuing, but for the purposes of the current proposal I need to make two claims. The first of these is weak but highly consensual in psychology, and the other somewhat stronger. The moderate claim is that higher-order mental phenomena such as perspective, intention, explanation, meaning and so on are important in their own right because they are subjectively experienced phenomena and therefore they are proper objects of study for a cognitively based science of psychology. As I say, this rationale is often seen as being entirely reasonable by most psychologists, defining as it does the very reason for existence of their field. However, I also propose a further rationale which is more controversial.

This claim is that higher-order mental phenomena and social interaction are mutual preconditions for each other – a point first made clearly by Mead (1934; see also Stryker, 1997). In other words, although a strictly computational account of the isolated organism may suffice to provide descriptions of cognitive processing, such an account will necessarily be deficient when extended to an account of two or more persons who are linked through social interaction. This is partly because social interaction depends upon the exchange of **symbolically** realizable mental phenomena (i.e., thoughts that we are capable of both thinking and expressing whether that be in the form of words or not), but also because the forms of social action which are achieved through social interaction rest upon shared forms of thinking. Genuine collective action involves people acting in terms of perspectives that they share. My argument is that people tend to coordinate their behaviour with others to the extent to which they share perspectives which have led them to develop closely matching explanations or interpretations of their common situation.

Let us return to the example of the sporting crowd. By and large, crowd members only coordinate their actions and beliefs with other people who support the same team. Of course, exceptions can occur when the crowd unites against the police or stadium officials or when the crowd spontaneously forms 'Mexican waves', but the most striking phenomenon is the contrasting behaviour and beliefs of two opposing groups of supporters.

Of course, the effects of communication and social interaction can be *described* in terms of the effects that these factors have on the neural states of individual minds. Social psychologists do not need to posit some mysterious essence in which social psychological phenomena are constituted. The creation of symbolic communication is presumably based on combinations of **sub-symbolic** patterns of neural activation within a communicator's mind. These symbols are then, we assume, decoded into sub-symbolic patterns of activation within the listener's mind. The fact that all terms in the process can be expressed neurologically does not, however, reduce the need to consider the causal role of higher-level mental phenomena because of the possibility that the pattern and forms of thinking are determined by social interaction.

In other words, it is argued here that the way we think is determined by social factors because thinking exists in the form it does primarily *in order to allow social interaction*. This view stands in stark contrast to many approaches in cognitive science, a point which can be explicated with an analogy. I argue that attempting to account for thinking without making primary reference to social interaction is like attempting to account for the behaviour of the share market without reference to motives for making profits and avoiding loss. Of course, such accounts of the stock market are possible, but they are by no means conventional, and are rarely seen to be *fully* satisfactory. The difference in the state of affairs in cognitive science is that it is routinely seen as *entirely* appropriate to develop formulations of thinking which do not refer to the social factors which provide the material conditions that enable thinking. There have, of course, been important exceptions in psychology and social theory and in this regard the work of Mead (1934) stands out even amongst a list of other impressive thinkers such as Asch, Bruner and Vygotsky. Recently Scheff (1993) has attempted to integrate Mead's work with that of Minsky (1986) on the society of mind, and one implication of such a successful integration would be an elaborated theory of socially mediated cognition.

What does it mean to say that social life and cognition are mutually enabling preconditions for each other? I will make a more detailed presentation of this idea later, but to foreshadow the argument I will briefly mention just three points. The first, which has already been mentioned, is that the existence of conscious thinking is essential for complex social interaction. We experience conscious symbolic thought for the purpose of communicating with other conscious, symbol-using beings and the forms that thought take have evolved to facilitate communication and the coordination of behaviour.

Secondly, the flow of conscious thought as the mind rapidly moves from one focus of attention to another is essential for varying perspectives, particularly perspectives that are shared or contested by other people whose behaviour also shows remarkable complexity and variability. We could not coordinate our behaviour with other people unless we each had a dynamic intellect that was capable of adopting new perspectives but which also experienced flow and variation in importance and continuity.

Thirdly, the existence of coordinated social behaviour implies that common constraining mental processes exist (in separate minds) which enable shared perspectives to be developed. In other words, complex mental processes which play a determining role in collective behaviour may be shared even though they are not directly communicable in symbolic terms. What is more, much of the regulation of collective behaviour can be considered to follow automatic non-conscious processes (cf. Greenwald and Banaji, 1995).

These are particularly challenging ideas. The suggestion here is that coordinated behaviour depends upon common perspectives but that these perspectives are not directly communicated. The implication is that the nature and scope of psychological functioning should be attuned in such a way to enable the mind to converge or diverge from the contents of other people's minds. This is despite the fact that people (a) have limited access to the operation and contents of their own minds, (b) have a strictly limited ability to communicate these contents to other people, and (c) are completely incapable of transferring the operation of psychological *processes* to other people.

The staggering feat by which people are able to coordinate thinking despite limited access and limited communicability may be the most remarkable achievement of human intellect. The achievement of this coordination and consensus provides the rationale for the next foundational assumption.

---

cognitive choice A term used by Turner et al. (1994) to refer to the selective representation of phenomena from the vantage point of the perceiver.

computational approach An approach to the mind that considers mental life as involving computations performed by neural processing units in the brain.

propositional approach An approach to the mind that considers the mind to be based on a complex hierarchy of logical structures.

reductionism A philosophical position that holds that because a higher-order phenomenon is based on the action of lower-order elements, the higher-order properties can be explained in terms of those lower-order elements. For example, the belief that the mind can be explained by reference to the activation of cells in the brain is a reductionist thesis.

sub-symbolic representation A representation involving perceptual elements that have no symbolic or linguistic representation. An example might be the perception of the texture of a wall pattern. The information is processed by the mind without the elements being (or needing to be) thought of as having distinct or discrete names.

symbolic representation Forms of representation which involve experienced symbols which have some form of correspondence to aspects of reality which can be expressed in language.

C. Social consensus and coordinated action

I adopt here the argument of Tajfel (1977) that the feature of social behaviour which most keenly demands explanation is not so much its diversity, but the fact that so many *different* people come to act in the same ways. By and large, social psychologists have developed three accounts for common behaviour: common language, common experience and shared group memberships.

These three accounts have different traditions and adherents. The role of language as enabling common reactions and behaviour stems from work in linguistic philosophy (e.g., Wittgenstein, 1974), critical social theory (e.g., see Billig, 1997) and research on **linguistic relativity** (e.g., Whorf, 1956). All of this work suggests, to a greater or lesser degree, that language systems constrain or shape thinking. We think in the same way as do our fellow language users because our language gives us words to express our thoughts.

We struggle to think things that we cannot say. As Billig puts the case strongly: 'The remarks are the thoughts: one need not search for something extra, as if there were something extra lying behind the words, which we should call the "thought"' (1997: 45).

Other accounts of coordinated behaviour have been developed in terms of shared situations and experience. This is to say, people behave in the same way as do others because they encounter the same stimulus conditions or share past experience with those others. Although there is a great deal of merit in this argument, it also runs into considerable difficulty when we consider the issue of behavioural and environmental complexity. Put simply, the enormous diversity of possible interpretations of situations along with the enormous number of different behavioural reactions to even simple situations suggest that other processes must serve to narrow the range of interpretive options and enable similar interpretations.

It is for this reason that the approach favoured here looks at the group as the source of social consensus. Indeed the primary social psychological function of groups can be seen as providing common perspectives through the development of social norms, and the key theoretical significance of the group concept for social psychology is in explaining collective behaviour.

The modern instantiation of these ideas develops out of the social psychological interactionism of Gestalt-inspired theorists such as Lewin, Sherif and Asch. Lewin (e.g., 1951) posited a field theoretic account of social behaviour where behaviour was seen as a function of the lifespace of the individual (the famous equation: behaviour = function[person, environment]). A critical part of the lifespace is the social environment, which in part comprises group memberships. These group memberships, which were made tangible for the individual by the experience of common fate, were conceived by Lewin to be inseparable from the person and the account of their behaviour.

The latter idea was developed and expressed in perhaps its most cogent form by Asch (1952). He rejected the idea of oppositions between the individual and the group and considered them to be mutually creative and complementary processes. Indeed Asch considered the group to allow the individual to go beyond his or her capabilities. Importantly, Asch rejected the prospect of mental events and processes that were not within individuals' minds. Rather he saw the task for social psychology as being to explain how a field within the individual mind came to be socially structured.

Sherif (1936) also played a crucial role by experimentally demonstrating how group norms can form. In particular, he showed that people who made judgements in a group setting mutually developed perceptual standards (judgements of the apparent movement of a point of light in a darkened room) and that these standards persisted when the group was no longer present. The revolutionary importance of this study was that it provided an experimental demonstration of the social mediation of cognition at a very early stage in the history of social psychology.

There were many important developments of these ideas in the late 1940s and the 1950s but for a variety of reasons (see McGarty and Haslam, 1997) they lost force within social psychology. However, the proposal of social identity theory (SIT) in the 1970s (e.g., Tajfel and Turner, 1979) ensured that the importance of the group in structuring psychological experience was restored to a high level of prominence in certain areas of social psychology.

It is impossible to underestimate the importance that the intergroup perspective of Tajfel and his colleagues had in leading them to conclude that group memberships powerfully influence perspectives and interpretations. This is because groups help generate both divergence and convergence. As I have been discussing here, what is remarkable about social behaviour is that different people behave in the same way in the same situation. However, we would not be aware of similarity between people unless there were some comparison standard that was different. Logically speaking it makes little sense to say that two things are similar unless we can also say that they are different from some other thing. Thus when we consider intergroup behaviour we see immediate comparison standards because of the processes which lead group members to conform to their own group norms and diverge from the perceived norms and standards of other groups. Unless we compare two or more groups we are unable to perceive similarities and differences and, in particular, if we study just one group in isolation we risk not seeing that the shared perspectives that develop within the groups are often developed in contrast to those of relevant outgroups. This is a point that was well understood by Sherif (1967) in interpreting his summer camp studies where groups of boys who were brought into conflict developed negative stereotypes of the outgroup, parallel to the development of social norms that assisted the group in engaging in conflict.

A theoretical understanding of the ways in which group members differentiate from outgroups and converge to the norms of the ingroups was provided by Tajfel and colleagues' early work on the categorization process (e.g., Tajfel and Wilkes, 1963). This process was conceptualized as a sense-making process whereby people differentiated between categories in order to make them coherent, separable and clear – a process which McGarty and Turner (1992) refer to as imbuing the categories with **differentiated meaning**.

This idea builds on the earlier ideas of Bruner (e.g., 1957) that perception involves an act of perception that allows the perceiver to go beyond the **information** given. The **categorization effects** perspective of Tajfel and colleagues gave this idea a more specific meaning. They argued that when we perceive categories we give them meaning by accentuating differences between them and accentuating similarities within them. The power and relevance of this idea for social perception was that these categorization effects are also applied by group members to *their own standards and norms*. Groups develop standards which are systematically different from the standards of relevant other groups and, through processes of mutual social influence, their members converge on those local standards.

During the 1970s the idea of categorization also became increasingly important in cognitive psychology. Moreover, this cognitive psychological tradition – as embodied in the work of Rosch (1978) but also E. E. Smith and

Medin (1981) and many others – had a strong influence on social cognitive psychology.

Social identity theory at the same time made a great deal of progress in specifying the conditions for collective behaviour by focusing on intergroup processes. The main ideas involved were categorization, identification and comparison. On the basis of the identification of shared social category memberships, group members were able to establish social identities which enabled them to perceive themselves positively by comparing their group with other groups, in the same way that individual people derive positive self-esteem by making favourable comparisons with others (Festinger, 1954).

Social identity theory, however, did not deal explicitly with social influence processes or provide an account of variable self-perception. These issues and others were addressed in self-categorization theory (SCT: Turner, 1985; Turner et al., 1987) which also drew on the cognitive work on categorization. The title of this theory is quite expressive: it is a theory of the way people categorize *themselves*, and thus categorization is not just something we do to other things and people.

An important precept of the theory is that the self is hierarchically organized so that self-perception can be located to a greater degree at an individual (personal) level or a group (social) level or a superordinate (human) level. On some occasions we view the world and ourselves from the perspective of a unique individual and at other times we perceive ourselves to be a member of a group and to share that perspective with other fellow ingroup members. Thus, at times we think in terms of 'I' and 'me' and at other times to a greater degree as 'we' and 'us'. The changes in perspective are driven by context such that categorization is largely driven by the fit between the objects being categorized and the category which is currently accessible (in terms of the perceiver's current intentions and past experience). The extent to which a categorization is being applied at some point in time is said to be the current **salience** (Oakes, 1987) of that social categorization.

The evidence for the role of this hierarchical variation in social perception has been rapidly amassed, especially in the areas of social influence and social stereotyping. A typical piece of research from a self-categorization perspective might involve demonstrating that people in different experimental conditions will react differently to the same stimulus when a different context is made relevant to them. The change in context drives a self-perception to a different level. For example, S. A. Haslam et al., (1995b) showed that Australian university students had a more positive stereotype of Australians when they judged Australians and Americans in an explicit intergroup context than when they rated Australians alone. The interpretation of this finding is that the explicit intergroup context makes people see themselves in social categorical terms so that the positive aspects of the ingroup are prominent in contrast to the negative features of the outgroup.

Above all, self-categorization theory can be seen as a framework for explaining how collective behaviour results from shared perspectives and shared understandings of a situation. As such the theory deals intimately with the relationship between stereotyping and social influence. Illustrative of this work, in recent times there has been explicit empirical work on the consensual development of social stereotypes (e.g., work on **consensualization** by S. A. Haslam, 1997; S. A. Haslam et al., 1996b; 1998).

These ideas allow a reconciliation in terms of the framework that I have proposed above. If background knowledge constrains category use then shared background knowledge will constrain common category use. Similarly, the use of shared common categories should serve to constrain knowledge. Semin quotes Vygotsky in addressing these matters:

> In order to transmit some experience or content of consciousness to another person, there is no other path than to ascribe the content to a known class, to a known group of phenomena, and as we know this necessarily requires generalisation. Thus, it turns out that social interaction necessarily presupposes generalisation and the development of word meaning, i.e., generalisation becomes possible with the development of social interaction. (1997: 296)

Given that social context provides the basis for mutual constraints between background knowledge and category use, the third element in the system should also be constrained. Consensual category use therefore should involve shared knowledge leading to the use of common categories which in turn leads to perceiving the same set of objects to be equivalent. Consensual knowledge develops, however, from knowing that the use of the same categories leads to perceiving the same objects to be equivalent. For example, a novice rock collector may come to learn the names of a set of minerals. This abstract knowledge only becomes useful knowledge though by watching an experienced collector apply these names to specific objects. The objects then come to be perceived to be equivalent and are then *known* to be equivalent. Category learning can thus be conceived of as learning covariations between category membership and similarities and differences between objects.

The two basic forms of consensual categorization are shown in Figure 1.3. In the upper form, knowledge which is shared with other people constrains the categories that are used so that stimuli are seen to be equivalent to each other. In the lower set of relations, common category use leads to perceived equivalence which leads to alterations in the current contents of knowledge. Much of this knowledge will be consensual but not all of it need be. Furthermore, not everybody would necessarily notice that the category use is common. Thus two people could use categories consensually but only one of them be aware of the categorization. You, the reader of this book, can accept or reject the categories of constraint relation that I advocate here. If you agree with me then you will be aware of the consensus between us but I will probably not be unless you inform me.

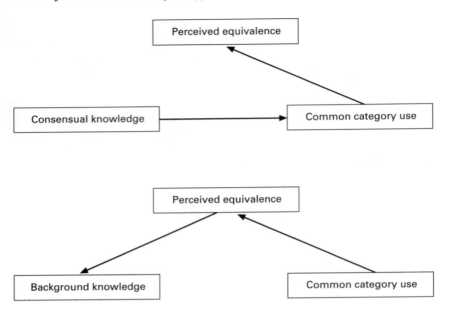

FIGURE 1.3 *Two possible constraint relations between knowledge and shared category use*

categorization effects The effects of categorization on judgement which were identified by Tajfel and Wilkes (1963) are the accentuation of perceived differences between categories and perceived similarities within categories.

consensualization The process of mutual influence whereby people's beliefs come to be both similar to other members of their own group and different from those of outgroup members. These differing views are often reflected in contesting or competing views of reality.

differentiated meaning Meaning which makes the members of categories separable, coherent and clear by virtue of their being seen to be different from the members of other categories.

information Uninterpreted or under-interpreted potential inputs to the mind. Generally, these are inputs which have not yet been linked to other cognitive elements or have been weakly linked to those elements. In everyday language we might say that a pamphlet contains 'bus timetable information'. To the extent that we internalize that information we can be said to have *knowledge* of the bus timetable. If, however, we simply learned the numbers in the bus timetable without associating the numbers with times in the day, it would still be appropriate to refer to our possession of *information* about the timetable.

linguistic relativity The idea that language influences the way people think about the world. This is also known as the Whorfian hypothesis (after Whorf, 1956).

salience A term with many different usages in social psychology. These include (a) perceptual prominence, (b) relevance or importance and (c) in self-categorization theory, the extent to which a category is psychologically switched on, activated or deployed in some setting.

D. Fluidity of psychological constructs

The idea of variable perspectives is of central importance for self-categorization theory. SCT assumes that perspectives are highly variable, that is, that people have enormous opportunities to interpret a complex environment in different ways. In part, the fluidity of mental structures can be seen as an appropriate response to a complex environment that affords many different interpretations, but this is only part of the story. In fact, mental fluidity is demanded by the existence of two other facts of social life, the implications of which are still not all that widely recognized (even within social psychology). I will address these arguments in greater detail later but for the time being I will merely summarize the nub of each idea.

The first point relates to social influence. A vigorous research tradition over the last century has established that people can experience genuine changes in their opinions following the exposure to persuasive arguments by relevant others, or even mere exposure to the positions of other people (see Turner, 1991, for a review). Assuming only that the opinion constantly refers to the same thing (not always a convenient or valid assumption), the existence of opinion *change* implies that mental structures can be fluid. The question is left open, however, as to how much fluidity there is in the absence of influence attempts.

The second and related point is that the existence of social consensus (which we discussed in the previous section) demands the existence of **mental flexibility**. This sounds rather paradoxical. Why is it necessary to posit the possibility of variability within individuals in order to explain the existence of consensus or consistency across individuals? The answer is that unless individuals were capable of changing their opinions they would never be able to come to agree. They would instead be forced to remain forever locked in irreconcilable disagreements. It follows that genuine social consensus rests not so much on starting at the same position but on creative attempts to view the world in new but valid ways.

Even though the facts of social influence and social consensus imply the need for mental flexibility, this idea has been the topic of a great deal of debate in the recent social psychological literature, particularly in relation to stereotyping. This is because many stereotyping theorists have adopted the view that stereotypes are enduring, rigid mental structures which arise owing to limitations in individuals' processing capacities (see Chapter 5 and also Oakes et al., 1994). To the extent that the sharedness of these stereotypes is addressed in social cognitive work (from the perspective I refer to as the biased processing approach in Chapter 4) it is normally seen to arise from the common experience of individuals in confronting an overwhelmingly complex environment.

Recently, however, the idea of mental flexibility has received stronger endorsement from social cognitive psychologists (e.g., Carlston and E. R. Smith, 1996; Uleman et al., 1996). Part of the reasons for this change can be attributed to the rise of **connectionist** ideas in social psychology. As Read et al., (1997) explain, connectionist ideas are well suited to addressing changes in complex mental structures over time.

Given that the prospect of mental fluidity is gaining wider acceptance it is useful to think about what form such flexibility can take. Broadly speaking there are four ways that this idea can be accommodated. These different interpretations of the concept of mental flexibility reflect different conceptualizations of mental organization (though some of the following approaches can be reconciled with each other).

Mental flexibility can result from the creation of new mental elements. That is, the contents of the mind may be altered because those contents are created anew for each occasion to deal with new circumstances. An example of this sort of flexibility is provided in the literature on stereotype formation (e.g., Hamilton and Gifford, 1976; McGarty and de la Haye, 1997; see Chapter 8). Following exposure to members of a social group, people develop mental structures which guide their perceptions and judgements of those groups. As I will detail in the chapters to come, authors such as Oakes et al., (1994) argue that mental entities such as social categories have the potential to be of very short duration though they also acknowledge the possibility of longer-term constraining entities such as background theories (cf. Murphy and Medin, 1985). The chief source of stability in mental life according to this approach though is the existence of stable contexts and social relations.

Mental flexibility can also be accounted for by the possibility that mental structures are switched on or off (or turned up or down). This is what is envisaged by Higgins (1996) when discussing the principles of mental accessibility. Mental structures such as knowledge about particular things can be highly activated at some times and relatively dormant at others. The *apparent* contents of the mind will thus vary from occasion to occasion.

Yet another possibility is that existing concepts are altered. Mental flexibility can be accounted for by positing the existence of some mental structure which becomes altered through the action of psychological processes. This idea is inherent in much of the literature on attitude change. Attitudes are often assumed to be relatively stable mental structures which are capable of being changed by persuasion (Hovland et al., 1953). Similarly, in the domain of self-concept change the self is often viewed as an enduring mental structure that changes gradually as a consequence of identity-threatening events and behaviours (see for example, Markus and Wurf, 1987).

Still another possible way for accounting for mental flexibility is to assume that elements which have a continuing existence are combined in different ways. This idea lies at the heart of E. R. Smith and Zárate's (1992) **exemplar** model of social judgement. Exemplars are representations of stimuli which are stored in a stable form at the time of encoding but categories are formed by recombining those exemplars in different ways. Thus the higher-level mental constructs such as impressions, categories and judgements are inherently fluid because they are created afresh for each cognitive situation even though the lower-level elements are highly stable. In Smith and Zárate's (1992) formulation there are no fixed categories. Every time we categorize some set of objects we combine the exemplars in a new way.

It is obvious from even this necessarily brief overview that there are many different meanings and usages of the idea of mental flexibility, and it is also obvious that there are compatibilities and incompatibilities between various usages. The assumption that I make is that we need to consider all of these bases for flexibility in psychological theorizing. In order to do this fruitfully though, it is necessary to specify the language that we use for this sort of psychological theorizing more clearly. I will suggest that recent connectionist developments in cognitive science are useful in this regard, and, as E. R. Smith (1996) and Read et al., (1997) have argued, these developments are particularly important for social psychology.

It also seems apparent that there must be some constancy in all this mental fluidity. Complete fluidity or total variability actually suggests a form of stability. In order for change to be noticed it must be sufficiently long-lasting to be detected. Thus, a random pattern such as white noise is highly variable but can also be perceived to have a repetitive sameness. One point of constancy is the flow and the experience of **historical continuity** of the perceiver. The crucial role that the flow of conscious thoughts plays as an organizing principle in cognition is a theme that I will return to on more than one occasion.

Acknowledging the fluidity in mental life is also very important for establishing the appropriate methodological strategies for testing social psychological theories. Experimental techniques are most appropriate for investigating dynamic mental processes which can be changed over a short period, whereas surveys are most appropriate for investigating stable and enduring psychological constructs (for a full discussion of this see Haslam and McGarty, 1998). Thus before we can decide on the appropriateness of methodological techniques we need theories which specify the speed of the effects we are interested in. As we will see in the chapters to follow, the focus of experimental social psychology on research sessions which last for periods of 60 minutes or less may create specific requirements for social psychological theory. For example, manipulations of the salience of social categorizations, which involve creating a feeling of identification with some group, are often expected to have effects that last for the duration of an experimental session. To explain how this could occur we need to posit the existence of a psychological process or structure that could endure for at least that length of time.

Returning to the theoretic model we can see that the constraint relations that I have specified imply relative amounts of dynamism for the various elements. Category use and perceived equivalence are clearly dynamic, fluid things. Even though we may deploy different aspects of knowledge at different times, and that store of knowledge may be augmented through learning, the elements available to be sampled may nevertheless have a relatively enduring existence.

---

connectionism An approach to cognitive science which conceives of the mind as being made up of many different elements that are connected to each other. The activation of some units will therefore have consequences for the states of other units.

exemplar A member of a category. The term is used at different times to refer to both an encountered stimulus and the representation of that stimulus in the mind.

historical continuity The continuing existence of an entity over time, and in particular, the continuity of those entities which are known or can be expected to maintain an existence over time.

mental flexibility The idea of change in mental phenomena. Such flexibility can take a number of forms involving: addition to existing mental entities, modification of existing entities, replacement of existing entities, varying sampling from a pool of available entities, and new combinations of existing entities.

E. Conscious and non-conscious processes

It is a curious feature of recent social psychological theorizing that the area is criticized for neglecting both conscious psychological processes and unconscious ones. For example, authors such as Moscovici (1993) and Greenwald and Banaji (1995) have decried the absence of treatments of the unconscious. Paradoxically though, there is not much work in social psychology which explicitly addresses vivid conscious representations either. This might reflect the effect of Nisbett and Wilson's (1977) caution that perceivers do not necessarily have access to the psychological factors which cause their behaviour.

It probably seems barely credible that both could be neglected: surely social psychological theorizing must focus on one or the other? However, much social psychological theorizing has subsisted in a gloomy half-light where we seldom seek to differentiate between mental events in terms of whether they are accessible to the conscious mind. Partly this stems from the behaviourist past of much of social psychology. Given the ambiguity about the prospect of individuals' access to their own mental states, the easier path has often been to theorize about processes without clearly stating whether they are conscious or non-conscious, and this has in fact been a fruitful strategy. As Bargh (1994; 1996) argues, multiple dimensions are necessary to differentiate between conscious and unconscious processes. A problem persists though because certain features of conscious mental activity make it of great importance for understanding the social mediation of cognition.

Conscious and non-conscious mental events appear to have a different character, and it is important to make the distinction for theoretical and methodological reasons, but it is nevertheless possible that conscious and non-conscious mental activity are distinct outgrowths of a single explanatory system. A good reason for entertaining this possibility is the social psychological observation that a great deal of coordinated activity seems to arise from shared understandings. For example, we can apply grammatical rules in much the same way as other people without being able to articulate those rules. Nonetheless where we do know the rules explicitly we can explicitly vary our usage in some instance.

In terms of the constraint relations model we can apply a conclusion similar to that in the previous section. There is no reason to assume that all elements (category use, knowledge and perceived equivalence) are equally accessible to the conscious mind. In particular, it is safe to assume that much of the long-term knowledge that is *available* in the mind will vary in its *accessibility* (for a fuller discussion of these ideas see Chapter 4 in this volume and Higgins, 1996).

How to approach this book

This chapter has given the briefest sketch of the ideas and issues that I am seeking to reconcile here. I therefore need to present these ideas and issues in much greater detail. This process is carried out in the remainder of Part I where I deal with a number of developments in the treatment of the categorization process in cognitive and social psychology. Chapters 2 and 3 deal with a series of topics in categorization research, mainly in areas of cognitive psychology. These chapters attempt to provide a dense, detailed and up-to-date treatment of the aspects of contemporary categorization research that I think are most relevant to social psychology. To aid comprehensibility I have tried to put most of the major approaches in constraint relations terms. The material is difficult but many of the issues which I cover in some detail are also major topics in social psychology in their own right. You will observe also that many of the difficult questions about categorizations – positions that I think researchers must almost inevitably take a stance on – are present in the cognitive literature.

In Chapters 4, 5 and 6 I outline some alternative approaches taken towards categorization in social psychology. In Chapter 7 I try to put these approaches in oppositional terms by stressing their competing treatments of some of the unresolved issues from Part I as well as some new issues which are of more specific interest in social psychology.

Part II involves a more selective examination of issues that relate to categorization in social psychology using the assumptions that I have outlined in Chapter 1. In these chapters I attempt to provide my own answers to what I see to be key problems in the study of categorization.

2 Categorization and Cognition I: Introducing Category Function and Structure

In this chapter and the next I will discuss literature drawn from both cognitive and social psychological approaches to categorization. This strategy is practicable because the disagreements and controversies that occur in this field are not between cognitive and social psychologists as such (though of course social and cognitive psychologists have different priorities and interests) but between proponents of different approaches to categorization that span both social and cognitive psychology. The intention here is to give the merest flavour of a vast body of research, a reasonably detailed summary of which would fill many volumes the size of this one, though at the same time I hope to provide enough signposts for the reader to access the specific details that are not included here. In Chapters 4, 5 and 6 I will focus more specifically on research that deals with social categorization.

I need to make two more global points before commencing this review. The distinctions that I make between the section headings in this chapter are questionable because there is inevitably overlap between them. In reality, the structure and representation of categories cannot be discussed separately from the functions of categories – even though I would argue that a number of research programmes have attempted to do precisely that. The structure of this review is thus an attempt to capture these different research priorities, particularly where I see strong implications for social psychology.

I have also tried to identify in each section in Chapters 2 and 3 one or more critical branches or choice points. These are issues where I feel that researchers have to make choices because one's stance on the issue will have strong effects on one's understanding of the categorization process. These choice points are by no means the most bitterly contested issues in the field, as they often involve meta-theoretical debates. The most hotly contested issues on the other hand tend to relate to issues that are more readily addressed by empirical studies.

In other words, I am trying to single out the big-picture questions in the cognitive psychology of categorization that are relevant to the issue of social thinking. Answers to these questions have already been proposed in many cases: the problem is not so much that there is no answer but that there is more than one answer that has wide currency in the literature. In the chapters to come, I will expand upon the sort of answers to these questions that I tend to favour; for the moment though I merely want to suggest that a perspective needs to be taken on each choice point.

A. The functions of categorization

In an intriguing short paper Barsalou (1990) sketched the categorization process in an elegant manner that is worth revisiting. He distinguished between the domains of *access* and *inference* in categorization. Access relates to the detection of featural information about some stimulus. This information is then transferred to a categorization system which activates possible categories and decides which of many possible categories applies to the stimulus. Inference, on the other hand, relates to what we actually do with the category, once the decision is made to categorize a stimulus in some way. The cognitive aspects of this process involve making inferences or drawing conclusions about the stimulus, including deciding how we will act towards it. The inference domain of categorization therefore relates to the functions of categorization (why we do it and what we do it for, rather than how we do it), and Barsalou points out that, despite some exceptions, the questions of inference have largely been a focus of interest in social psychology rather than cognitive psychology (which has focused more on questions of access). In line with Barsalou's observations Krueger and Clement (1994) note that cognitive psychologists commonly use reaction time measures (which, I submit, are good measures of access) and social psychologists use judgemental measures (which require inferences). Barsalou argues plausibly that these divisions of labour do not aid progress in the study of categorization.

Issues of both access and inference can be encapsulated in the form of constraint relations (Figure 2.1). Deciding on the category membership of a stimulus refers to the constraints of perceived equivalence and background knowledge on category use. If we know that a stimulus is similar to other blades of grass and we have previously used the categorization grass/not-grass in similar circumstances then we will be more likely to apply it again.

Drawing inferences involves the constraining effect of category use on

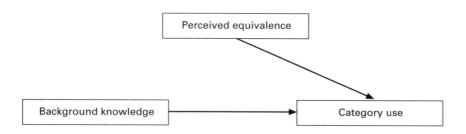

FIGURE 2.1   *Constraint relations involved in access to categories*

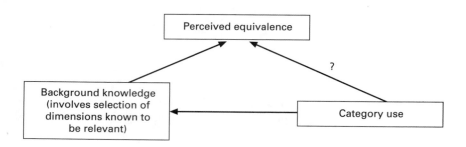

FIGURE 2.2   *Constraint relations involved in inferences from categories*

perceived equivalence and background knowledge. Recognizing that an object is a blade of grass means that we can expect relevant similarities and differences and we can also store knowledge about category assignments for future reference. The word 'relevant' creates an immediate ambiguity. Does category use have a direct constraining effect on perceived equivalence? The idea of relevance implies a selection process so that effects occur on dimensions known to be relevant.

This raises the possibility that the effect of category use on perceived equivalence is mediated by background knowledge. For our immediate purposes though, Figure 2.2 should suffice. The question mark on the link between category use and perceived equivalence conveys the doubt about the possibility of the direct effect.

Categorization emerged most clearly as a central process in social psychology in the work of Allport (1954) on prejudice, but his concerns were soon to be echoed in the writings of a range of other authors. The relevance of categorization to this was that Allport argued that prejudice was based on the perception and accentuation of differences between groups.

To illustrate this idea consider the statements often attributed to white bigots that 'all blacks (or Chinese) look alike' or 'those Jews are all the same'. Such statements carry with them two powerful ideas. The first of these is that perceiving people as group members is associated with small perceived differences within groups. That is, treating someone as a group member makes it difficult to perceive the unique qualities of the individual. If we make the familiar leap in psychology that our perceptions enable certain sorts of action then we have the seed of an explanation of prejudice. If people cannot differentiate between members of a group perceptually they cannot treat them as distinct individuals.

However, the simple statement that 'all blacks look alike' also conveys a prior unspoken assumption. To say that all blacks are alike also assumes not only that blacks are similar to each other but that they are different from other groups. Otherwise the bigot would say that 'all people are the same' or even that 'blacks look like me'. In other words, social categorization has the immediate effect of drawing attention to differences between groups as well as similarities within groups. It was recognized by Campbell that these categorization processes could apply to judgements that did not have a physical, perceptual basis:

> One important aspect of the general syndrome of social stereotyping is *enhancement of contrast* or the exaggeration of relative differences between social groups. Thus if on intelligence tests in New York City schools Jewish students test slightly higher than white Christian students, and Negro students slightly lower, these small differences are exaggerated in social stereotypes about the students into the judgments that Negroes are 'dumb' and Jews are 'smart'. (1956: 350)

Allport (1954) also provided a functional explanation for the categorization process. We categorize because the amount of information that we would otherwise be required to process would overwhelm our capacity.

1   Categorization forms large classes and clusters for guiding our daily adjustments. The argument is that we have so many daily experiences that we need to type them. Open-mindedness literally cannot occur, as we handle new experiences in terms of existing categories. Allport quotes Bertrand Russell: 'A mind perpetually open will be a mind perpetually vacant' (1954: 20).
2   Categorization assimilates as much as it can to the cluster. We tend to categorize things and events into the most general categories we can get away with in everyday life.
3   Categories enable us quickly to identify a related object. Categories are automatically linked to perception. Their function is to facilitate perception and behaviour, even though we can make mistakes while using these categories.
4   The category saturates all that it contains with the same ideational and emotional flavour. Allport argues that there are intellectual categories which we call concepts (*chair* would be an example). There are also concepts which are associated with feelings (or connotative meanings), and these concepts include group memberships.
5   Categories may be more or less rational. Categories generally contain a kernel of truth but they are only rational if they have a high probability of being true. Allport suggests that irrational categories (ones with a low probability of being true) form as easily as rational categories.

In terms of the model of constraint relations both Allport and Campbell were arguing for reciprocal relations between perceived equivalence and category use. When Allport says that a category saturates all it contains with the same ideational and emotional flavour, or Campbell says that stereotyping enhances contrast, they are arguing that using categories leads to a perceived equivalence of their members. Less explicit in these passages, but also contained in their work, was the idea that the categories we can use are constrained by the experience of certain things being like some and different from others.

An early example of this emphasis is contained in a paper published by Campbell (1958) that is still widely cited in research on the perceptions of groups. Campbell used the term **entitativity** to refer to 'the degree of having the nature of an entity, of having real existence' (1958: 17).

The explicit assumption in Campbell's definition of entitativity is that it is a continuous variable. That is, groups can be more or less entitative. This idea resonates with a crucial concern (that I will address in the second section of this chapter) that categories have more or less fuzzy boundaries rather than all-or-none defining features.

Campbell's analysis centred on identifying the sources of such boundaries in the perception of social groups. In his view the characteristics that made groups more entitative were the **Gestalt** principles of visual perceptual organization: **proximity, similarity, common fate** and **pregnance**. That is, he asserted that people would judge some **social aggregation** to be more like an entity (i.e., more 'groupy') if its component parts were close together, were perceptually alike, moved together in the same direction, and constituted a good, continuous (i.e., well-formed) figure.

Probably the most important developments in the study of the functions of categorization occurred in cognitive psychology but had an immediate and significant effect in social psychology. This work is summarized in the publication in 1957 of Bruner's magnificent paper 'On perceptual readiness'. Bruner chose to open his paper with the statement 'Perception involves an act of categorization', demonstrating the importance he attached to this sense-making process.

The sequence underlying perception is that we move from the recognition of cues to the inference of the class identity of the stimulus. Categorization is defined as assigning an input to a subset. A category is a rule for classing objects as equivalent. Categorization achieves **cognitive economy** by translating the myriad stimuli in the physical environment into usable entities. It is selective and contextually dependent: 'It [cognition] does not turn base metal into gold but turns physical stimuli into knowledge, a much more valuable transformation' (Bruner, 1983: 66).

The functions of categorization as a sense-making process appear clearly in Bruner's (1957) principles of **veridical perception**, many of which involve categorization. The following are held to be the general properties of perception. These properties define the sense-making role of categorization in perception as follows:

1   Perception is a decision process: it involves deciding what a stimulus is. This is the most obvious of the properties.
2   The decision processes in perception involve **discrimination** between stimuli. Stimulus information makes it possible to sort the stimuli into categories of best fit (i.e., the categories in which the stimuli are most appropriately placed).

3 There is a chain of inference from the detection of cues to the inference of identity. This chain of cue utilization has the following stages: isolating an object from the background stimulation; cue searching involving fitting cues to category specifications; tentative categorization with further searching for confirming cues; and final categorization with reduced cue searching. Thus a butterfly collector searching for a rare species would first of all distinguish a small flying object from the background. The next stage might involve identification of the object as an insect, and would be associated with a search for general cues which would place it in the category *butterfly*. The tentative categorization would be supplemented by further cue searching (involving, for example, colouring and markings) before making the final categorization 'This is [is not] species X.'

4 A category may be regarded as a set of specifications about which stimuli can be grouped as being equivalent.

5 The **accessibility** or **perceptual readiness** of categorizations varies. This variation in perceptual readiness makes perception consistent with past experience and current intentions. All butterflies may be equivalent for most of us most of the time, but this is manifestly untrue for the butterfly collector.

6 Veridical perception involves coding of stimulus inputs such that one may go from a cue to categorical perception, and then make inferences about other properties of the object. In order to perform this, perception requires the learning of categories and category systems appropriate to relevant events and objects. Perception has a representative function in that we can infer the nature of objects and events, and go beyond them to the correct prediction of other events.

7 The veridicality of perception depends upon the match between the relative accessibility of appropriate categorizations, and the objects and events that the person is likely to encounter. This also implies that perception is of varying veridicality. It is not an exact representation of the world.

The statement of the principles of veridical perception is neatly encapsulated in Bruner's proposition that the capture of a stimulus by a category depends upon the interaction of the relative accessibility of the category and the **fit** between the input and the category specifications. In other words, the stimulus will be assigned to the category which is perceptually ready (in terms of past experience and current intentions) and which has specifications which match the stimulus.

The constraint relations between components of the categorization process can be conceived as in Figure 2.3. Fit and accessibility constrain category use but they do this in interaction rather than independently. These relations suggest that the interaction between fit (perceiving stimuli to be equivalent) and the subset of background knowledge which is currently accessible determines which category is used.

Bruner's principles also acknowledge two other important constraint rela-

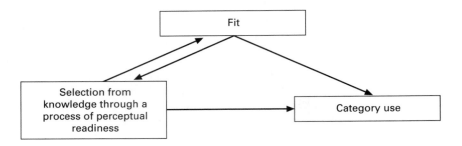

FIGURE 2.3   *Constraint relations relating perceptual readiness and fit to category use*

tions. Principle 4 is a somewhat weaker statement of the idea that we have seen prefigured in the work of Allport and Campbell that categorization constrains perceived equivalence. For most of the last 40 years this idea has been taken more seriously by social than cognitive psychologists.

Finally, we can discuss the idea of multiple chains of inference in constraint relations terms. This is the idea that the detection of cues shared by members leads to category formation which in turn leads to inferences about other category members (Figure 2.4).

Although Bruner (1957) is sometimes cited as the source of the idea that categorization is an overly selective process by which distorted perceptions are developed through the loss of unique information, this is a misrepresentation of the thrust of Bruner's work. Bruner's entire approach to cognition was motivated by the belief that perception involved going beyond the information given to create new knowledge. This is a point that was more recently echoed by Medin (1988) who suggested that the problem perceivers normally face is having too little information rather than too much. Bruner's work on the relationship between perception and cognition is an important and enduring contribution to the study of categorization. The 1957 paper could and should be read by every student of categorization with surprisingly little need

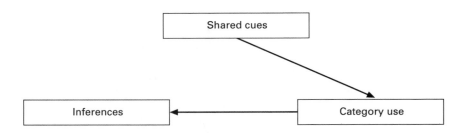

FIGURE 2.4   *Constraint relations for inference derived from Bruner's work*

for an update on the key points.

The ideas of motivated or goal-directed categorization have had several resurgences in interest in the cognitive and social psychological literatures. Key social psychological approaches are considered further in Chapters 4, 5 and 6.

Recently, there has been a revival of interest in cognitive psychology in the functions of categorization. This has been sparked by Anderson's (1991) approach to adaptive human categorization. The nub of Anderson's argument is that features of the environment imply that it is rational (in something like the economic sense of rationality) for people to categorize. A related idea has been picked up in social psychology by Fiedler (1996) and I will discuss Fiedler's intriguing BIAS model in Chapter 8. Anderson's idea is that the complex structure of the environment that confronts people suggests that the goal of categorization is *prediction*. In more precise terms this means minimizing the mean squared error of prediction in a Bayesian inference scheme. This involves setting up categories which are distinguished in terms of expectations about their members. Rational categorization involves setting up the categories that will use prior information and incorporate new information to predict most efficiently. These processes are particularly useful where there is clear separability between categories, but there is random variation of features within the categories. This is an environment which Anderson focuses on because of its application to species of organisms. The constraint relations follow the form shown in Figure 2.5.

Anderson's formulation assumes that knowledge is a response to a complex environment. In other words, categorical information reduction is a precondition for knowledge production. Recent work by Anderson and Fincham (1996) supports the rational approach and shows that participants' categorization behaviour is sensitive to within-category correlations.

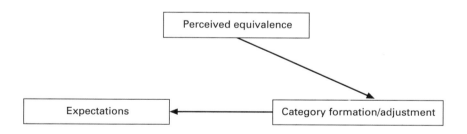

FIGURE 2.5 *Constraint relations for expectations in Anderson's formulation*

There is no real disagreement in the literature that categorization is a goal-directed cognitive activity which functions to make sense of reality. Despite this consensus the choice point that emerges in the discussion of the functions of categorization is therefore one that existed in the 1950s and remains a lively topic of interest to this day:

- Is categorization driven by an undersupply of knowledge? Under this view categorization is creative in that it allows us to go beyond the information given by translating that information into knowledge.

  or

- Is categorization driven by an oversupply of information? Under this view categorization is designed to reduce information that would otherwise confuse us and overwhelm the capacity of the mind.

I can illustrate this conflict with a simple example. Imagine you were to look at a brick wall and see a wall rather than many individual bricks joined together. Do you perceive the wall as a coherent whole, ignoring the individual elements, because you do not *need* to pay attention to the individual bricks (because they are not relevant) or because you *cannot* pay attention to the individual bricks (because you do not have the cognitive resources)?

In fact, almost all categorization theorists would agree that relevance does determine the level at which categorization occurs (whether we see a wall or individual bricks). The real debate is over the degree to which our experience of reality is structured by the need to have *more knowledge* or *less information*. We will see this issue and others that bear upon the functions of categorization emerge time and again in the pages to come, and especially in the review of social psychological literature.

accessibility The extent to which some mental construct is ready to be used by the mind. In Bruner's (1957) usage it is related to current intentions and past experiences, as they change the needs and values of perceivers. Higgins (e.g., 1996) distinguishes the concept from availability which relates to the existence of the construct in the mind.

cognitive economy The mind's management of its available mental resources. The explicit assumption in a *cognitive miser* approach is that these resources are strictly limited and are readily dissipated by the cognitive challenges presented by the environment.

common fate A Gestalt principle that holds that elements are more likely to be perceived as part of a whole if the same events occur to them.

discrimination In a cognitive or perceptual sense this refers to telling the differences between objects. In social psychology and in everyday language the term also commonly means treating people or groups differently.

entitativity The extent to which some set of elements is perceived to be a group or a whole.

fit The degree to which elements match the specification of a category.

Gestalt A German word with many meanings including 'a whole' or 'meaningful unit' (basis of Gestalt psychology).

perceptual readiness Another name for accessibility. Oakes et al. (1994) instead refer to perceiver readiness to make it clear the construct is a property of the person and not of the perceived category.

pregnance A Gestalt principle relating to goodness of form.

proximity A Gestalt principle relating to the physical or other distance between elements. It is distinct from similarity.

similarity A Gestalt principle relating to the degree to which elements are perceptually alike.

social aggregation A term used to distinguish some set of people who may be perceived at some time as a group.

veridical perception Perception that is accurate or true to life.

B. Category structure and representation

Despite the fact that Bruner's work was in what we would now call cognitive psychology the categorization process did not become a central topic in cognition until the 1970s following the work of Eleanor Rosch and colleagues on category representation.

The view of categorization that dominated psychology until the 1970s was called the **classical view of categories**. This was traced to a work attributed to Aristotle (it is doubtful that this work was actually written by Aristotle). The classical view was that categories had all-or-none boundaries. That is, a category could be said to exist where a line could be drawn around the members of a category that made them clearly separable from members of other categories. These boundaries would correspond to a set of defining features.

The problem with this view was first clearly articulated by Wittgenstein (1974). He pointed out that even very simple categories like the concept 'game' did not have all-or-none defining features that could be simply written down. There were no common elements that connected the Olympic Games with non-competitive children's amusements like ring-a-ring-a-rosy. Yet people used the concept readily and effectively in their everyday lives.

The important implication of this result was that it seemed to demonstrate that categories did not have the all-or-none nature that was implied by the classical view. Categories were not just grab bags: it was not a question of whether a member of a category was in or out, it was a matter of how 'in' it was. In other words, categories had a structure which psychologists needed to be able to explain. Lakoff (1987) summarizes the evidence that the classical view of categories does not hold for natural object categories (even for the biological category species) or for mental representations of categories.

To help move beyond the classical view Rosch and colleagues proposed the idea of **level of abstraction**. The same object could be categorized in a number of different ways which differed in their inclusiveness. A chair, for example, could be classified as a piece of furniture, a man-made object, or a particular type of chair (e.g., a kitchen chair). At different times any of these possible classifications could be appropriate but certain categorizations would be more prevalent. This level of abstraction was termed the **basic level**, and this is the level at which the object was most likely to be spontaneously mentioned when someone was asked what an object was.

Research also showed variation in the **internal** (i.e., how the members of a category are organized) and **external structure** of categories (how they relate to other categories). For example, Rips (1975) showed that differences in the internal structure of categories led to asymmetries in inferences. Subjects were given a scenario in which a particular species of the bird population of an island was afflicted with a disease. Subjects were more likely to infer that ducks (a non-typical species) would catch a disease if robins (typical) had it, than that robins would be affected if ducks had the disease. The implication is that the subsets *robin* and *duck* had different relations to the superordinate category *bird*, and that this structure affected judgement.

Variations in the external structure of categories were demonstrated in the work of Tversky (1977; Tversky and Gati, 1978; see also Medin et al., 1990; 1993) who showed asymmetries in judgements of the kind 'How similar is A to B' compared with 'How similar is B to A' when A and B are countries. For example, Mexico was seen by American students to be similar to the USA, but the USA was *not* seen as similar to Mexico. The implication appeared to be that the categories used for comparison affect categorical judgements.

All of this work showed that categories could not be seen as having a simple classical structure. The research imperative then became to determine the nature of category structure (E. E. Smith and Medin, 1981). The two general suggestions made in the literature were the **probabilistic** view and the **exemplar** view. My review of this material follows the pattern of the 1981 review by Smith and Medin, in which they attempt to map out the **epistemological functions of categorization**; cf. Rey's (1983) critique that Smith and Medin ignore the **metaphysical functions of categorization**, and E. E. Smith et al.'s (1983) reply.

The most straightforward version of the probabilistic view takes the evidence on goodness-of-example (**typicality**) ratings and specifies that categories are represented in terms of an abstract summary (often the **prototype** or best example). Category membership under this view is based on the level of similarity between the stimulus and the abstract summary. It is said to be probabilistic because category organization is based on the probability of a member matching the abstract summary.

The exemplar view maintains that categories are represented in memory as sets of *exemplars* or known instances of the category. The particular features of the probabilistic and exemplar views will be considered below, but before we do this, it is useful to note some points made by Rosch on the implications of her work for category structure.

Rosch (1978) warned that to speak of a prototype, as such, was a grammatical fiction. It was more precise to speak of variations between category members in their *degree of* **prototypicality**. To posit a single fixed prototype was simply to relocate the problems raised by Wittgenstein about fixed category boundaries.

Furthermore, Rosch argued that the existence of prototypes in itself does not demand any *particular* model of category processing, learning or structure (representation), though they do provide constraints in that they rule out certain models (such as the classical one). Lakoff (1987) suggests that this is a clear reversal of Rosch's thinking in the early and mid 1970s. Her work at that time did suggest that prototypes constitute mental representations, and that typicality effects directly mirror category structure. Rosch also suggested that we must focus on both the internal and external structure of categories. These warnings should be borne in mind as the models below are considered.

The probabilistic view of category structure

According to Smith and Medin (1981) the basic premises of the probabilistic view are that (a) categories can be represented in terms of some abstract summary, and (b) categories do not necessarily have a set of defining features. The first assumption is the distinctive one, but in fact it is vague without the further specification of the type of probabilistic model utilized. The three kinds of probabilistic view discussed by Smith and Medin are the **featural approach**, the **dimensional approach** and the **holistic approach**.

The featural and dimensional approaches describe categories in terms of properties (either features or dimensions). These two can be jointly contrasted with the holistic approach which does not make use of properties and instead uses holistic patterns or templates.

The featural approach has three basic assumptions:

1 Concepts and categories are assumed to be represented in terms of an abstract summary which is not necessarily realizable as an instance (i.e., the ideal chair may not actually exist).

2 Categories are represented in terms of their salient features (i.e., in Smith and Medin's usage, those features which are conceptually or perceptually prominent). Thus *four-legged* is a salient feature of chairs but it is not true of all chairs (and is therefore a non-necessary feature). This introduces the idea that features can vary in both (a) their salience with respect to the concept, and (b) the probability that any instance will have the feature (for the category *bird* flying has a high salience, but has a probability less than 1.0, i.e., not all birds fly).

3 A stimulus will be assigned to a category when it has a critical number of features (weighted by their salience and probability). This is the general processing assumption of the featural approach. For example, an instance may need only fly and have feathers, wings and warm blood to be categorized as a bird (though note again that not all of these are true of all birds).

The basic change from the classical view is the acknowledgement that many properties are used for categorizing (including non-necessary properties), and these properties need only be generally true of the category. The featural approach accounts for the problems noted for the classical view in a straight-forward way. These problems were (a) the absence of defining features, (b) the difficulty defining features have in accounting for ambiguous cases, (c) variations in typicality, (d) **family resemblance** (higher typicality follows from the presence of frequent properties, such as barking in dogs), (e) non-necessary properties can be used to define category membership, and (f) the existence of **nested categories**. Points (a), (b) and (e) are basic premises of the probabilistic view. Variations in typicality (c) and family resemblances (d) depend upon the proportion of shared features between instances. The only other point that needs addressing is point (f). Smith and Medin (1981: 70–2) argue that the featural approach can be consistent with all of the available evidence on nested categories. All that is necessary is that the right weights are attached to particular features (see the third assumption of the featural approach above). For example, *chicken* will be seen as more similar to the distant superordinate *animal* than to the immediate superordinate *bird*, if features like *feathers* and *wings* are given low weight. However, this can necessitate *ad hoc* assumptions about the feature weights making the approach unconstrained (i.e., the weights can be continually changed until the model fits the available data).

Models which Smith and Medin describe as featural include Collins and Loftus's (1975) **spreading activation** model, **cue validity** models (a cue validity is the distinctive probability that a feature belongs to a given category as opposed to relevant alternative categories), and the feature comparison model of E. E. Smith et al. (1974).

The main problem Smith and Medin raise with the featural approach is that a set of features does not represent much of the knowledge people have about concepts. We not only know that category members share features, but we also know that particular features occur together. We know that wings and feathers occur together more frequently than wings and fur, and this is represented in our conceptual structures. Rather than just having *lists* of features we need to posit *networks* of features. Other problems include the lack of constraints incorporated in the general featural model. It seems that the weights of particular features can be varied arbitrarily to make the model work.

The second approach subsumed within the probabilistic view is the dimensional approach. This has one distinctive assumption with two parts (Smith and Medin, 1981: 102):

1   Any dimension used to represent a concept must be a salient one, some of whose values have a substantial probability of occurring in instances of the concept.
2   The value of a dimension represented in a concept is the (subjective) average of the values of the concept's subsets or instances on this dimension.

The second part of the assumption allows for quantitative variation in properties. This is the crucial difference between the featural and dimensional approaches. Instead of categories being represented in terms of all-or-none features they are seen as having properties which vary on continuous dimensions. These dimensions can vary in their importance (and can have weights assigned to them). Both approaches see concepts as being represented in terms of central tendencies, but under the dimensional approach the central tendency is the average of the instances' (or subsets of instances') values. Under the featural approach it is a representation in terms of the modal properties of the concept.

There is an additional analytical assumption commonly made in the dimensional approach. This is that concepts and instances having the same relevant dimensions can be represented as points in a **multidimensional metric space**.

For a space to be metric (i.e., allowing measurements to be made in the same way as they are in physical space) three assumptions must be met. These are minimality, similarity and triangular inequality (Birnbaum, 1982; Lingle et al., 1984):

1   *Minimality*: The difference between any point and itself should be minimal and equal to the difference between any other entity and itself:

$$\delta(x, y) \geq \delta(x, x) = 0$$

2   *Symmetry*: The difference between any two entities should be equal to their reversed difference:

$$\delta(x, y) = \delta(y, x)$$

3   *Triangular inequality*: The distance between any two points should not be greater than the combined distances between each and a third entity:

$$\delta(x, y) + \delta(y, z) \geq \delta(x, z)$$

The metric assumptions, while not necessary for the dimensional approach, do in fact appear in most models based on this approach. They also allow us to calculate probable category membership on the basis of a computation of distance in the metric space.

The first of these models that Smith and Medin consider is the simple distance model. An instance is categorized as a member of a category if it is less than some threshold distance from the category centre (i.e., an average distance on the relevant dimensions). A category can therefore be represented as a circle (where there are two dimensions) bounding all of the instances within the threshold distance. An example of this is shown in Figure 2.6.

A further (processing) assumption is that the closer an instance is to the category centre, the faster and more accurately the stimulus will be categorized as a member of the category. This implies that some instances of a concept will be less typical. A simple distance model of this form was used by Rosch et al. (1976b).

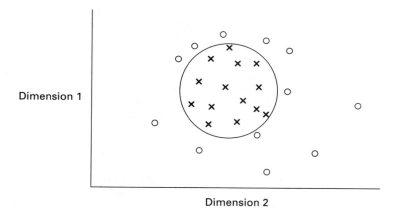

FIGURE 2.6   *The simple distance model*
Note: The crosses are instances which are considered to be part of the category because they lie
within the threshold distance. The circles are outside the category.

This sort of model can account for many of the conventional findings in
1970s categorization research (which were problematic for the classical
model) except for findings by Rosch and Mervis (1975) that contrasting concepts influence categorization. In other words, people might not just compute
the simple distance between the concept and the instance, but also take into
account the comparative distance between the instance and other contrasting
categories. This gives rise to the comparative distance model which assumes
that an instance will be categorized as a member of a given category to the
extent to which the distance between the instance and the category is less than
the distance between the instance and any other category. The model further
assumes that the closer (relatively) the instance is to the closest category, the
faster and more accurately it will be categorized. Effectively, the fixed threshold of the simple distance model has been replaced by a contextually
dependent distance. Such a model was proposed by Reed (1972).

In Chapter 3, some of the problems with the idea of similarity as a basis
for invariant metrics are considered. For the moment though I would note
that a long tradition of research questions the possibility of psychological
organization being based on stable similarity judgements. For example,
Livingston et al. (1998) have shown that multidimensional similarity spaces
can vary as a function of learning. In the light of this evidence the metric
assumptions are questionable.

The last approach to the probabilistic view is the holistic approach. Under
this view categorization occurs by a process of template matching, where
templates are images of concrete objects (the ideal chair or coffee cup: see
Ullman, 1989). This approach would seem to be easier to apply to visual
images than to more abstract concepts or categories. Having said that, models
such as associated systems theory (Carlston, 1994) and the dual-process
model of impression formation (Brewer, 1988) in social psychology emph-

asize the importance of visual information in categorical representation, and Goldstone and Barsalou (1998) emphasize the perceptual basis of *all* knowledge.

The exemplar view of category structure

The third view of categorization is the exemplar view. The exemplar view maintains that categories are represented, to some extent, not by abstract summaries but by a set of instances. This does not negate the possibility that categories involve some form of summary information, but holds that the exemplars play the dominant role in representation and processing. The critical assumption of the exemplar view (according to Smith and Medin) is that the representation of a concept consists of separate descriptions of some of its exemplars.

This contradicts the probabilistic assumption of abstract summary representations in that an abstract summary does not play the primary processing role. Exemplar-based representations of categories involve less abstraction than probabilistic or classical representations. There are enormous differences between the various exemplar-based models.

One such exemplar-based model is the context model of Medin and Schaffer (1978). Under this model category representation is strategy-based. Representations are limited to that particular set of exemplars which are currently being attended to. Thus the categorization of any given instance depends crucially upon the range of other stimuli taken into account at that time. The processing assumptions of the context model (which could also be applied to other models) are:

1 An entity is categorized as an instance of a concept if it retrieves (i.e., when the entity is presented it triggers from memory) a criterial number of the exemplars of that concept before retrieving a criterial number of exemplars of any contrasting concept.
2 The probability of retrieving any specific exemplar is a direct function of the similarity between the target stimulus and that exemplar.

Under the context model similarity is computed multiplicatively. This involves multiplying the differences between stimuli and exemplars on relevant dimensions (as opposed to simply summing these differences). Results obtained by Medin and Schaffer (1978) suggest some advantages for multiplicative similarity computation (for certain stimulus materials) over the additive approach.

To understand the implications of this model, it is useful to consider some of its characteristics. First, a great deal of information is assumed to be stored in memory in a form that is similar to perceived stimuli. Secondly, the retrieval of that information is assumed to be described by many simultaneous simple mathematical operations. This feature makes computer simulation of such models attractive. Thirdly, there are no higher-order structures referred to that might determine the operation of the categorization process.

That is, apart from the rules for identification and categorization and the category labels associated with the stored exemplars, there is nothing somewhere else in the mind that can be called a category.

Hintzman (1986) added yet another element to the picture by extending Bower's (1967) idea of **multiple memory traces** to the categorization literature, an idea that is also incorporated into Smith and Zárate's (1992) exemplar model of social judgement. The multiple-trace conceptualization holds that each perceived exemplar can be stored as a set of values on different dimensions. Similarity between two exemplars is thus defined not by a comparison between two numbers representing their positions on one dimension but by comparing two ordered sets of numbers. The easiest way of summarizing mathematical operations involving sets of numbers is to treat them as vectors. This enables categorization theorists to use matrix algebra to summarize large sets of operations.

The exemplar approach to category structure has also been adopted by social psychologists such as Smith and Zárate (1992) and Linville and colleagues (1989). Linville et al. argue that views of ingroups and outgroups are based on an exemplar representation whereby people store information about individual people (exemplars of a social category). Linville et al. proposed that this storage explained the **outgroup homogeneity effect**, because people have a more finely differentiated view of groups of which they are members owing to greater familiarity with those groups.

Smith and Zárate (1992) spelled out an exemplar model of social judgement in some detail. They suggested that perceptions of groups are derived from weighted combinations of exemplars. The exemplars are stored in the form in which they are originally interpreted and then retrieved to make social judgements. These exemplars are retrieved automatically (with or without awareness or existence of prior conscious experience) by target stimuli which they are similar to. In this model similarity is defined by the perceiver's allocation of attention to stimulus dimensions and this similarity can be theory-dependent in that one's theories determine what is important to attend to. More generally, attention to stimulus dimensions depends on social, motivational and contextual factors. Note that aspects of Smith and Zárate's theorizing are captured in the constraint relations diagram showing categorical inference (Figure 2.2).

One assumption is that the self – or more particularly, one's social category memberships – serves as a basis for organizing social categorization processes (as per self-categorization theory: Turner et al., 1987). To take an example, when judging members of ingroups and outgroups more attention should be directed to individuating features of ingroup members as these distinguish the personal self from other ingroup members, and to the category-defining features of outgroup members as these distinguish the shared social self from the outgroup (E. R. Smith and Henry, 1996, found in a reaction time study that group memberships were processed in the same way as the individual self). Smith and Zárate do not rule out the existence of abstract category-level information but they do not see it as necessary to emphasize this type of knowledge to explain key differences in the representation of categories of ingroup and outgroup members.

Messick and Mackie (1989) concluded that neither exemplar nor prototype models have exclusive support in social psychology and some kind of **mixed-model representation** is best. They give two reasons for this (1989: 47). Strict prototype and exemplar models predict that judgements of the group and judgements of individual stimuli should be related. Park and Hastie (1987; also Judd and Park, 1988) found that this was not necessarily the case. Secondly, exemplar models deal with category variability in a more obvious way than prototype models but they have difficulty dealing with the finding we have already discussed, that some judgements do not seem to involve the retrieval of exemplars – particularly when judging cohesive, homogeneous categories. The best precedent for the mixed-model approach in cognitive psychology is the category density model of Fried and Holyoak (1984; but see Sloman and Rips, 1998, for an overview of work stressing combinations of abstraction or rule-based information and more specific information).

Park and Hastie (1987) suggest that the categorization of social objects is more likely to rely on abstraction-based information than the categorization of non-social objects. The first reason given by these authors is that while information about individuals remains available, more information is provided by many socializing agents about *groups* of people. Furthermore, social perceivers may not have had much contact with individual members of outgroups. While it would be difficult to argue with these suggestions, it should be noted that the same assertion could be made about many non-social objects (e.g., cars and species of animals). It is possible, however, to accept that the relatively novel stimuli and categories (such as geometric shapes) used in cognitive psychological *experiments* on categorization are more likely to be perceived initially in terms of instances rather than abstractions. This is because the categories are chosen precisely because they are novel and are associated with no prior knowledge.

Park and Hastie point to another difference in emphasis between cognitive and social psychological interests in categorization. Whereas cognitive models focus on the perceiver's ability to assign stimuli to a newly learned category, social psychologists are more commonly interested in the perceiver's decision to apply particular previously learned categories (the question of which categories are applied relates to the issue of category salience, an issue we will return to in the chapters to follow).

Park and Hastie's (1987) empirical work suggests that both abstraction and instance-based processes are implicated in categorization. They showed that participants formed estimates of the variability of group members, and that these estimates were influenced by whether the stereotype which they relate to was based on instances or abstractions. For example, in their second experiment participants were asked to develop an impression of a group of people. Those participants who were exposed to the group's traits (abstractions), before they were given examples of their behaviours (instances), developed impressions that the groups were much less variable than did participants who were exposed first to the behaviours and then to the traits.

Yet another approach to representation can be seen in Carlston's (1994) associated systems theory (AST) of person impressions. This approach holds that representations of people are based on the overlap of four primary and hierarchically organized mental systems: the visual system (visual appearances), the verbal system (personality traits), the action system (behavioural responses) and the affective system (affective responses). Particular impressions of people relate to the overlap of these systems, so that for Carlston categories represent the overlap of the visual system and the verbal system and are therefore distinct from, for example, evaluations of people and orientations towards people. Carlston and Sparks (1994) therefore draw the conclusion that categories and stereotypes do not involve action or evaluation, or even the self. To quote them: 'From the perspective of AST, stereotyping thus reflects target-based forms of representation with little self-reference or engagement.' As we will see in the chapters to come, this would appear to misconstrue the role of the self in stereotyping and cannot be considered to be a reasonable basis for understanding stereotyping (as Brewer, 1994, points out, social categorizations tend to involve self versus not-self categorizations). Having said that, the idea of representations involving the overlap of systems is a very attractive and promising suggestion. Unfortunately Carlston and Sparks reject the possibility of extending the model to consider further overlap between the systems. Until this is done the model would appear to be an inadequate treatment of categorization.

Finally, some authors (e.g., Barsalou and Medin, 1986; McGarty, 1990; Mullen, 1991) have raised the possibility of **variable representations**. The appeal of this idea is that the same category can be represented in one way at one time and in another way at another time. Thus a category could be considered as a set of exemplars at one time and as a coherent group at another time. This is clearly consistent with the dynamic approach to thinking that I discussed in Chapter 1. To illustrate how the variable representation model might work, consider the task of a perceiver who is at one time comparing individual members of a category and at another time comparing the members of two categories. In the first case relations amongst stimuli can be conceived of as similarities and in the second case they can be conceived of as differences (Turner et al., 1987; see also Haslam et al., 1995b, 1996c, and Chapters 5 and 8 of this volume, for an application of these ideas to social perception). A relation might change from being a similarity to a difference because there has been a change in the categorical representation from exemplar-based to abstraction-based.

For example, when we are looking for a misplaced pen (e.g., one which is a personal belonging) we can remain aware of the fact that it is a member of the general category *pen*, but know that is irrelevant for the task at hand. We should instead focus on the distinctive differences between it and other pens.

However, under conditions where we are just looking for something to sign a cheque with, the individual characteristics become unimportant and we focus on the general category of pens. It is under these conditions that we may be more likely to represent pens in terms of an abstract summary or prototype. This abstract summary can be used to distinguish pens from other alternative categories (e.g., pencils, chalk or crayons). That is, we use abstract summaries when we are interested in the general properties of the category members. It is not necessarily the case that we distort the difference between pens and pencils under these circumstances (though this is possible). We merely pick out those differences between the categories which are relevant to the situation (e.g., pencils and chalk can be easily erased, crayons are used by children and lack a fine point). The process envisaged is similar to the dimension selection process discussed by Smith and Zárate (1992).

The picture is more complex than this, however, because we can also instantaneously switch to a mixed-model representation if the task requires slightly more differentiation. When searching for any suitable pen we may scan the array of pens lying on the telephone table and retain the goal of finding *any* pen, but discriminate between the pens there in terms of whether they write, or leak, or are an appropriate colour. This implies that we do not necessarily distort the perceived similarities between pens (though again this is possible). We perceive a level of similarity which is appropriate for the task at hand. An illustration of this is readily available. Under some circumstances we can look at the same stimulus and see 'five pens'. Under other circumstances we see: 'my good pen, a red pen, a black pen, a blue pen that doesn't work, and the pen that someone left there'. Several of these discriminations involve memory of past experience with the stimulus.

The three different constraint relations are shown in Figure 2.7.

The purpose of these examples is to illustrate the possibility that category structure is flexible, and that changes in category representation reflect changes in the level of abstraction. We focus on exemplars when we are differentiating between individual stimuli, and we focus on abstract summaries when we are differentiating between categories. These are not dichotomous: we can perceive the same set of stimuli more or less in terms of abstract summaries or exemplars.

A wide range of approaches has been considered in this section. These approaches are summarized in Table 2.1

There is no real debate in the field that models of categorization need to incorporate some variability or mental flexibility. The question is really, how much variability? I would therefore single out this issue as the critical choice point for this section.

> • Do categories have relatively fixed and enduring representations with potentially variable content but a fixed form as (a) a set of exemplars, (b) an abstract summary like a prototype, or (c) some other representation?
>
> *or*
>
> • Do categories have a variable representation so that, at different times in different circumstances, people will have representations of categories that are more like exemplar or prototype representations?

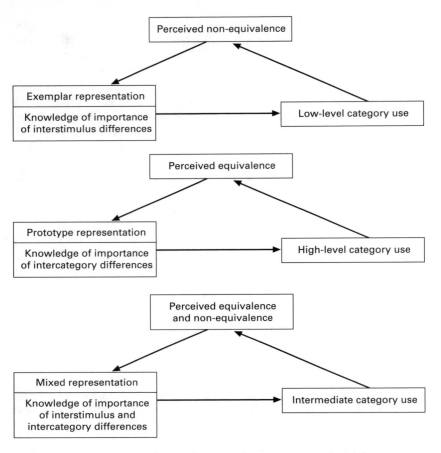

FIGURE 2.7   *Constraint relations for exemplar, prototype, and mixed-model representations*

TABLE 2.1   *Approaches to category structure*

Approach	Properties	Representative examples
Classical	All-or-none defining features	Aristotle
Probabilistic:	Abstraction-level representation	
featural	Based on features of stimuli	Collins and Loftus (1975)
dimensional	Dimensions used to distinguish stimuli	Rosch et al. (1976b)
holistic	Based on template of ideal member	Ullman (1989)
Exemplar	Information stored at the level of instances	Medin and Schaffer (1978)
Mixed	Abstraction and exemplar information	Fried and Holyoak (1984)
Variable	Changes from exemplar to abstraction	Barsalou and Medin (1986)

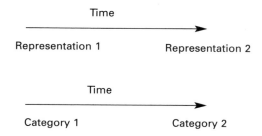

Time

Representation 1   Representation 2

Time

Category 1   Category 2

FIGURE 2.8   *Variability in representation or category*

If we do accept that representation is variable, a tension emerges. If categories have a variable structure then that implies they have a continuous existence. Two options are presented in Figure 2.8. Either different representational forms of the same category are adopted at different times or different categories are constructed at different times. Still another possibility is that certain aspects retain their existence and others change.

basic level The level at which an object is naturally or automatically categorized. This will tend to be the level at which an object is spontaneously named when a person is asked what an object is. Thus the basic level for pieces of furniture is assumed to be at the level of *chair* and *table*.

classical view of categories The view that categories have all-or-none defining features that enable clear boundaries between categories.

cue validity The extent to which some feature of a stimulus is correlated with category membership.

dimensional approach An approach to the probabilistic view of categorization whereby categories can be differentiated in terms of the positions of their members on relevant dimensions.

epistemological functions of categorization Those functions of categorization that involve knowledge about how people understand the world. This is the function that psychologists are normally concerned with.

exemplar view The view of categorization which holds that categories are stored in terms of a set of instances that belong to that category.

external structure The relations between a category and other categories. These structures are often thought to be hierarchically organized (like a tree diagram).

family resemblance The extent to which members of a category share similar features or positions on a dimension.

featural approach An approach to the probabilistic view which defines differences between and within categories in terms of the degree of shared features.

holistic approach An approach to the probabilistic view that is most relevant to perceptual categories whereby category membership is defined in terms of a degree of match to some template.

internal structure The organization of the members of a category *as* members of that category.

level of abstraction The idea that categorization schemes have a hierarchy that varies in inclusiveness. Thus the category *furniture* includes the category *chair* which in turn includes the category *armchair*. These differing levels of inclusiveness might be referred to as the superordinate, intermediate and subordinate levels, one of which *could* be the basic level.

metaphysical functions of categorization The functions of categorization relating to determining how the world is. This relates closely to scientific procedures of classification.

mixed-model representation The idea that some categories are represented in terms of abstract summaries and others in terms of sets of exemplars.

multidimensional metric space A space defined by multiple dimensions in which distances between points in that space can be described in terms of some consistent measurement system.

multiple memory-trace models A model of category representation which assumes that exemplars are encoded in terms of multiple characteristics. The traces could include the category label as well as information specific to the stimulus such as the shape, size and aesthetic beauty of a painting.

nested categories Categories contained within other categories. The nested categories can be said to be at a lower level of abstraction or to be less inclusive.

outgroup homogeneity effect The commonly reported finding in social psychology that the perceived similarity of outgroups is higher than the perceived similarity of ingroups.

probabilistic view The view of category structure which holds that categories are based on an abstract summary (or prototype). Category membership is defined in terms of the likelihood of a match between a stimulus and the abstract summary.

prototype Either (a) an exemplar which is most typical of a category or (b) an abstract ideal summary of a category that need not correspond to any actual exemplar.

prototypicality Similar to typicality but also conveying the idea of the degree to which the exemplar is similar to the ideal or best summary of a category.

spreading activation An idea popular in many cognitive metaphors for mind that the activation of some mental structure sets in train processes whereby related or connected structures are activated.

typicality The extent to which some stimulus or exemplar is a good example of a category.

variable representation The idea that categories do not have a fixed structure but that their structure changes with circumstance.

Conclusion

In this chapter I have tried to provide an introduction to the functions of categorization and the structure of categories. It is fair to say that most of the recent interest in cognitive research on categorization has related to the latter. Indeed, much of the relevant research in the past 20 years has been directed to differentiating between prototype and exemplar models of categorization.

Having said that, there is a new emphasis in categorization research on the reasons for categorization and this provides the first of the critical choice points that I suggested. If categorization is seen to result from the need for less information or from the need for more knowledge we end up with quite different views of the process. Of course partial reconciliations are possible: most theorists who see categorization as being driven by a need for information reduction would argue that information reduction actually makes knowledge production possible. That is, people are only able to develop categorizations which help them to understand a buzzing, whirring, confusing world by simplifying that world.

Similarly, if we see categories as having fixed structures that are relatively invariant despite changes in context then we will have a completely different view of the nature of the categorization process to the one we would adopt if we assume that category structure is flexible. To take just one example from social psychology: extending the idea that social categories are relatively fixed implies that to change stereotypes people need to *learn* exemplars which disconfirm their stereotypes (e.g., as envisaged in some of the arguments of Rothbart, 1981). If the categories on which stereotypes are based are highly flexible, however, then strategies involving the learning of new exemplars will be less likely to have long-lasting effects.

These examples illustrate the immediate relevance of issues in the study of categorization for social psychology. We will consider further issues in categorization, many of which stem quite directly from the issues of function and structure that I have discussed here, in the next chapter. Partly this involves addressing the question of what underpins the formation and use of categories.

3 Categorization and Cognition II: Category Learning, Formation and Use

A. Similarity-based approaches to category learning

So far I have talked about the functions and structure of categorization without addressing the processes by which these categories are formed. Category learning is in fact one of the most important continuing concerns in the cognitive psychology of categorization (see e.g., Estes, 1991; Fried and Holyoak, 1984; Lassaline and Murphy, 1998; Medin and Schaffer, 1978; Nosofsky, 1986). Many of the issues and developments in category learning arise out of research done in the 1980s and 1990s that attempted to distinguish between exemplar and prototype models (with respect to the details of this debate as it relates to the interests of both social and cognitive psychologists the review by Lingle et al., 1984, will repay a close reading).

In constraint relations terms there are two direct routes for category learning: similarity-based category learning and theory-based learning. The first assumes that people form categories by detecting equivalences amongst stimuli and then store those categories for future use. The second assumes that the detection of similarities (or perceiving equivalence) depends upon pre-existing knowledge.

In relation to the first type, Estes (1991) reviews developments in category learning including his own stimulus sampling model (Estes, 1950). He agrees though that the modern approach to category learning begins with Medin and Schaffer's (1978) exemplar memory model (also referred to as the context model) that we discussed in Chapter 2.

Estes (1991), however, raises some difficulties with this model. Nosofsky (1984; 1986) found that it was necessary to change the parameter values in order to account for both identification and categorization performance, and this research led to a generalization of the model by Nosofsky (who later extended the generalized model and showed that Anderson's rational model was a generalization of his own generalized context model). Similarly, Estes's earlier work found that the model worked well for recently perceived exemplars, but that a decay parameter was necessary to account for exemplars that had been perceived in the past. Inclusion of this parameter seemed to be a reasonable extension from findings in other memory situations.

The next stage of development in the field involved simple connectionist approaches to categorization. Gluck and Bower (1988) proposed a connectionist architecture to deal with simple categorization situations. The models assume **layers** of interconnected **nodes**. These layers can be **input layers, output layers** or **hidden layers**. The links between nodes are called **associative weights**. When a stimulus is presented to an input layer, the nodes which are relevant to the input will be selectively activated and these will in turn activate nodes in the next layer. The actual output produced by the system will be a sum of the activation received by the output layers; the actual value of this activation gives the probability of a particular response.

In the Gluck and Bower architecture the input layer relates to the feature set used to generate category exemplars. Imagine that we have two categories of people and four features: short, tall, studying and working. Presenting the system with a stimulus with the features *short* and *studying* will activate those features which will in turn activate nodes in the output layer that the features are linked to. The associative weights are updated on each presentation by feedback which teaches the system whether the categorization was correct or incorrect. Note that for ease of description I have given the features symbolic names but the units in connectionist systems need not (and in general are not) things that we can represent easily in symbolic terms.

Imagine a naive system that is to learn some categories about which it currently knows nothing (Figure 3.1). Imagine that the first stimulus has the features *short* and *studying*. Only two responses are possible and these are equally likely because there is no prior information. Imagine that it responds 'category A'. The system will then receive the feedback that the categorization is 'correct' or 'incorrect'. If it is correct the associations between category A and these features will be incremented, so that next time a stimulus with the same features is received, category A will become still more highly activated and that response will be yet more likely. If, on the other hand, the feedback 'incorrect' is received the association between category A and these features will be decremented. In a system with only two output nodes this will mean that category B will be more likely to be activated by a similar stimulus in the future.

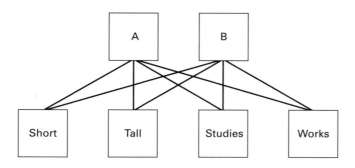

FIGURE 3.1   *Example of a simple connectionist network for categorization*

Such a network performs better than the context model in simple categorization tasks but it does not work where there are correlations between features within categories. To deal with this situation a middle layer must be added which captures covariations between features. Both of these layers are connected to the output categorization layer.

One additional feature of connectionist networks that I should address here is the issue of **back-propagation**. So far, I have described networks that proceed in a forward direction (called **feedforward**) so that nodes in one layer activate those in subsequent layers. Back-propagation allows for nodes in different layers to have reciprocal influences. In categorization terms the clearest analogy is to think of categories being formed by features, but the interpretation of those features is then influenced by newly formed categories. As we will see, in relation to similarity judgements and a range of other issues, this is a vital issue in the analysis of the categorization process.

Although there are some similarities between the exemplar and connectionist accounts they are in fact quite different conceptually. The exemplar models assume that individual stimuli are stored in their entirety. The connectionist models assume a **distributed representation** that does not rest on the storage of unique pieces of information.

The connectionist account appears very useful for category learning from the ground up, but Holyoak and Spellman (1993) have identified a number of limitations with connectionist models that are particularly pertinent with respect to the discussion of categorization. These limitations do not rule out connectionist accounts but rather suggest that they must be complemented by symbolic accounts.

First, simple connectionist accounts lack constituency relations. The lack of meaningful relationships between elements implies that connectionist accounts cannot deal with the systematic nature of human thought. Thus connectionist accounts do not tell us how distributed representations are **bound** meaningfully to objects in the world, or to contexts or roles in the world.

Secondly, simple connectionist accounts have problems in dealing with relations generally. The knowledge that we derive from categories allows us to think thoughts that are related to those categories (going beyond the information given). To quote Holyoak and Spellman:

> More generally, it seems characteristic of thinking that if each concept in a set of potential constituent concepts is understood, and a relation structure (such as a frame for a predicate and its arguments) can be instantiated by one assignment of the constituent concepts, then the thinker can also instantiate the relation structure with other permissible assignments of the concepts. (1993: 270)

This important idea needs to be unpacked. The example Holyoak and Spellman use involves the sentences 'The girl loves the boy' and 'The boy loves the girl.' If we understand the first sentence then the second sentence should also be easy to understand. Without the existence of symbols and knowledge that takes the form of abstract rules it is difficult to understand why this should be true.

Thirdly, these points are compounded when we deal with multiple-task contexts or with **multiple-place predicates**. Connectionist models deal well with one-to-one relations between objects and predicates but they struggle to deal with one-to-many or many-to-many relationships between objects and predicates because of the need to keep track of the multiple roles played by **arguments**. If a category is learned in one context by a network in contrast to some other category then in order to match the power of human relational thinking it must be able to draw inferences from those categories that will be valid under different roles. That is, a system that assigns 'girl' to the category 'loved by boy' must be *ready* to assign 'boy' to the category 'loved by girl' or 'not loved by girl' as well as being able to draw inferences of the form 'boy knows girl' without *automatically* inferring that 'girl knows boy'.

In this regard the proposal for category learning by Nosofsky et al. (1994) is intriguing. Their RULEX model (RULE-plus-EXception) proposes that people learn simple rules as well as remembering occasional exceptions to those rules. The model proposes that rules are formed from the construction of a decision tree on the basis of a stochastic combination of individual stimuli. The model provides a good account of basic effects in category learning.

An interesting feature of the model is that it assumes that a common process of rule formation underlies classification learning but that the particular rules which are obtained will vary markedly from person to person. The implication of this model is therefore that there should be large individual differences in categorization behaviour. This suggests a paradox in the analysis of categorization: even though the same processes may operate in the minds of two different perceivers the outcomes of the categorization process may be very different. From a social psychological perspective therefore we need to pay very close attention to the existence of consensus in categorization behaviour. This is because coincidence or the common operation of the same mental processes is unlikely to provide a good account of what is going on and thus other constraints such as the social context must be considered (see also Haslam, 1997).

It is worth noting that this approach is consistent with Anderson's (1991) rational approach to categorization that I mentioned in Chapter 2. However, the model does not assume the same massive demands on memory that are required by purely exemplar-based approaches. The model is therefore an important development in the categorization literature.

The relative merits of connectionist models which include or exclude symbolic elements are a major current concern in the contemporary cognitive psychological literature on categorization. I identify this as the choice point for this section:

> - Can models based on connectionist (and specifically, sub-symbolic) principles provide an adequate account of category learning?
>
> *or*
>
> - Should any account of category learning include the provision for symbolic elements which permit the encoding of abstraction-level information? We also need to ask to ask: what psychological role do categories play once they are formed?

To be fair, in order to model the processes that social psychologists are interested in, the connectionist principles would need to be considerably more sophisticated than those discussed in this chapter. Having said that, some candidates already exist in terms of models of constraint satisfaction (e.g., Thagard, 1989; see Chapter 10 of this volume).

arguments In a technical sense, what is operated on in a function. Thus in the function $y = f(X)$, X is the argument of the function f.

associative weight The connection between two nodes in a connectionist network. Positive weights increment the activation of the receiving node, negative weights decrement the effect. The weights can be considered to have one-way or two-way effects.

back-propagation The transmission of weights back from subsequent layers to lower layers in a network. For example, a link from an output layer to an input layer would be an example of back-propagation.

bound (binding problem) The binding problem relates to the issue of establishing the connection between a representation of some thing and the role or meaning of that thing. The problem becomes particularly acute when we consider things with multiple roles or changing roles.

distributed representation The sort of representation envisaged in connectionist systems where the representation of some thing is distributed across an array of nodes rather than being localized in some particular place.

feedforward systems Connectionist systems that have no back-propagation. The associative weights involve one-way connections between lower-level layers and subsequent layers.

hidden layers Layers between input layers and output layers. They are hidden from external view in that they do not correspond directly to observable stimuli or responses.

input layers Layers of nodes that are activated by stimulus events or at least the starting conditions of the network.

layer A set of nodes that have connections of the same quality with nodes in other layers. Thus a particular hidden layer might be defined by all nodes having connections with one or more nodes in the input layer and one or more nodes in the output layer.

multiple-place predicate A predicate is a function which takes arguments. In the expression Apple[RED], 'Apple' is the predicate and 'RED' is the argument. A multiple-place predicate is a predicate with more than one argument. Thus, Marriage[HUSBAND, WIFE] is a multiple-place predicate.

nodes A unit of a connectionist system that is connected to other units by associative weights.

output layers A layer in a connectionist system that is associated with a response or finishing state of the system.

B. Theory-based approaches to category learning and use

Now that the similarity-based approaches to category structure and learning have been summarized it is useful to look at different theories of category formation and use. According to Medin and Barsalou (1987) three major theories of category formation have been proposed in the realm of cognitive psychology/science.

I will term these the **ecological approach** (Neisser, 1987), the **experiential-realist approach** based on the ideas of kinaesthetic image schemas and idealized cognitive models (ICMs) (Lakoff, 1987), and the **theory-coherence approach** (Murphy and Medin, 1985). In fact there is some overlap between these approaches. For example, all to some extent draw upon the notion of perceivers' models of the world, and all of them should be seen in the context of the 'Roschian revolution' (Neisser, 1987: vii) in the study of categorization (i.e., all borrow from concepts developed by Rosch and her co-workers in the 1970s).

The ecological and other perceptual approaches

The ecological approach applies what Neisser (1987) describes as the most complete theory of perception, i.e., Gibson's (1966; 1979) ecological theory, to the study of categorization. The environment is made up of a number of structures which can be detected optically. These optical structures include aspects of stimulus information which are termed **invariants** (i.e., they remain constant despite motion by the perceiver). Under this view the perceptual system is seen as resonating to the invariants. That is, perception is based on the detection and direct pickup of these invariants. There is held to be a direct correspondence between the structures present in the environment and that which is perceived. We are aware of and perceive reality, and this is what is termed **direct perception**.

An important type of invariant posited by the theory is **affordances** for particular organisms. These affordances are relationships between some aspect of the environment and possible actions by the organism. Thus a chair affords sitting for a human but not for a whale, a fallen tree branch affords shelter for a beetle but is a tool for a chimpanzee, and so on. There are infinitely many affordances, but only some of them are ever perceived.

In Neisser's view categorization is less direct than perception in the same way that thinking is less direct than seeing. Categories are dependent upon cognitive models about the world. These are cultural assumptions that establish the real (social) meanings of words (in as much as they signify concepts). An example due to Fillmore (1982) is *bachelor*. This concept might be classically defined as a man who has never married, but in fact the term conveys a general set of social practices that rule out certain possible category members. For example, the model of bachelors does not normally include Catholic priests.

In Neisser's view, whereas perception involves the detection of immediately apparent invariants, assigning instances to a category involves the use of complex cognitive models about the nature of the stimulus. He acknowledges that these models are often incomplete, but at the same time he acknowledges the existence of what Putnam (cited in Neisser, 1987) refers to as the **linguistic division of labour**. That is, it is the duty of some expert to have the definitive and complete cognitive model of something (examples of these experts include dictionary writers, judges and scientists depending upon the subject matter). It is generally sufficient for us to know that somebody has access to these cognitive models, rather than for us to have the models at our fingertips. One does not need to understand the workings of the internal combustion engine to drive a car. However, Neisser rules out the possibility of a perceptual division of labour: 'we can and must see for ourselves' (1987: 18). Thus categorization is regarded as less direct than perception, and categories are regarded as relationships between objects and cognitive models, in the same way that affordances are relationships between objects and possibilities for action.

Neisser also assumes the existence of the hierarchy of categorization that was proposed by Rosch et al. (1976a). Categories vary in their inclusiveness: for example, *feminists*, *women*, *females* and *humans* are examples of categories of increasing inclusiveness. Categories at a higher level of inclusiveness are said to be *superordinate*, those at a lower level are said to be *subordinate*. Of particular interest is the *basic level* of categorization. This is a level which is near the middle of the hierarchy and has a number of important characteristics.

Members of basic-level categories tend to have a very similar appearance. For example, *chair* is a basic-level category which is subordinate to the category *furniture*. All members of this category look very similar (as opposed to the members of the category *furniture*). Secondly, basic-level objects are used in very similar ways (our physical interactions with them are similar). Thirdly, they seem to have many describable perceptual attributes. Research has shown that basic-level objects are identified most rapidly, that they can be treated as a Gestalt whole without attribute analysis, and that the basic level is the level at which objects are spontaneously named (Mervis and Rosch, 1981).

Basic-level objects are categorized by appearances. This sits comfortably with the ecological approach adopted by Neisser in that categorization is shown to depend upon direct perceptual properties and affordances. However, the other levels of categorization are also important. There are many things which cannot be judged just on appearances. These objects are categorized in terms of properties other than their physical appearances (i.e., on the basis of more complex cognitive models, as with the example of bachelors).

The recognition of the existence of this superordinate structure led Neisser to posit that categorization begins at the basic level (where it is dependent upon appearances and affordances which are perceptually given). Categorization moves beyond this to superordinate categories based on **idealized cognitive models** which involve knowledge about objects which is not directly given (or is beneath the perceivable surface).

When we frame the ecological approach as a constraint model the relations in Figure 3.2 apply. Set (a) shows how superficial similarities in appearance lead to the formation of basic-level categories which are then stored. Set (b) shows how the perception of less superficial similarities which are detected

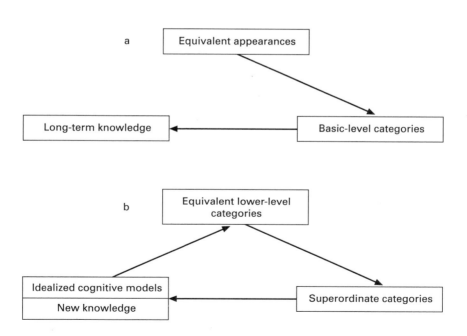

FIGURE 3.2   *Constraint relations derived from Neisser's ecological perspective*

through the application of idealized cognitive models leads to the formation and storage of superordinate categories.

Although they do not specifically adopt an ecological perspective, a number of writers in cognitive and developmental psychology adopt a strongly perceptual approach (e.g., Goldstone and Barsalou, 1998; Jones and Smith, 1993). There are some variations in these authors' work but an important element is that category use is heavily constrained by perception. By this, these authors mean that the categories which are created dynamically in working memory are grounded in perceptions of reality. In particular, Goldstone and Barsalou (1998) hold out the prospect of an eliminative standpoint which suggests that all knowledge is perceptual (in this regard the authors cite Barsalou and Prinz, who in turn follow British Empiricist philosophers in seeking to eliminate non-perceptual knowledge from their account). In any case Goldstone and Barsalou argue strongly for a perceptual grounding for all concepts (a view consistent with that of Jones and Smith). As these views were derived as a counterpoint to some developments in the theory-coherence approach I will consider their specific ideas in more detail below.

The experiential-realist approach

Another approach to category formation uses concepts similar to those in the previous one. The ideas of a basic level, the adaptiveness of perception, and the role of theories and cognitive models in categorization are used, but at the same time some of the most basic assumptions in the previous view are rejected. This approach is the one suggested by Lakoff (1987), and is based on a philosophical position referred to as *experiential realism.*

Lakoff rejects what he refers to as the **objectivist** thinking which underpins much scientific and non-scientific thought. The objectivist view, which can be closely linked to classical logic and mathematical thought, has given rise to, amongst other things, the classical view of categories. Lakoff argues that recent research on categorization has falsified this view (e.g., through the demonstration of the existence of variations in typicality within categories), but the objectivist approach is customarily accepted as a fundamental set of truths which are seldom questioned.

At the centre of the objectivist view is the idea that meaning is based on correspondence. That is, concepts are otherwise meaningless sets of symbols which derive meaning through association with structures in the world. In the objectivist view (which Lakoff acknowledges is very broad: he does not claim that all objectivists share all of the positions which he attacks) the mind is a mirror of the world, and categories are internal representations of external reality (this is the **correspondence view of meaning**). Categories in the mind *are* categories in the world, and both categories in the mind and categories in the world have a classical structure.

Lakoff (1987: 370–1) lists the following aspects of an objectivist view:

1   Categories in the mind (i.e., conceptual categories) are symbolic structures which correspond to objective categories in the world.
2   Categories in the world (i.e., classes) must be capable of being objectively characterized in a way which is independent of the observer.
3   Categories in the mind can only exist for corresponding real world categories.
4   Categories in the mind must have a structure which is identical to real world categories, otherwise they would not be true representations.
5   Given the above, the classical structure of real world categories must be matched by a classical structure in conceptual categories.

Lakoff argues that this view is wrong for both real world categories and categories of the mind, and for the relationship between these two. If the classical view is wrong for conceptual categories then it becomes impossible for the classical view to provide the mechanism for correspondence between real world and conceptual categories.

An example of the classical structure not holding for real world categories is the biological category of *species*. The question of what constitutes a species in biology cannot be objectively answered but depends upon the particular biological theory one subscribes to. Thus species is a category of the world but *it does not have a classical form.*

Lakoff believes that it is possible to show that human conceptual categories are dependent on the observer, in that they are partially determined by observers' mental and physical properties. Examples of these mental properties are imaginative thought processes such as metaphor, metonymy (i.e., a subset of a category standing for the whole) and mental imagery. An example of the determination of conceptual categories by physical properties is the way perceptual colour categories are shared by people of all cultures (suggesting that we all share the same neurophysiological perceptual mechanisms) even though the number of words that cultures have for colours varies markedly (Heider (i.e., Rosch) and Olivier, 1974).

Lakoff argues at length that the doctrine of meaning through correspondence (i.e., that things acquire meaning through correspondence with their mental representations) has been shaken to its core by Putnam's theorem, which has the implication that meaning cannot be given by direct association with real world objects (at least not in terms of the theories of meaning demanded by the objectivist approach to semantics).

The negation of the objectivist account suggests to Lakoff an alternative view which he refers to as experiential realism (Lakoff and Johnson, 1980). Under this view (Lakoff, 1987) the existence of the objective real world is not questioned, but it is not seen as directly given, or as directly psychologically effective. Lakoff writes: 'On the experiential account, meaningful thought and reason make use of symbolic structures *which are meaningful to begin with*' (1987: 372, emphasis in the original).

There are two kinds of thought which are directly meaningful. These are basic-level concepts and **kinaesthetic image schemas**. The former are directly meaningful in that they reflect our perceptual motor experience and mental imagery (cf. the characteristics of the basic level on which Neisser focuses: a basic-level object like a chair or tree would be directly meaningful). Kinaesthetic image schemas relate to the way space is (and our bodily movements in it are) preconceptualized.

This latter point requires some explanation. According to Johnson (cited in Lakoff, 1987) a great deal of our experience is structured in terms of spatial functioning before concepts even exist. For example, we understand our bodily experience in terms of *containers*, or at an even more basic level in terms of in–out relationships. We experience our bodies (and by implication ourselves) as containers and as things in containers (rooms, places, cities, personal relationships, groups etc.). There are hundreds of literal and metaphorical uses of in–out relationships in language. As is illustrated by this example, these kinaesthetic image schemas are held to be so basic that their presence is not always immediately obvious.

Another example of a kinaesthetic image schema is that the human body is a whole with parts, and we treat other objects as also being wholes with parts. We treat objects as having centres (which are important) and peripheries (which are less important). These image schemas are associated with a basic logic which is held to be naturally consistent, and provide the basis for other categorizations and metaphors (we refer to something which is less than crucial as 'peripheral' or we say that we are '*out* of luck').

Thus there is a dual basis by which directly meaningful categorizations are built up. Those which are not directly meaningful are built up from the imaginative capacities of metaphor and metonymy (leading to the formation of idealized cognitive models about these more complex categories). At the same time reality provides a constraint on the sorts of conceptual structures which can be built up on the basis of directly meaningful concepts (basic-level concepts and kinaesthetic image schemas).

Lakoff deals with the ecological position of Gibson and finds it unsatisfactory as an account of the results of categorization processes (he suggests that it cannot account for categories but only for individual phenomena). However, the ecological view, as adapted by Neisser, is very similar in parts to the experiential-realist account suggested by Lakoff. Both approaches focus on the basic level as being governed by perception and bodily functioning, and suggest the importance of higher-order cognitive models (indeed the constraint relations for the role of basic-level categories are identical to those given earlier for the ecological approach). It might even be argued that Lakoff and Johnson's kinaesthetic image schemas are simply particularly common affordances. There are also, however, clear differences in the latter approach's focus on imaginative thinking and the idea that even the basic level is not completely constrained by appearances.

The theory-coherence approach

The last general approach considered in this section is that inspired by Murphy and Medin (1985). Although I class it as a theory-based approach the thrust of the work is to stress the importance of both theory and similarity. Murphy and Medin's ideas also provide the inspiration for the constraint relations treatment that I have introduced here. These authors stress the role of people's theories and the perception of category coherence in categorization (see also Medin and Barsalou, 1987; Medin and Wattenmaker, 1987). The question they raise is: why do *particular* categories form? Out of all the possible categorizations that can be applied, why are particular ones seen as informative, useful and psychologically coherent? The answer that they propose is that categories are psychologically coherent to the extent to which they fit in with perceivers' theories about the world.

An example due to Rips and Handte (cited in Medin and E.E. Smith, 1984) involves the categorization of a disc approximately 5 inches (125 mm) in diameter as a coin or a pizza. Participants were more likely to categorize the object as a pizza even though the object was equidistant (in terms of the linear distance) from the norms for the two categories. It seems therefore that the knowledge people have about categories determines their utilization independently of 'raw' or absolute similarity (assuming such a construct exists). In this case people obviously know that coins are set by law and custom (in our culture) to particular sizes and do not vary beyond a certain range. Similarly, Carey (1982) observed that 4-year-olds were more likely to attribute the possession of a spleen (described as a greenish thing inside people) to a worm than to a mechanical monkey (the latter being perceptually more similar to people). Both these examples indicate that something other than absolute perceptual similarity must govern category formation and use.

Murphy and Medin (1985) argue that previously proposed theories of categorization are insufficient to explain **conceptual coherence**. In other words, theories based on processes such as similarity and attribute matching do not adequately explain how categories form or how conceptual structure works. They argue that other mechanisms (e.g., attributes or perceived correlations of attributes) which have been suggested as constraints on categories are insufficient to account for conceptual coherence. On the contrary, they suggest that category representation depends upon correlated attributes plus underlying principles which determine the attributes that are attended to. Thus categorization does not arbitrarily cut the physical environment at its edges. We do not simply notice that wings and feathers occur together more often than wings and fur, but we attend to that particular correlation because it matches our understanding of which animals are birds. That is, we have a theory that birds are warm-blooded creatures with wings and feathers which often fly, and that theory serves to constrain the category *bird*.

This is only one of the characteristics which distinguish similarity-based approaches (as discussed in the previous section) from theory-based approaches, but it is this idea which is at the core of the theory-based approach. Murphy and Medin acknowledge that the sorts of intuitive theories which underlie category coherence need to be specified more completely. They believe that there are two components to conceptual coherence: the internal structure of a concept and its external structure (i.e., how it fits into the overall knowledge base).

These ideas were taken further in Barsalou and Medin's (1986) work on concepts. These authors advocate a change from a view of concepts as static, neatly organized packets of knowledge to the idea that the representation of categories varies dynamically with experience and current context, and that they serve to generate useful expectations, regardless of whether these have a high probability of being true (cf. Allport, 1954) or have other criteria which suggest conventional logical adequacy. For example, it will be vitally important to remember that snakes can be poisonous when we encounter a snake, even though most snakes are not poisonous. Context specificity improves prediction but it also represents an argument against static representations, and suggests that we need to understand relations between concepts (cf. Thagard, 1989; 1992).

The subsequent work of Medin and colleagues on these topics can be divided into two related pools. There is one set of work which addresses the insufficiency of similarity-based approaches to categorization. The other set of work articulates a theory-based approach (or demonstrates the powerful constraining effects of background knowledge on category use, e.g., Hayes and Taplin, 1992, 1995; Lin and Murphy, 1997).

With respect to theory-based approaches Medin (1989; see also Gelman and Medin, 1993; Medin and Ortony, 1989) developed the concept of **psychological essentialism**. He argued that people believed that objects had essences which distinguished them in kind from other objects. In other words, a dog is different from a cat even if it is surgically altered to look like a cat. These essences are used as organizing principles. Medin does not claim that psychological essentialism is a philosophically plausible approach; he argues nonetheless that it is one that people adopt as a means of making sense of regularities in the world.

This idea has been applied to social psychological phenomena by Rothbart and Taylor (1992). These authors argue that social categories are similar to categories of natural objects in that people believe social categories have features which make them appear as if they have a coherent core that binds the category together. However, artificial object categories do not seem to have this essential nature.

Continuing on the theory-based theme, Wisniewski and Medin (1994) have demonstrated that the features that are used in categorization are determined by the theories and expectations about the data that perceivers bring to a learning situation (see also Cho and Mathews, 1996, for a somewhat different approach). Furthermore, features involve the instantiation of abstract expectations about categories. They give, as an example, learning to use artificial objects. The process of learning involves expectations about the intended function of an object. Artefacts will be expected to have been designed to have some functions; learning to use them involves identifying that function and carrying it out (instantiating it). Indeed, when we see some new gadget our first question is often 'What does it do?' This question can

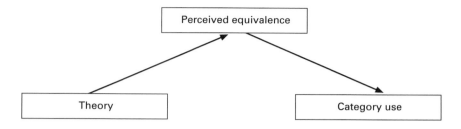

FIGURE 3.3 *Constraint relations emphasized by Wisniewski and Medin*

only be generated on the basis of a theory about gadgets that generates expectations that they will have functions. The answer that something is a 'tachistoscope' is of no value unless we know what tachistoscopes do. These principles would also apply to Semin's (1997) discussion of a language in terms of cognitive tools. When we hear a new word we assume that it will have a meaning, that it will have illocutionary force, and so on.

Wisniewski and Medin (1994) suggest that people's knowledge of the world helps to determine the features that are used to derive similarities. However, their results and interpretations suggest that knowledge does much more than just select features. People with different knowledge actually select different types of features (e.g., more or less abstract features) and engage in searches for different types of features. In terms of constraint relations the model can be articulated as in Figure 3.3.

One problem with this overview is that the other links are by no means excluded in Wisniewski and Medin's work; they are just de-emphasized. The central message of their work is that knowledge-driven and data-driven processes interact and mutually influence each other. Perhaps most importantly, the features which are considered to be equivalent are not stable but change with the type of knowledge that is activated. For example, Wisniewski and Medin describe 'pockets' and 'collars' as features of pictures of clothing that would not normally be seen to be equivalent. They become equivalent when it is *known* that the drawings do, or should, show *detail*.

Supporting evidence for Wisniewski and Medin's analysis can be found in the work of Schyns and Rodet (1997) who showed in a perceptual learning task not only that features were grouped to form categories but that features are constructed in order to form new categories. That is, category formation involves feature creation and not just feature grouping (as is routinely assumed in similarity-based approaches to category learning).

The other related arm to Medin and colleagues' work builds on the suggestion of Murphy and Medin (1985) that similarity is an insufficient principle to constrain category formation. Some of the arguments against a mere similarity approach have already been presented. The key problem is that perceived similarity changes in context-dependent ways and with knowledge and experience, and this is represented by the link between knowledge and perceived equivalence in Figure 3.3. That is, similarity is not a raw material that can be dug out of the environment in the way that sand might be mined from a beach; rather it must be sought out, refined and processed like a rare and valuable mineral.

To take one illustrative example, Medin et al.'s (1993) experiment 1 involved ambiguous pictures of shapes that shared features with each of two contrasting categories of unambiguous figures. The results showed that both sets of unambiguous figures influenced the interpretation of the figures in mutually exclusive ways. In other words, the category presented defined a context-dependent standard for comparison. A category thus provides a base for comparison which helps determine which dimensions are used to determine similarities and differences. This can be contrasted with approaches that assume that similarity is a **primitive** from which categories are wrought.

The spirit of these authors' insights can be captured in Medin et al.'s analogy that similarity is not so much a chameleon (i.e., an elusive changeable creature, citing Goodman) but two chameleons chained together:

> The entities entering into a comparison jointly constrain one another and jointly determine the outcome of a similarity comparison. (That is, paradoxically, two chameleons may behave in a more orderly manner than one.) Thus similarity is changeable and context-dependent but systematically fixed in context. (1993: 272)

Recently, the idea that entities which are compared constrain each other has been articulated in a number of ways. This work is considered in the following sections.

Structural alignment and thematic integration

Some of the work derives from Gentner's (1983) structural alignment hypothesis (this work has been updated by Gentner and Medina, 1998, who stress the importance of comparison as a bridge between similarity and abstraction). The motivating insight behind the application of this idea to similarity judgement was that although similarity was not constant it nevertheless seemed to be lawful. That is, when people said two objects were similar they appeared to select systematically those dimensions or features which enabled that judgement. Similarity was derived not from fixed qualities but from the way perceivers structured the situation, and in particular the way they aligned the situation for the purpose of *comparison*.

If we need to decide whether two objects are similar it makes sense to focus on those qualities which allow us to compare them readily and to ignore those qualities that are irrelevant. An important assumption of the structural alignment hypothesis is that perceived equivalence (in my terms) or analogy (in Gentner's terms) can arise from perceiving shared attributes (single-place predicates, e.g. Scales[FISH]) or relations between objects (multiple-place predicates, e.g., Same skin texture[FISH, CROCODILES]). This argument was extended to similarity by Medin et al. (1990) who argued that there was a consistency in similarity judgements that derived from structural alignment. When people saw entities as sharing relationships they could see them as similar despite the fact that they did not share attributes. Thus, a duck could be seen as being like a fish when attention is drawn to the fact that they are *both* aquatic despite mismatches in features such as one having scales and the other having feathers.

The distinction can also be seen in the following example. An angle of 60° between two lines is a feature of an isosceles triangle; the fact that all internal angles are the same involves a relation between features. An isosceles triangle shares the feature of a 60° angle with certain other shapes but it also shares the relations 'all internal angles the same' with rectangles and 'three internal angles' with all triangles. Clearly though, the distinction between attributes and relations starts to break down because the relation 'three internal angles' can also be treated as an attribute with the object 'triangle' as a predicate.

The structural aspect of the structural alignment hypothesis refers to the hierarchical structure of relations and attributes. Alignment means that higher-order relations (relations which take other relations as arguments) constrain matches on relations which in turn constrain matches on attributes. Thus, matches on the higher-order relation Moves[WALKS, SWIMS, FLIES] constrain the lower-order relation 'walks' which in turn constrains the attribute 'legs'.

I am ambivalent about the need for the attribute–relation distinction on top of an attribute–category distinction because most of the relations that Medin and colleagues refer to are categorical relations involving shared category memberships. 'Aquatic' can be seen as a feature of fish and as a feature of ducks; the fact that they are both aquatic can be seen to be a relation between fish and ducks, but only when they are perceived to be equivalent because they share a category membership. Still other relations convey the quality of entitativity (or being like an entity: Campbell, 1958; see Chapter 8) such as 'A is like B', 'A is near B', 'A has changed in the same way as B' and 'A and B are part of the same larger thing.'

Nevertheless, the usefulness of the attribute–relation distinction for understanding constraints on similarity is suggested by Bassok and Medin's (1997) research in which they argue that semantic dependencies between nouns denote attributes of objects and semantic dependencies between verbs denote relations between objects. They had participants judge the amount of similarity between two simple statements of the form 'The carpenter fixed the chair' and 'The electrician fixed the radio.' Such statements were perceived to be similar because the participants reasoned that the statements shared the relation 'Professionals repairing broken items.' This was consistent with the structural alignment hypothesis. However, participants also saw the statements 'The carpenter fixed the chair' and 'The carpenter sat on the chair' as similar because they reasoned that both statements related to a single process of fixing the chair and then ensuring that the repairs were successful (if the perceived temporal order of the statements was reversed, presumably the participants would have seen sitting on the chair as part of the process of diagnosing or even creating the fault).

Bassok and Medin (1997) argued that *thematic integration* was important as well as comparison. Rather than automatic similarity-based processes where category use automatically dominates perceptions, people may rely on a bidirectional process of rule-based inference. The apparent dominance of the similarity-based approaches may reflect the inference-poor environment of many tasks in psychological experiments. The chance of coming up with a thematic integration that allows perceivers to make useful inferences about a set of abstract geometric figures may be much lower than that of coming up with a thematic integration of a set of sentences (or if thematic integrations do emerge for the abstract figures they may be highly idiosyncratic and not detectable in the averaged data for participants).

Bassok and Medin's (1997) data and their discussion of them are intriguing and informative. They appear to have correctly identified that thematic integration is an important determinant of perceived similarity. They may, however, have understated the case for thematic integration by positing it as an alternative to structural alignment. Indeed, in every case structural alignment may rest upon a thematic integration. I have already suggested that the relation–attribute distinction is tenuous, but it is also true that the relative inclusiveness of concepts depends on a thematic integration. For example, 'walks' can be an attribute of an object or a relation between an object and its environment. Similarly, 'moves' can be an argument of the relation 'walks' and 'walks' can be an argument of the relation 'moves'. A thematic integration is required before the relations A = Fixed[CARPENTER, CHAIR] and B = Fixed[ELECTRICIAN, RADIO] can be contained within the relation Repair Activity[A, B]. If additional background information (such as that the workers were members of a charity or were employed by the same company) were provided a different thematic integration would suggest the higher-order relation might be Acts of Kindness[A, B] or Same Billing Code[A, B].

The problem is perhaps clearest with social categories. During a war, there are relations involving friends versus enemies and both friends and enemies can be divided into soldiers and civilians. The point is that the friend–enemy distinction can contain or be contained by the soldier–civilian distinction. Which of these relations contains the other will depend upon the thematic integration that is employed. The Geneva Convention can be seen (in part) as a thematic integration that demands that enemy civilians and soldiers be treated differently at times of war. The problem of defining attributes in social categorical systems will be considered in Chapter 10, but for the time being I simply want to raise the possibility that the relative inclusiveness of categories is ambiguous: the hierarchical structure that is imposed in some situation is not independent of the interpretation (thematic integration) of the situation. The Geneva Convention is a thematic integration that demands that friend–enemy be treated as a more abstract categorization than soldier–civilian.

Problems also emerge in relation to the mass–count distinction (e.g., Wisniewski et al., 1996). Some nouns can be differentiated in terms of continuous qualities (mass relations) and others can be differentiated in terms of discrete entities (count relations): we talk of 'much' water but 'many' cars. Wierzbicka (1988) has suggested that things which enable count relations tend to exist as individuated, separate entities. Wisniewski et al. (1996) have found that structural alignment is less important than thematic integration for things which allow mass relations.

In summary of this subsection, the attempt to provide specificity via structural alignment may be similar to the effort to define similarity as a fixed abstract quality. Structural alignment may itself follow ubiquitous thematic integration. Upon closer inspection the structural principles are themselves changeable, and may have the goal-directed *ad hoc* character that Barsalou (1987; 1991; 1993) has reported.

Consensual categorical systems

Medin et al. (1997) carried out intriguing research on the development of different categorical systems by groups of experts. The impetus for this research was the attempt to find whether perceived covariation between objects in the world led to the formation of common categorical systems, or whether those systems diverged owing to the different background knowledge, theories and goals that the different experts brought to bear.

The stimuli considered were trees and the experts were taxonomists, landscapers and park maintenance workers. The results showed highly consensual categories for each of the three groups but both overlaps and differences. They found that the difference between maintenance workers and landscape workers was that the latter sorted trees into goal-derived categories based on their particular needs (i.e., landscape use) whereas maintenance workers relied more heavily on the shape of the trees. The taxonomists largely reproduced the scientific classification.

This research is probably the clearest single demonstration of a relatively complete set of constraint relations. Knowledge and perceived equivalence constrain category use, but perceived equivalence is also constrained by knowledge, in that different groups' thematic integrations (in Bassok and Medin's, 1997, terms) led to differing levels of perceived similarity. The clear evidence of different consensual categorical systems is also an important contribution (see Chapter 9).

Medin et al. (1997) may, however, have missed the goal-directed nature of *all* the categories used. The landscape workers' categorical systems were described as goal-directed and utilitarian because they related to what these workers wanted to *do* with trees. This appears entirely correct, but the taxonomists' categorical system can be seen to be equally goal-directed and utilitarian. Taxonomists are also involved in doing things with trees but the work they do is intellectual rather than physical. Scientific taxonomies *are* goal-directed pursuits – the goal being to understand the nature of reality. The utility of such categories is that they serve to cut nature at those joints which are useful for scientific purposes (e.g., determining the likelihood of the spread of a disease between trees). The accepted scientific taxonomy is not the only possible scientific taxonomy, but it is a useful taxonomy because it serves the scientific goals of description, explanation and prediction. The pre-eminently useful feature of this system is that it helps to explain the production and reproduction of entities (organisms) which have covarying features. That is, scientific taxonomy serves the goal of explaining why there are different types of trees and why trees reproduce other trees which are similar to them. This goal does not apply to maintenance workers' or landscapers' categorical systems which are designed to serve other goals. The idea that taxonomies are outcomes of the categorization system rather than determinants is considered in Chapter 10.

Linear separability

Wattenmaker (1995) has examined the concept of **linear separability** as a constraint on the categorization process (see Medin and Schwanenflugel, 1981). This work stems from a long tradition of research on linear separability which had a particular focus on the importance of linear separability for prototype models.

Linearly separable categories are categories that can be defined on a set of dimensions to be non-overlapping. That is, it is possible to draw a line between the two categories. Note that in Figure 3.4 the categories overlap on both dimension 1 and dimension 2 when we look at them one at a time, but the categories are separable if we take them together. Imagine the circles are sofa beds and the crosses are lounges, and dimension 1 is the number of times someone sleeps on the piece of furniture and dimension 2 is the number of times someone sits on it. People sit and sleep on both, but the two types of furniture are clearly separable if we compare both uses.

Wattenmaker (1995) argues (following Wattenmaker et al., 1986) that whether or not linear separability constrains categorization depends on the

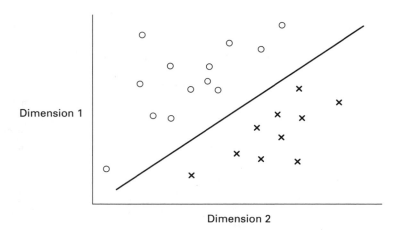

FIGURE 3.4 *Example of two linearly separable categories*

compatibility between linear separability and activated knowledge (for a view leading to rather different conclusions see D. J. Smith et al., 1997, who show that linear separability is important for large, well-differentiated categories). For example, defining category membership by summation is compatible with linear separability; knowledge that emphasizes interactions or relations will be incompatible with linearly separable knowledge structures. The question Wattenmaker poses is whether social and object categorizations are differentially compatible with linear separability.

He focuses on three features: flexibility, interpretation of features and form of representation. He suggests (following Lingle et al., 1984) that social categorization is much more flexible than object categorization and that reasoning schemas for inconsistencies are easier to develop for social than non-social categories. I would note that this makes sense owing to people's capacity to change their behaviour, including changes in behaviour in response to the way people expect themselves to be categorized by other perceivers, a power not shared by other objects. He also suggests, in line with the above, that social categories readily allow flexible interpretation of features and that exemplars of social categories seem less accessible and are less central in concepts and that social categories appear abstract and inferential. Wattenmaker argues that all of these features suggest that linearly separable categories will be more compatible with knowledge about social categories. To this I would add that linear separability is also commonly argued to be a *consequence* of social categorization – an idea considered in the next section, which is a restatement of the idea that category use constrains perceived equivalence.

Formally, linearly separable categories can be expressed in terms of additive functions. That is, it is possible to come up with a mathematical rule to draw a line between the categories that involves adding the weighted score of the members on dimension 1 to the weighted score of the members on dimension 2 and so on. In Figure 3.4 the rule is: dimension 1 – dimension 2. The circles always have higher scores on this function than the crosses. Thus the mathematical rule that defines circles can be expressed as 'higher on dimension 1 than on dimension 2'. In Figure 3.5 no straight line can be drawn to separate the circles from the crosses. This roughly follows the rule that 'the product of dimension 1 and dimension 2 is higher for crosses than circles' or 'high on dimension 1 AND high on dimension 2'. Non-linearly separable categories can involve such interactive terms or products of weighted scores on the two dimensions.

Wattenmaker (1995) has assembled an impressive amount of evidence that summation sorts (i.e., additive rules for classifying objects) are more widely used for social than object categorizations and that this preference is associated with specific knowledge differences and not the global nature of processing. He also showed that participants generated more and varied alternative explanations for social categorizations, and that participants made fewer errors in learning linearly separable structures with social stimuli.

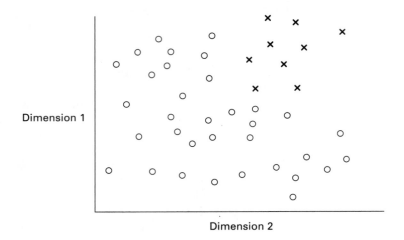

FIGURE 3.5   *Example of two categories that are not linearly separable*

Responses to and developments on the theory-coherence approach

The theory-coherence approach to categorization has prompted some responses, criticisms and developments. For example, Jones and Smith (1993) question whether categories have the essentialist cores that Medin (1989; Medin and Ortony, 1989) and colleagues assign to them. Instead they argue, as do many others, that categories are created dynamically in working memory. Part of their argument against psychological essentialism is that people's verbal reasoning about categories is far more diverse than would be expected from the essentialist stance. Indeed they argue that reasoning about essences is another example of a task-specific assembly of knowledge that does not require the *prior* existence of the essence. For example, when people are asked to say what a 'skunk' is they draw on biological theories, but Jones and Smith believe that the essences that people describe under these circumstances are created in an *ad hoc* manner for the purpose of answering the experimenter's questions. This is a point that we will return to a number of times in the chapters to come.

Barsalou (e.g., 1991; 1993) also argues that *ad hoc* goal-derived categories are commonly used which violate the correlational structure present in the environment. A striking example of such a goal-directed category is 'children, insurance policies and photographs'. These objects seem to have no logical connection until the category 'things to take out of the house during a fire' is invoked. Barsalou also argues that such goal-directed categories can be learned and become enduring over time.

Sloman and Rips (1998) summarize the recent research on the importance of similarity- and rule-based processes in categorization and other domains. They conclude that there are four views in the field about the role of similarity as an explanatory construct (these are termed the strong, weak, feeble and no role). However, the weight of opinion in cognitive psychology suggests a role for both similarity- and abstract-rule-based processes (and this view includes that of writers included in the special issue of the journal *Cognition* edited by Sloman and Rips, such as Gentner and Medina, 1998, and Smith et al., 1998).

Goldstone and Barsalou (1998) argue that perception and conception have become disassociated in philosophy and psychology. Their position represents a more detailed version of the critique developed by Jones and Smith (1993) in the developmental literature and I will deal with this more recent view in considerably more detail. Goldstone and Barsalou argue for a reunification of perception and conception, arguing that both conceptual processing and similarity are grounded in the same perceptually based representations. That is, these authors accept the existence of a distinction between abstract conceptual processing and perceptual processing but argue that both types of processing share the same perceptual representational system to a large extent (the authors consider two alternatives – all knowledge is perceptual and all knowledge is influenced by perceptual processing – but do not argue strongly for either).

The core of the argument is that conceptual processing uses representation and processing mechanisms drawn from perception rather than substantially separate systems. In this their approach differs from conventional theories of concepts. Consider the constraint relations formulation (that I have developed largely for the purposes of describing these conventional theories of concepts). The constraint relations formulation places perceptual similarity in a different 'box' to background knowledge. If we eliminate the possibility that background knowledge and perceived equivalence are the same thing then it is possible that we are making a conceptual error by drawing a line between knowledge and perception (Figure 3.6).

On the contrary, Goldstone and Barsalou conceive all conceptual processes to be mediated through perceptual mechanisms and (possibly) all knowledge to be represented in perceptual forms. This is an argument for strong mediating links involving knowledge and perceived equivalence:

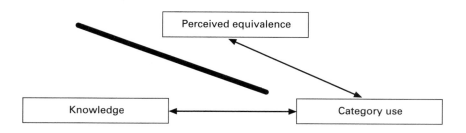

FIGURE 3.6   *Separation in constraint relations questioned by Goldstone and Barsalou*

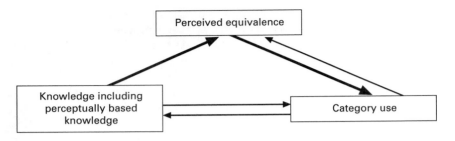

FIGURE 3.7 *Additional constraint relations emphasized by Goldstone and Barsalou*

indeed part of the evidence that Goldstone and Barsalou use to support their argument is that perceptual similarity is not stable but becomes attuned to conceptual demands. The examples used suggest that Goldstone and Barsalou are primarily referring to the visual modality of perception. These authors' position can be seen as a full constraint model, but this does not do justice to its richness and some important variations from other ideas in the literature. In Figure 3.7 the thick arrows represent the primary causal links anticipated.

Goldstone and Barsalou seek to show how perceptual knowledge is irreplaceable in forming concepts. The chief bases of their argument are as follows.

PERCEPTUAL SYSTEMS ALLOW ANALOGUE REPRESENTATIONS   When we want to understand something it is useful if we can understand it in a form that preserves its physical properties. That is, rather than converting an object's properties into symbolic representations and performing computations on them it is convenient to preserve an analogue representation of the object's appearance. Goldstone and Barsalou use the example of a representation of a couch that has to be moved through the door. If we were to imagine the couch being picked up and rotated then, providing that we do this accurately, we can be confident about conclusions drawn. However, even abstract concepts can be represented in analogue form and these representations have benefits because other properties 'free-ride' on the representation. The machine analogies that Goldstone and Barsalou use are reasonably complex, but a simple example of such an analogue representation might be representing time by the shadow cast by a sundial. Although it is *designed* to tell the time a property that 'free-rides' on the sundial is that we can tell the direction of the sun from it.

OVERALL SIMILARITY   Goldstone and Barsalou suggest that similarity often involves integration across many properties so that overall similarity is computed. They argue that this holistic similarity computation occurs rapidly and involves parallel processes. The strong assumption therefore is that overall similarity has a distinct explanatory role. They therefore reject the arguments of Goodman and others that similarity is superfluous (i.e., to say two things are similar is to say no more than that they have some property in common). Rather Goldstone and Barsalou argue that overall similarity serves important psychological functions and that overall similarity is constrained by perception. That is, two things cannot be seen to be similar at an overall level unless they have similar appearances. This view can be seen as a reiteration of the ecological approach's commitment to a basic level in categorization which is constrained by similar appearances. However, the authors suggest that these benefits are generalized to other conceptual structures. They suggest that taxonomic categories are structured by overall similarity that allows efficient inferences: the similarities between birds allow us to make inferences about the attributes of a stimulus that is assigned to the category *bird* (see Chapter 10 for a contrary view).

DERIVED SIMILARITY   Goldstone and Barsalou suggest that just as similarity can constrain categorization, so categorization can constrain similarity, but the effects of categorization on similarity are weaker. These authors cite recent cognitive research as evidence for this (see Goldstone, 1998) rather than the social psychological research considered in Section C of this chapter. However, they argue that such perceptual learning is slow to change and involves relatively small changes. They contrast this with the hyperflexible conceptual system which is highly context-dependent.

ABSTRACTIONS ARE DERIVED FROM PERCEPTION   The authors argue that abstract information involves or is based around perceptual information. They suggest that, even where categories are organized around theories, these theories themselves are based on perceptual information and in particular perceptual similarity.

PERCEPTUAL SIMULATION   The authors argue that the available evidence suggests that people use perceptual simulation (like the analogue representation of moving a couch) in conceptual tasks where they are presented only with linguistic materials. This conflicts with standard theories which assume that reasoners use symbolic representations for such tasks.

SHARED PROCESSES BETWEEN PERCEPTION AND CONCEPTION   Goldstone and Barsalou make a number of cogent arguments about the close match between processes that are clearly involved in perception and those that seem to underpin conceptual processing. The examples they cite include selective attention, blurring/filtering, binding, sub-categorization, matching across sensory modalities, and productivity (creating structures from lower-level units).

The implication of the work on and responses to the theory-coherence approach is thus that similarity is derived from context-specific comparisons that derive from developing understandings of relations between objects. The core message of this work is therefore an updated, elaborated and in specific ways a more sophisticated presentation of ideas that had been developed earlier by Tajfel, Turner and others in social psychology: we see objects to be similar when we *understand* that they are related. Ramifications of these ideas for social psychological issues are discussed in Chapters 5, 6, 7 and 8 (see also Berndsen et al., 1998). The choice point I identify for this section emerges as an issue in all three approaches:

- Is categorization primarily based on structure in the world which constrains us to perceive certain similarities?

  or

- Is categorization primarily based on theories which inform the perceiver about *which* similarities and differences are relevant, which in turn become the basis for theories?

The difference between these two ideas can be put in the form of the constraint diagrams in Figure 3.8.

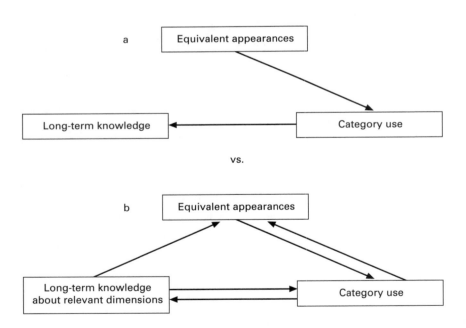

FIGURE 3.8   *Contrasting constraint relations for (a) similarity and (b) theory/similarity approaches*

affordances Relationships between objects in the environment and possible actions by the perceiver.

conceptual coherence The idea that concepts hang together in a meaningful and intelligible way. It was to explain this that Murphy and Medin (1985) proposed the theory-coherence approach.

correspondence view of meaning The objectivist idea that concepts have a universal meaning by virtue of the direct association with things in the world. This is a very old idea in analytical philosophy. It has been challenged by idealist and/or linguistic approaches. The former tend to the view that concepts have no fixed meaning; the latter imply that concepts have no meaning that is independent of a language system.

direct perception The pickup of information directly from the environment.

ecological approach An approach to perception, and more recently categorization, which posits the direct pickup or perception of invariant features of the world.

experiential-realist approach An approach to categorization that proposes that categories can be based on directly meaningful symbolic structures.

idealized cognitive models Models that underlie concepts and give meaning to those concepts. The knowledge contained in these models is not directly perceivable by inspecting the surface features of the object. Thus, for people in modern societies the idealized cognitive model of a coin is not limited to its shape and size but extends to an understanding of the role of money in a trading economy.

invariants Perceptual features of the world that remain unchanged despite changes in the observer.

kinaesthetic image schemas Symbolic structures that are directly meaningful by virtue of the way they preconceptualize space in terms of the movements of our bodies through space.

linearly separable categories Categories which can be separated by a function based on adding weighted values of members on dimensions.

linguistic division of labour The idea that we do not know the meaning of all concepts but that we expect experts in our society to have meanings of specific concepts available when necessary.

objectivism The philosophical view underlying the correspondence view of semantics which holds that there is a lawful underlying objective reality. Its opposite is subjectivism, which implies that reality is different for all people.

primitive The most basic element or building block for some process.

psychological essentialism The intuitive philosophical standpoint, held to underlie categorization behaviour by Medin (1989) and others, that natural objects have core features (essences) which make them distinct from objects that belong to other categories. This idea is intended to explain how people think and not how the world is. Rothbart and Taylor (1992) have extended this idea to social categories.

theory-coherence approach The approach to category formation and use which proposes that categories are constrained by background theories which give a coherent meaning to those categories.

C. Categorization effects

An enduring concern in social psychology is the possibility that categorization produces changes in judgement and we saw this emphasis in the work of Allport (1954) and Campbell (1956) mentioned at the start of Chapter 2. Such changes in judgement are most interesting if we assume that they reflect changes in the perception or understanding of things in the world as a result of those things being categorized. They are specifically interesting here because categorization effects provide evidence of the relatively unexplored constraint in cognitive work in categorization: category use constrains perceived equivalence. At one level, it would seem remarkable if category use did not constrain equivalence, but nevertheless the research on the effects of categorization on judgement has been patchy, and has been concentrated largely within social psychology (but there is increasing interest in learned categorical perception in cognitive psychology: Goldstone, 1995; 1998; Livingston et al., 1998).

The reasons to expect categorization effects are easy to see. As Lassaline and Murphy (1998) observe, categories should be easier to learn if there is high similarity within categories and dissimilarity between categories. If perceptual similarity is itself variable, but is tuned to conceptual demands (Goldstone and Barsalou, 1998), then increasing perceptual similarity should serve to make it easier to learn categories.

Tajfel and Wilkes (1963) applied earlier work on the estimation of the magnitudes of objects (e.g., the sizes of coins of differing values) to develop an understanding of the processes by which people learned associations between category labels and positions on quantitative dimensions and then used that categorical information as a basis for the judgement of those objects. Thus Tajfel and Wilkes (1963) argued that when people come to learn that Swedes are taller than Italians they can use the knowledge of that difference as a basis for estimating heights. The effect of this knowledge will be to accentuate perceived differences between groups (known as the **interclass effect**) and accentuate perceived differences within groups (the **intraclass effect**). The processes involved could also be termed intercategory **contrast** and intracategory **assimilation** effects, or accentuation effects.

The first direct test of the accentuation hypothesis was conducted by Tajfel and Wilkes (1963) who used the case of two classes (a biserial classification) correlated with the size of a set of stimuli. The stimuli were black lines drawn on white cardboard. There were eight lines varying by a constant proportion of 5 per cent. The categories used involved labels (the letters A and B). In the classified experimental condition the four shorter lines were labelled A and the four longer lines were labelled B.

After the categorization was made salient (participants had been shown that one set of lines was longer than the other) the participants were asked to judge the stimuli. They were presented in a random order between six and eleven times. It was found that participants in the classified condition over-estimated the judged differences between the shortest B line and the longest A line (compared with people who judged unlabelled stimuli). This was interpreted by Tajfel and Wilkes as demonstrating an accentuation of differences between classes. It should be noted that they did not test whether the A lines were judged to be (on average) shorter, and the B lines to be longer, than they really were. There was no clear evidence for a reduction of intraclass differences (there was a non-significant tendency).

Tajfel and Wilkes also tested for the effects of familiarity (or past experience with the categorization) and salience. The term 'salience' was used by Tajfel and Wilkes (1963) to refer to subjective importance or relevance. Salience was manipulated in two ways: either simultaneously or successively. In three versions of the experiment the subjects were shown the stimuli before the experiment: they were arranged so that the longest B stimulus was adjacent to the shortest A stimulus. The subjects were able to walk around and look at the lines for as long as they wanted. In the successive presentation of the stimuli the subjects were shown the cards one at a time in order from the smallest to the largest. It was hypothesized that the simultaneous presentation would be more salient and lead to stronger categorization effects. It was found that the interclass and intraclass effects were no stronger in the salient conditions.

Familiarity was manipulated by retesting the participants. This occurred either one week later (between sessions) or in the same session. In the same session it was measured by presenting the stimuli to the subjects a further five times (that is in addition to the six presentations which were standard).

It was also found that there was no difference due to past experience between sessions. It was found that there were stronger interclass and intraclass effects with past experience within a session. This suggests that subjects may have been more likely to use the categorization following extensive exposure to it.

I have lost count of the number of researchers who have told me that they attempted without success to replicate Tajfel and Wilkes's results using the original labelled line-judgement paradigm or minor variations on it (Livingston et al., 1998, cite the unpublished thesis of Richardson in this regard). It is troubling but not surprising that these unsuccessful replications do not appear in the published literature. More surprisingly though, replications of the results using the original paradigm are also absent despite the fact that the paper is very well known and widely cited.

The attitude judgement studies conducted by Eiser and other workers in this field provide one important class of evidence on accentuation effects. In these studies statements expressing attitudes towards members of social groups are expressed. The original interest in these studies was the effect of **own position** on the rating of attitudes, as it had earlier been assumed (by Thurstone, 1931) that ratings of attitudes would be independent of own position. The conclusion from a long tradition of research on this point is that attitudes do depend upon own position (see Eiser, 1980, 1990, for a review).

Some of the studies in this tradition have looked at the effects of classification on judgement. The study by Eiser (1971) of attitude judgement introduced a new area for research on categorization effects. The experiment involved the judgement of a set of statements reflecting attitudes towards the non-medical use of drugs: 32 of the statements were permissive and 32 were restrictive. The subjects were told that the statements came from newspapers. The task of the subjects was to rate the statements on an 11-point scale from *extremely permissive* to *extremely restrictive*.

In the control condition the participants were simply asked to judge the statements. In the experimental condition, however, the permissive statements were ascribed to one newspaper (given the fictitious name *The Gazette*) and the restrictive statements were ascribed to another paper (*The Messenger*). ` This study was a replication of Tajfel and Wilkes's (1963) study, the main difference being that the stimuli were attitude statements. The newspapers, of course, did not actually exist but the subjects were told that the fictitious names were used to 'control for any personal biases' (Eiser, 1971: 5). Another feature of this experiment was that the participants were asked to express their agreement or disagreement with the statements, half before rating (the *salient condition*) and half after rating the statements (the *non-salient condition*). In this way they could determine the participants' actual views on the issue (these were classified as being either restrictive or permissive towards the use of drugs).

An accentuation of interclass differences was found but the reduction of intraclass differences was not significant. There was a slight tendency for a reduction of intraclass differences but variation between participants was very high.

The conventional finding in attitude judgement (as expressed in the accentuation theory of Eiser and Stroebe, 1972) is that judges with extreme positions use their own position as a cue for organizing judgements. They accentuate the differences between statements associated with own position and alternative positions. This effect, however, only applies when the language associated with own position is evaluatively congruent. Judges do not accentuate differences between groups of statements when the terms used to describe their own positions are negative.

McGarty and Penny (1988) demonstrated accentuation effects using political attitude statements. It was found that left-wing participants (who evaluated the labels for their positions positively) showed more contrast between a group of right-wing attitude statements and a set of left-wing attitude statements than did right-wing participants (who tended to evaluate the terms for their own positions less positively).

These findings can be explained in terms of accentuation theory (Eiser and Stroebe, 1972), social identity theory (McGarty and Penny, 1988) or self-categorization theory (Haslam and Turner, 1992; 1995). From an SCT perspective the explanation is straightforward. The differing language used to label the regions of the attitude judgement scale serves to make different categorizations salient. The evaluative language can reduce the congruence (normative fit, see Chapter 5) between the statements and a social identity as, for example, a right-winger. Self-categorization and social identity theories assume that a positive self-concept is part of normal psychological functioning, and that objects associated with the self tend to be evaluated positively. Note that in another context the left-wing terms could have been evaluated negatively, resulting in more contrast between the statement groups for the right-wing judges. To take two extreme examples, the comparison between statements labelled 'fascist' and those labelled 'progressive' is more likely to make a moderate left-winger's social identity salient, whereas a comparison between statements labelled 'conservative' and 'loony left' might be more likely to increase the normative fit of a social categorization for a moderate right-winger. The point is that the variation of contrast between categories depends on the evaluative language used to the extent to which it makes *different social categorizations salient*.

Haslam and Turner bring this idea into sharp focus in their hypothesis 1:

> any stimulus will be perceived to share the same social category membership as a stereotyper to the extent that that stimulus is perceived to be less different from the stereotyper's own position than from all others that are psychologically salient for the stereotyper. (1992: 255)

They argue further that variable self-perception will result in assimilation of the stimulus towards own position when the stimulus is perceived to be psychologically interchangeable with self, and to be contrasted away from own position when the stimulus is seen to belong to a non-self category. In a series of studies Haslam and Turner showed that the perception of a target person was assimilated towards own position when the perceiver and the target shared a category membership, and contrasted away from own position when the perceiver and a target belonged to different social categories.

These ideas were used further to provide an account of differing judgements of extremists and moderates. As I noted above, most theories of social judgement anticipate that people with extreme positions will show greater accentuation than moderates (with the caveat that under certain circumstances, extremists will show no more accentuation than moderates). Under Haslam and Turner's application of SCT the greater accentuation shown by moderates than by extremists is due to the fact that extremists will tend to be more clearly different from other people. However, Haslam and Turner (1995) showed how this prediction could be reversed where the distribution of comparison positions was skewed towards the positions of the extremists. Their empirical investigations on this point generally supported this prediction.

Haslam and Turner (1995) draw the conclusion that this is evidence that the same psychological processes of categorical judgement apply for moderates and extremists (rather than separate, deficient processes for extremists).

Categorization effects using an attitude judgement task have also been obtained by McGarty and Penny (1988) and by McGarty and Turner (1992). We found an accentuation of both interclass differences and intraclass similarities using a task involving the judgement of political attitudes classified by authors compared with unclassified statements. McGarty and Turner (1992) also found that judgemental confidence was higher when judging classified than unclassified statements.

However, not all studies show that classification leads to increased contrast between categories. The experimental conditions used by Manis et al. (1986) and by Eiser et al. (1991) both produced assimilation between categories.

Krueger and colleagues have conducted a number of studies which have looked for evidence of categorization effects. Krueger et al. (1989) investigated categorization effects in a category learning paradigm. This research investigated what happens when a categorization that is already well learned is challenged by new information that suggests that previously detected differences are bigger or smaller than they were before.

Participants learned a sequence of 48 three-digit numbers, of which half were associated with one category and the other half were associated with another. The dependent measure was the estimate of the mean for each category.

In the test phase the same stimuli were presented again for one category accompanied by a new series of 24 stimuli for the other category which either increased or decreased the mean for that category. The question was whether participants' perceptions of increases and decreases in the categories would match the changes in the means of those categories. A change which decreased the mean of a larger category would decrease the differences between the categories, and one which increased the mean of a larger category would increase intercategory differences. Thus if participants were particularly attentive to information which increases intercategory differences the effect of reducing category differences should be less than the effect of increasing intercategory differences. On the other hand, if people ignore information which suggests a reduction in differences between categories then the reduction of intercategory differences should have little effect on the perceived differences between categories. The results of Krueger et al. (1989) and subsequent research by Krueger (1991) suggested that the effect was greater when the mean differences were enhanced rather than reduced (see also Krueger, 1992).

In a follow-up experiment Krueger et al. (1989) surprisingly found that inducing expectations of differences had no effect on the estimates of category means. They associated the categories with the weights in pounds of marathoners (lighter) and sprinters (heavier) but found no changes in the categorization effects.

Krueger and Clement (1994) investigated accentuation effects in a series of interesting studies. A very important aspect of this work was that Krueger and Clement sought to evaluate the predictions of models based on specific prototype and exemplar theories of category judgement. They contrasted the prototype theory of Huttenlocher et al. (1991, developed in relation to spatial location) with the exemplar model of Smith and Zárate (1992). Huttenlocher et al. (1991) argue that memory and knowledge about categories consist of knowledge about category prototypes, category boundaries and individual exemplars (each component of which is associated with error and uncertainty). To the extent that there is high uncertainty about the stimulus, the prototype will be used as a default value. The implication is that this prototype model predicts the intraclass effect (increased homogeneity within categories) but not the interclass effect.

On the other hand, the exemplar-based model of Smith and Zárate (1992) holds that there is no separate memory trace for the abstract summary or prototype, but in developing an impression of a category people form a weighted average of the known values of exemplars, giving most weight to exemplars which are very similar to the target. This model predicts the intraclass effect to the extent that attention to the category label leads to (a) more exemplars being assigned to the category with that label and (b) greater weight being given to same-category rather than other-category exemplars.

Krueger and Clement (1994) actually contrast the predictions of these models with accentuation theory for single-, two- and multiple-category cases. They argue that accentuation theory predicts clear categorization effects in the two-category case and state that accentuation theory predicts the interclass and intraclass effects under these circumstances. They argue that the prototype model predicts the intraclass effect regardless of the number of categories and that the exemplar model predicts categorization effects with two or more categories. Their overview can be schematized as in Table 3.1

TABLE 3.1   *Overview of Krueger and Clement (1994)*

Approach	Single category	Two categories	Multiple categories
Accentuation	—	Interclass and intraclass	Ambiguous[1]
Prototype	Intraclass	Intraclass	Intraclass
Exemplar	—	Interclass and intraclass	Interclass and intraclass

[1]The paper is ambiguous about the predictions of accentuation theory for multiple categories.

The empirical studies reported by Krueger and Clement (1994) involve the effect of a pre-existing categorization (month of the year) on the estimation of maximum and minimum temperatures on given days. The months provided a classification scheme which was known to the participants and which provided expectations about temperature. Relative to actual changes in temperatures the interclass effect was defined as the overestimation of between-month differences and the intraclass effect was defined as the underestimation of within-month differences. The overall level of accuracy was quite high (with overestimation in four months and underestimation in three others). In experiment 1 they showed categorization effects involving a reduction in dispersion in categories that could be interpreted as a contrast away from the category boundary and assimilation to the category central tendency.

Experiment 2 was an attempt to compare the predictions of the three different models by examining categorization effects in single-category (considering March, April *or* May) and multiple-category cases (considering March, April *and* May). They found more overestimation in the multiple- than the single-category case; however, they also found that the mean within-subjects correlation between the actual and estimated temperatures was .89 in the multiple-category condition. They do not report the correlation in the single-category case, but this result would seem to militate against the claim that categorization produces distortion. The overall results obtained in this study tended to support the exemplar rather than the accentuation theory approach.

Krueger and Clement's work is a timely reminder that the original accentuation theory account needs to be updated and the psychological factors which control categorization effects need further specification. It also seems to be the case that, although these authors have taken the very distinctive step of seriously attempting to address the question of the degree of distortion created by categorization, their data do not provide much evidence of such distortion. Indeed, Krueger and Clement make the intriguing observation that categorization effects improve prediction despite the loss of information (cf. Anderson, 1991).

Recently, Livingston et al. (1998) have examined the idea of whether the accentuation effects anticipated by Tajfel and Wilkes (1963) are of the same nature as categorical perception effects. Categorical perception effects relate to the perception of discrete categories in a continuous band of stimulation. The most obvious example is seeing bands of colour in a rainbow even though the rainbow is constituted by the (continuous) spectrum of visible light (see Harnad, 1987). Categorical perceptual effects are referred to as expansion (interclass) and compression (intraclass) effects and there is good reason to believe that the mechanisms in the categorical perception of, for example, bands of colour in a rainbow are innate (see e.g., Heider and Olivier, 1974, on the similarity of the perceptual judgements from cultures using completely different colour spaces).

The question addressed by Livingston et al. was whether categorization effects based on category induction procedures were of the same form as categorical perception effects. They observed considerable difficulty in reproducing these effects with stimuli that differed on a single dimension (they noted also the difficulty that Richardson had had in replicating the Tajfel and Wilkes, 1963, line judgement effects in an unpublished doctoral dissertation). However, in research using multiple dimensions they did obtain compression effects. In their fourth experiment, participants viewed the genitalia of day-old male and female chicks (the participants were told that they were actually looking at the larynxes of monkeys). The participants rated the similarities of pairs of stimuli either after being trained in the difference between the two categories or not. The effect of training was a compression or intraclass effect (stimuli classified A or B were seen as more similar to each other but not more different from stimuli differently labelled) and the dimensional structure of the similarity space changed. Goldstone describes research in this field in the following way:

> In sum, there is evidence for three influences of categories on perception: (a) category-relevant dimensions are emphasized, (b) irrelevant variation is de-emphasized, and (c) relevant dimensions are selectively sensitized at the category boundary. (1998: 590)

In summary, the evidence for the categorization effects that were originally outlined by Tajfel and Wilkes (1963) is far less clear than one would expect for phenomena that are believed to be so pervasive. Few social psychologists explicitly question the existence of the categorization effects but this is not due to overwhelming evidence for the effects, and the very patchy evidence of the intraclass effect with non-social stimuli appears puzzling. The evidence in the cognitive psychological literature strongly suggests that perceptual contrast effects involve multiple dimensions whereby differences on dimensions that are relevant to differentiating between stimuli become highly prominent and differences on irrelevant dimensions are ignored.

Nevertheless if we accept that categorization effects do actually occur we have to ask what their significance is. By far the most common view in social psychology is that categorization effects represent judgemental distortions or changes in the response language without any underlying changes in perception (Birnbaum, 1982; Eiser, 1986, 1990; Upmeyer, 1981; Upshaw, 1984; Upshaw and Ostrom, 1984). An example (due to Eiser) of context effects understood from this view would be where somebody says an elephant is large in one context (when compared with an ant) but says it is small when compared with a planet. The argument is that the perceiver's impression of the physical size of the elephant does not change even though the language used to describe the elephant has changed. Eiser refers to the interpretation of context effects as changes in the response language as the **semantic view** and it is based on the principle of absolute judgement (Upshaw and Ostrom, 1984): differences in judgements of stimuli correspond to a scaling of differences in the stimulus information.

The other broad view is that context effects reflect genuine changes in perception (the **perceptual view**). This approach has been championed for context effects generally by Helson (1964) and Sherif and Hovland (1961) and for categorization effects in particular by Haslam and Turner (1992; see Chapter 5), McGarty and Turner (1992) and Oakes et al. (1994).

Although the possibility of semantic effects is a very strong one, when it comes to explaining certain findings we run into problems if we adopt this view exclusively. Many treatments of categorization from Bruner onwards maintain that using a category leads to a perceived equivalence of members (either directly or through long-term knowledge). If we take the semantic view that categorization effects are not evidence of this process, then we must conclude that either the process does not occur or there must be some other form of evidence for it.

If we adopt the second view, that there can be perceptual effects which involve changes in the understanding of the entities categorized and the relations between them, then categorization effects take on a profound significance. The most important implication of the idea of categorization effects for cognition stems from the prospect that they reflect changes in category representation. When perceivers accentuate similarities and differences, are they also perceiving stimuli in terms of abstract summaries or prototypes? If they are, as some approaches to categorization such as self-categorization theory suggest, then this would be a very important implication indeed. As yet though we are not in a position to draw firm conclusions about the implications of categorization effects for category representation.

Even from this necessarily brief review it is possible to enunciate a choice point as well as two important unanswered questions. In no particular order of importance these are:

- Are categorization effects true changes in perception implying a variable representation ?

  or

  Are categorization effects distortions about categories?

- Why is the intraclass effect weaker with non-social information?
- Can categorical perception effects be equated with categorization effects?

assimilation effect Perceiving or judging two elements to be more similar to each other in one setting than other.

contrast effect Perceiving or judging two elements to be more different to each other in one setting than other.

interclass effect The accentuation of differences between members of different categories as an effect of categorization. This effect has some similarities with what Sherif and Hovland (1961) referred to as a *contrast* effect.

intraclass effect The accentuation of similarities between members of a category as an effect of categorization. This effect has some similarities with what Sherif and Hovland (1961) referred to as an *assimilation* effect.

own position The attitudinal position favoured by some person.

perceptual view The view that context effects in judgement can reflect changes in perception.

semantic view The view that context effects in judgement reflect changes in the response language used in different contexts.

Conclusion

Research on category formation and learning represents the cutting edge of contemporary work on categorization. It has replaced the continuing emphasis on the nature of category representation as the focus of intellectual energy in cognitive work on categorization.

A very large proportion of this work is comfortably described in terms of the constraint relations framework which I have introduced here. This should come as no surprise because the idea of constraints on categorization is an important emphasis in the work of Medin and many others.

The constraint relations framework does, however, suggest some areas have been underexplored. The constraints which are currently receiving the most attention are the constraints of knowledge on category use and knowledge on perceived equivalence.

Perhaps the area that has received the least attention is the study of the effects of category use on the perceived equivalence and non-equivalence of category members. This has been a research priority in social psychology (where as Krueger and Clement, 1994, observe, categorization researchers use judgemental measures) but less so in cognitive psychology (where researchers are more likely to use reaction time measures). Somewhat paradoxically though, many of the social psychologists who do study categorization effects believe that these effects are relatively superficial changes in responses rather than genuine changes in perception. That is, many of the people who do study categorization effects believe that they are of relatively limited importance to the categorization process.

This paradox emerges from common assumptions in social psychology about the functions of categorization and its distorting effects on perception. To move towards its resolution we need to consider social psychological treatments of categorization in more detail. The next three chapters are devoted to mapping out some key social psychological approaches.

4 The Categorization Process in Social Psychology: Biased Stimulus Processing and Knowledge Activation

In this chapter I intend to examine a number of organizing principles which derive from work with a social cognitive orientation. In some, but not all cases, these approaches are closely based on ideas developed in cognitive psychology.

The structure I adopt in relation to each approach is to state the fundamental principles of each view, signpost the historical antecedents of that view, and then tease out some implications of the principles. I will also provide very brief illustrations of some recent work or updates of both of the views considered and then suggest how a combination of these views represents a mainstream consensus about categorization in social psychology.

As a rough summary, the social cognitive literature on categorization can be seen to be organized around the following three principles: (a) categorization involves biased stimulus processing, (b) categorization involves the activation of previously stored constructs, and (c) categorization is constrained by motivational and evaluative concerns. In terms of the constraint framework these insights represent a focus on the relationships between category use and perceived equivalence in the first case and the relationships between long-term knowledge and category use in the second case. The motivational and evaluative concerns reflect a further set of constraints outside the six that I have discussed so far (or at least controls on these constraints).

A. Categorization as biased stimulus processing

We have already touched on the motivation for this approach in relation to the cognitive miser metaphor. What I want to do here is present this approach in a rather more general light as an account of how the categorization process works in relation to social stimuli. The fundamental principles of the view can be presented as in Figure 4.1.

The **cognitive load** created by the demands of a complex environment, combined with perceivers' processing **capacity limitations**, create conditions of overload. Overload is dealt with by categorization which is a form of selective (biased) and over-generalized perception which inevitably leads to error and

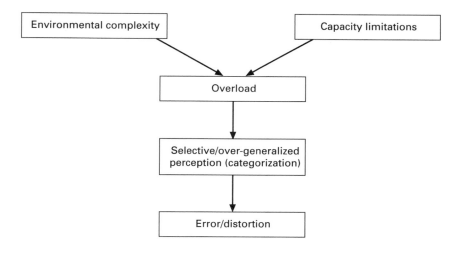

FIGURE 4.1   *The biased stimulus information processing approach*

distortion because individuating evidence which necessarily conflicts with the generalizations is ignored.

The first decade of research on the biased stimulus information processing approach is best summarized in the volume edited by Hamilton (1981). Chapters by Rothbart (1981), Taylor (1981) and Wilder (1981) are particularly useful for articulating certain themes in this work. The foundations for the biased processing view lie in cognitive psychological work in the 1960s which suggested the metaphor of the human mind as an information processing device with a fixed level of processing capacity.

Yet other antecedents for this view include the work of authors such as Allport (1954) and Tajfel (1969) on categorization and stereotyping. These authors took the view that the social environment makes extreme demands on attention owing to the large number of individual people that we all encounter. An adaptive response to this situation is to treat individuals as indistinguishable from other members of the same group, because it would take too much effort to distinguish between all of them. Selective generalizations thus represent a solution to the problem of overload.

The final antecedent that I will consider is the idea of attributional error. This reached considerable prominence in social psychology in the 1970s (see the book by Nisbett and Ross, 1980, for an excellent guide to this research). Research in the early 1970s had established the existence of attributional biases such as the **actor–observer effect**. It seemed to be the case that many judgements that people made were characterized by errors and biases so that, for example, people were overly attentive to stimuli that were very **available**, and to possibilities that seemed **representative** (Tversky and Kahneman, 1974).

Having identified the immediate antecedents of the approach it is useful to point out some of the key concerns. I will identify five as being important to understanding a wide range of ideas within the approach.

Distinctiveness

Research on the development of negative stereotypes of minorities showed how the biased processing approach could be used. Hamilton and Gifford (1976) argued that stereotype formation develops from the phenomenon of **illusory correlation**. Owing to the inability of people to store all of the information they encounter they are forced to take short-cuts. These short-cuts involve attending only to the information that is particularly attention grabbing by virtue of its **distinctiveness**. Owing to this selectivity, impressions of groups come to be based on a biased subset of all the available information.

Hamilton and Gifford (1976) had two further assumptions that made this explanation very important for social stereotyping. They reasoned that minority groups would be distinctive by virtue of their small size because members of small groups are only encountered infrequently. It was also reasoned that rare or infrequent behaviours would also be distinctive. Thus, rare or infrequent behaviours performed by a minority would be doubly distinctive and would have a disproportionately large effect on the stereotype because they would be overrepresented in memory. The full relevance of the account is apparent when the next step is taken. What sort of behaviours are distinctive (i.e., rare)? The plausible assumption was that, given that positive behaviours are socially desirable, negative or undesirable behaviours would be less common and more distinctive. If negative behaviours by minority members are particularly distinctive, and hence likely to be encoded in stereotypes, then the prospect exists for negative stereotypes of minority groups to form by a process of illusory correlation, whereby people develop an erroneously negative view of minority groups.

This explanation was initially put to empirical test in two studies by Hamilton and Gifford (1976; see also Hamilton and Sherman, 1989, and McGarty and de la Haye, 1997, for reviews; and Mullen and Johnson, 1990, for a meta-analysis). They showed participants statements which described behaviour by members of group A and by members of group B. Two-thirds of the statements were about group A members and one-third about group B members, and approximately two-thirds of the statements described desirable behaviour and approximately one-third described undesirable behaviour. In each group there was the same 9:4 proportion of desirable to undesirable behaviours. Nevertheless the participants developed a much more positive impression of group A than of group B. This finding was interpreted as support for the distinctiveness account but alternative accounts have been proposed more recently (Fiedler, 1991; McGarty et al., 1993a; E. R. Smith, 1991; see Chapter 8).

The distinctiveness account has been updated by McConnell et al. (1994) who have suggested an extended distinctiveness-based explanation of the illusory correlation effect. This model holds that illusory correlations form on the basis of encoding paired distinctiveness but that these perceptions can be modified by post-representational processes whereby stimuli are reinterpreted during the perception of a series of stimuli (but prior to the judgement of those stimuli). In this way stimuli which might not be salient at the time of presentation can become distinctive after other stimuli have been presented, because the distinctiveness of the stimuli may only become apparent after further stimuli have been presented. McConnell et al. (1994) use an example drawn from the work of von Restorff of perceiving a single nonsense syllable amid a series of numbers. If the syllable is presented early in the series then there will be no distinctiveness at the time of encoding. What the research seems to show, however, is that so long as such items are infrequent in the entire list, overall distinctiveness will appear, and that this can be the basis for illusory correlation. (See Hunt, 1995, though, who argues that von Restorff's work has been frequently misinterpreted to show that distinctiveness is an insufficient principle to account for memory advantages without being linked to other mediating processes.)

Another important early application of the distinctiveness idea was in the **who-said-what paradigm**. The study by Taylor et al. (1978) looked at the effects of sex and racial categories on stereotyping. Subjects viewed a (purported) discussion on slides (with an accompanying audio tape). Their task was to recall statements made by various members. It was found that subjects were more likely to misattribute statements to members of the same category than to members of the other category (the other sex or race depending upon the experiment). A number of other studies (e.g., Arcuri, 1982; Eiser et al., 1979; Howard and Rothbart, 1980; Nesdale et al., 1987; Oakes and Turner, 1986; van Knippenberg et al., 1994; van Twuyer and van Knippenberg, 1995) report similar results which are nevertheless open to widely different interpretations. The dominant result obtained from research in the who-said-what paradigm has been that errors (incorrectly attributing a statement to a source) are more likely to occur within than across categories. That is, results from the who-said-what paradigm are conventionally interpreted as showing that categorization leads to errors. The application of the distinctiveness idea was through the suggestion that these errors should increase when stimulus salience is increased by the solo or minority status of members of one group. Unfortunately, the measures used in the who-said-what paradigm are extremely sensitive to the relative and absolute sizes of the groups being compared. In the most extreme case, if there is only one member in the group then all misattributions are between-category errors. The who-said-what paradigm remains useful for investigating many other issues in the field of social categorization and memory, however.

Yet another development on the biased stimulus processing model of categorization is Mullen's (1991) prototype-exemplar model. This model suggests, as did Taylor et al. (1978) and Hamilton and Gifford (1976), that the salience of a group emerges from the distinctiveness or numerical infrequency of stimuli. Under this view salient groups (in this sense, statistically infrequent or minority groups) will be more likely to be represented in a coherent or entitative form. This will apply to minority groups or outgroups which will tend to be represented by means of an abstract summary or prototype representation. On the other hand, majority groups will be represented in a more differentiated form as a set of exemplars.

Although Mullen and colleagues have provided evidence consistent with the intriguing idea that there are different representations for ingroups/majorities versus outgroups/minorities (a view also consistent with the ideas of authors such as Park et al., 1991), the approach is nevertheless untenable. If the amount of attention directed to a group is a function of the salience of that group it makes little sense to expect that focusing more attention on a group will produce a less differentiated, prototype representation. In other words, Mullen's treatment of salience conflicts with a wealth of evidence which suggests that more attention leads to a more finely differentiated perception of targets. Some other definition of salience seems to be required.

Memory-based versus on-line processes

In an influential article Hastie and Park (1986) promoted the distinction between **memory-based** and **on-line** processing to account for some differences between memory and judgement. Memory-based processing involves storing a set of exemplars which are then retrieved to make a judgement. The exemplar model of social judgement (Smith and Zárate, 1992) provides a clear description of the ways in which this processing could work. On-line processing involves forming and adjusting representations based on new information as soon as new stimuli are encountered.

The following example illustrates the differences between the processes. Think of your impression of your summer holidays as a child. This impression could be based on an incrementally changing impression of what holidays were like which was formed long ago and gradually altered on-line, or it could be computed now in response to the stimulus of my example by retrieving memories of different holidays in different years and combining them.

The distinction between these two ideas raises important and interesting questions for social cognition. How plausible is it that many different impressions such as these are formed and stored? If the impressions are not stored on-line, how are the seemingly infinite number of exemplars needed for memory-based judgements retrieved and organized? Returning to the concerns raised in Chapter 2, is it even sensible to think of exemplars in this sense? Are impressions computed from some other form of network that doesn't need individual representation?

The distinction is, however, widely used in the social cognitive literature. Carlston and Smith (1996) have raised doubts, though, as to the primacy of on-line processing that is assumed by many authors.

Trait-based, relationship-based and group-based categorization

Most social cognitive research focuses on categories of persons which potentially correspond to social groups. However, Andersen and Klatzky (1987) introduced a distinction between categories of persons based on stereotypes and categories based on traits. Andersen and Klatzky's research suggests that stereotype-based categorizations were richer and better articulated.

On the other hand Hampson (1988; see also John et al., 1991) argues that categorizations based on traits are the primary bases for organizing information about persons. Hampson argues that the fundamental unit in perception is not the person but their behaviour. That is, what interests us about people is not *who they are* so much as *what they are doing*. Her analysis is that behaviour is dynamic and goal-oriented and that processing which leads to social understanding will be geared towards explaining events. From this perspective a hierarchical organization of categories which rests on traits at the superordinate level with persons and behavioural events at lower levels is necessary.

Finally, a range of different points have been made about interpersonal relationships as categories. Different authors use this idea to mean quite different things. Sedikides et al. (1992) have shown that relationships act like social categories. That is, perceivers can confuse two partners in a relationship in the same way that they confuse members of the same group. This must be distinguished though from the idea developed by N. Haslam (1994, following the work of A. Fiske) that the mental representation of different types of social relationship has a discrete (i.e., categorical) rather than continuous (dimensional) structure. The potential for confusion arises in everyday language. If we say that 'Jill always drinks the same beer' we *might* mean that Jill only ever drinks the same glass of beer (beer is a category), but we are more likely to mean that Jill always drinks the same *type* of beer (beer belongs to categories). We can distinguish the common point being made by Sedikides et al. and Haslam as being that 'A relationship is a category' and the distinctive point of Haslam (following Fiske) as being 'Relationships belong to different categories.'

Typicality and prototypicality

A number of researchers have emphasized the importance of typicality or prototypicality of instances in triggering category use. There is a wide variety of reasons for this emphasis. Some authors who have adopted an exemplar-based approach emphasize the importance of typicality because the most typical exemplars will be best related to other exemplars on average and will therefore be most likely to activate a wide range of other exemplars. Others assume that categories are organized around prototypes and that therefore information about typical instances is distinctively important in its own right.

One area where typicality of instances is particularly important is in relation to stereotype change (see e.g., Hewstone and Lord, 1998). If disconfirming instances are not typical of the stereotyped category then the prospect exists for the disconfirming instances to be ignored.

Rothbart and Lewis (1988) investigated some of these issues. In their experiments 1 and 2 the categories used were geometric shapes (triangles, rectangles, pentagons and ellipses). The subjects were shown an array of good and bad exemplars of these categories (e.g., an equilateral triangle was seen as a good example, and an acute triangle was seen as a poor example). The good and bad exemplars of each shape were of different colours. After a filler task the subjects were asked how many of each shape were of a particular colour. In experiment 1 it was found that subjects overestimated the frequency of the good exemplars and this was replicated in experiment 2 (where there were further controls for intraclass similarity).

In experiment 3 they used social categories. Their subjects were asked to judge the degree of political liberalism in a college fraternity on the basis of information about one member of that fraternity. These people varied in the extent to which they were typical of a stereotypical fraternity. It was found that as the typicality of the group member increased, stronger inferences were made about the political views of the fraternities. In other words, subjects' inferences about groups on the basis of their individual members depended upon the goodness of fit of those category members.

Categorization versus individuation

It is customary in the social cognitive literature to distinguish categorization from an alternative process called individuation. The formal status of this latter process varies from formulation to formulation. In some cases individuation is simply the absence of categorization: it is what happens to stimuli when the perceiver is not categorizing them (this is true of the Fiske and Neuberg, 1990, continuum model). In other cases individuation is understood to be distinctly different from categorization but the characteristics of this process have not yet been well articulated. An example would be Brewer's (1988) dual-process model, where categorization is top-down and involves effort minimization. Personalization is bottom-up, resource intensive and elaborative, and involves processes of inference. Brewer (1994) argues that Carlston's (1994) associated systems theory clarifies central distinctions that were not clear in the 1988 model, but Carlston and Sparks (1994) conclude that Brewer had misunderstood Carlston's model to be bottom-up when it actually involves bottom-up and top-down processes.

A suggestion by Bodenhausen and Macrae (1998a, citing Bodenhausen et al., in press) that advances consideration of the nature of individuation is that stereotyping (categorical responses) and individuation differ in the number of dimensions used to judge a person. Stereotyping involves judging someone on a single dimension and therefore individuation is defined as

> the simultaneous consideration of multiple stereotypes. If a sufficient number of distinct dimensions is activated, a personally unique constellation of attributes will define one's impression of the target. (1998a: 246)

This perspective implies that individuation is not a distinct process but instead involves multiple categorizations. This is an intriguing suggestion as to what individuation is, but it also implies a restrictive use of the term 'categorization' that is hard to reconcile with the discussion of the categorization process in general. If we assume, as I have done on the basis of the research reviewed in Chapter 3, that categorization involves the alignment of multiple dimensions, we cannot reserve the term 'categorization' or 'stereotyping' for the use of a single dimension.

The effects of both individuation and categorization can be understood in constraint relation terms as the constraint of category use on perceived equivalence. Using categories increases perceived equivalence and not using categories decreases perceived equivalence. These effects can also be understood as intracategory assimilation and intercategory contrast respectively.

A clear application of the categorization process occurs in the continuum model of impression formation developed by Fiske and Neuberg (1990: see also Verplanken et al., 1996, for a direct test, and Fiske et al., in press, for an update).

This model holds that impressions of people involve varying degrees of individuation and categorization. Categorization occurs in the model at a number of possible stages. Categorization is a primary process used to decide whether a person merits attention. This is the initial response that we might make when we encounter someone walking down the street. If it is decided that the person merits attention then we might apply other specific categorizations. If the available categorizations do not fit the stimulus information then the person may be individuated. In other words, there is a continuum from **categorical processing** to **piecemeal processing** and the more piecemeal the processing the more individuated the impression. Importantly though, to move along this continuum in the direction of individuated impressions the perceiver needs to be motivated to allocate attention to the target. Thus individuated perception is believed to be accurate perception, and the centrepiece of the model is that effort is required to achieve accurate perception. If there are insufficient cognitive resources to deploy there will be a concomitant reduction in accuracy.

The dual-process model of impression formation (Brewer, 1988) posits that rather than there being a continuum from categorization to individuation, categorization and individuation are two distinct processes. Under conditions of low cognitive resources the perceiver will tend to use category-level information. Thus despite some differences between the dual-process and continuum models they actually end up having very similar implications for categorization.

The resource ideas in the continuum model have been applied to research on power by Fiske (1993). Fiske argued that powerful people stereotype more than powerless people because powerful people are busy and have less time to form accurate individual impressions. A summary of representative research on this topic appears in the chapter by Fiske and Morling (1996). These authors conclude:

> People always have to budget their limited capacities to meet the many demands on their attention. They pragmatically use cognitive strategies that meet their motivational goals with the resources they have. People's dependence on or rejection of default categories apparently results from the tradeoff between capacity limits and control motivations, whether this tradeoff is necessitated by social structure, personal needs, or both. (1996: 340)

This quote highlights two points on which the biased processing view has been updated since the 1970s. First, there is an increasing concern with motivation and emotion (highlighted in the volumes of the *Handbook of Motivation and Cognition* edited by Sorrentino and Higgins: the Fiske and Morling chapter appears in the third volume of that handbook). One aspect of this focus on motives relates to **control motivation**. The suggestion is that a desire for control or mastery implies that we must make sense of the world (E. R. Smith and Mackie, 1997, highlight this as one of three crucial motivational principles in social cognition). Effective control over the environment implies that we need to attend to those aspects of the environment which could affect us. Fiske and others suggest that interdependence with other people increases the need for control and this motivates greater accuracy in perceivers as they wish to have accurate impressions of other people on whom their own fate may depend (Ruscher and Fiske, 1990). Thus, interdependence entails a loss of control for which perceivers compensate by developing accurate impressions.

Although Fiske and colleagues have been strongly involved in this development, their contribution to a second development is more distinctive. This involves a concern with social structure as a determinant of cognitive processing. The clearest example of this has been in relation to the relative amounts of power held by individuals. The analysis of power builds on the earlier work on interdependence. Fiske and colleagues argue that powerful individuals are less dependent on their subordinates than subordinates are on superiors, so the powerful will be less strongly motivated to have accurate impressions of those others. This disparity in need for attention is normally correlated with the fact that the weak greatly outnumber the powerful, thereby creating overload for the powerful (they have more targets to attend to). Note that in all cases the assumption is the same as that made in the original continuum model: individually based perception is accurate perception and categorization leads to error.

Another major development in relation to the biased stimulus processing perspective is the recent work on cognitive busyness and the processing of category-consistent/inconsistent information by Gilbert and Hixon (1991), Macrae et al. (1993) and others. In different places these authors have argued that mood depletes processing resources, that arousal affects processing resources (following the inverted U-shaped relationship made famous in the Yerkes–Dodson law) and that under conditions of low availability of cognitive resources there will be high levels of categorization. In particular, Gilbert and Hixon (1991) argue that cognitive load (busyness) increases stereotyping providing that the stereotype has already been activated.

For the purposes of this overview, Spears and Haslam's (1997) summary of the work on cognitive load is difficult to improve upon. Research in the cognitive miser tradition shows, or purports to show, that as load increases people adopt a group-level impression of others and are more likely to rely on stereotype or expectancy-congruent information and less likely to rely on stereotype or disconfirming information.

Work that has specifically focused on the categorization process within this very broad tradition includes a study by Pendry and Macrae (1996). Participants were motivated to pay attention to a stimulus person (by being told that they would be asked to account for the impression they formed to another person). **Priming** of a sub-category with which the stimulus person shared features only occurred under conditions of high motivation. That is, participants responded more rapidly in a lexical decision task (deciding whether a stimulus was a word or a non-word) to trait words which were stereotypical of the sub-type *businesswoman* than to words which were stereotypical of the category *woman,* but only when participants were highly motivated (accountable) and not when they were asked to pay attention to the target's height.

Unfortunately the study confounds motivation with the dimension that was attended to. That is, the more motivated participants were attending to the target's behaviour and the less motivated participants were attending to the target's height. Research by McMullen et al. (1997) shows why this is particularly problematic. McMullen et al. note that Kunda (1990) and others have argued that motivation affects categorization in two ways. It can bias judgements in a particular direction or it can lead perceivers to process information more carefully. Following Smith and Zárate (1992), McMullen et al. (1997) argue that motivation also leads to selective attention to dimensions that allow the categorization of stimuli. The dimensions selected can be appropriate (matching, for example, the demands of the experimental task) or inappropriate resulting in relative inaccuracy. The specific mechanism proposed for this by McMullen et al. (1997) is that motivation can lead people to construe the *sample space* in a way that is appropriate or inappropriate for the task. If the experimental instructions lead participants to focus attention on one dimension they may neglect other less important dimensions. This will result in **base-rate neglect** and relative inaccuracy.

This would appear to apply to Pendry and Macrae's study, where participants who were asked to focus on the target's height (or in another condition the clarity of the video) showed weaker priming. In McMullen et al.'s own research, subtle effects of motivation on attention are shown on conditional probability judgements. They show relative accuracy and minimal base-rate neglect when participants are primed to focus on a dimension that is relevant to the question actually asked.

The biased processing approach is shown in Figure 4.2 in constraint relations terms. Limitation on capacity is an additional variable that determines category use independently of the level of perceived equivalence and background knowledge. The need for an additional constraint points to a genuine tension. The other constraint relations imply that categories are being used for four purposes (reflecting the two direct links between category use and equivalence and two indirect links between category use and knowledge): (a) to capitalize upon perceived similarities and differences, (b) to identify those similarities and differences, (c) to capitalize on knowledge about the world, or (d) to establish knowledge about the world. The cognitive miser tradition overlays an additional purpose: categories are used to reduce the overload of information. This can be conceived of as an additional variable outside the constraint system that we have discussed so far: cognitive load causes category use. It is increasingly the case though that approaches within this tradition consider the constraining effect of background knowledge. Some of this work is considered in the next section and in Chapter 6.

The cognitive miser view can be reconciled with some approaches in cognitive psychology such as Anderson's (1991) adaptive model of categorization. Notwithstanding this, the highly developed cognitive miser view is unique to social cognition.

The current state of the field reflects a change from the cognitive miser metaphor to what is called the *motivated tactician* perspective. This is the idea that perceivers still use categorization and other tactics to reduce load but in forming accurate perceptions the social perceiver is best characterized as 'good enough' rather than 'bad' (Fiske, 1993). Interestingly, Uleman et al. (1996) reject the motivated tactician metaphor, preferring the idea of people as flexible interpreters, because the motivated tactician standpoint implies that people are driven by explicit, cognitive goals which involve deliberation. In contrast, they argue that people also engage in spontaneous cognition where motivation is often distal. Some of these elaborations are considered in the remaining sections of this chapter and in Chapter 6.

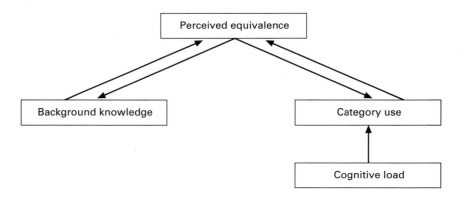

FIGURE 4.2   *Principal constraint relations in the biased processing approach*

actor–observer effect An attributional difference in that actors are more likely to perceive the world to be the cause of their actions but observers are more likely to see actors as responsible for their own actions.

availability (a) In Tversky and Kahneman's (1973) usage of the availability heuristic the term refers to the ease with which some stimulus or event can be brought to mind owing to its vividness or salience to help in problem solving. Plane crashes may be more available events than car crashes so the risk of death by plane crash may be overestimated. (b) In Higgins's (1996) usage, whether some information exists in memory.

base-rate neglect Ignoring information about the relative frequency of some event when deciding the likelihood of that event.

capacity limitations The limit on the mind's ability to process information. With the exception of short-term memory capacity it has been difficult to establish these limitations.

categorical processing Processing of stimuli at the categorical level. In Fiske and Neuberg's (1990) model categorical processing is necessarily prone to error and is the opposite of piecemeal processing.

cognitive load The demands on information processing capacity. The connotation of this term is that these demands threaten to overwhelm capacity.

control motivation Motivation to establish or maintain mastery or control over some aspect of the environment (often the social environment).

distinctiveness The extent to which some stimulus is perceptually prominent.

illusory correlation The erroneous perception of a relationship between variables which does not in fact exist.

memory-based processing Constructing impressions by recalling and combining a set of instances.

on-line processing Processing of a set of stimuli so that impressions are formed and updated as stimuli are encountered.

piecemeal processing Processing of stimuli at the individual level (opposite of categorical processing).

prime (priming) An event which stimulates the activation of knowledge. Priming of an alternative frequently results in faster responses towards that alternative.

representativeness In Tversky and Kahneman's (1974) usage of the representativeness heuristic, the extent to which some event is seen to be similar to (or representative of) a class of events.

who-said-what paradigm An experimental paradigm that involves presenting participants with a set of statements attributed to target persons and then asking participants to remember the source of those statements.

B. Categorization as the activation of stored knowledge

Whereas the biased stimulus processing approach makes formal use of the term 'categorization' a great deal of the time, this is somewhat less true of work concentrated on knowledge activation, use and representation. Although the terms *category* and *categorization* are used less frequently, categorization is nevertheless a central construct in this area (see e.g., Martin, 1985; Martin and Tesser, 1992; Schul and Burnstein, 1990).

A statement of the knowledge activation approach to categorization could take the following form. Elements of knowledge are stored so as to allow perceivers to retrieve related elements. Related retrieval in turn enhances the prospect of the development of enduring connections between those elements. Categorizations can thus be seen as networks of meaning built upon related elements. The process of categorizing can therefore be seen as both retrieving linked elements and deciding which elements are to be linked in the first place. A key principle of this view is that related elements of knowledge are more likely to activate related elements because of stored connections between them. Under this approach category membership is one determinant of relatedness.

Again many disparate elements in cognition and social psychology contribute to the foundations of this view. One prominent antecedent is the work of Bruner (1957) on construct accessibility: the idea that the extent to which knowledge is actively switched on at any given time depends on the perceiver's current intentions and past experience. In relation to this point, a long tradition in cognitive psychology has shown that intentions and past experience can prime perceivers in certain ways. In particular, perceivers can be expected to respond more rapidly to a stimulus if related stimuli have already been presented. Priming has also been shown at the categorical level, that is, presenting a category label can produce faster responses to members of that category.

Another major historical foundation for this work is cognitive work on representation. The most directly relevant traditions were discussed in Chapters 2 and 3. In particular the ideas of exemplar models of representation, category structure and distributed representation have all had an impact on this approach within social cognition.

One way to distinguish the field from the biased stimulus information processing approach is to focus on an idea that Higgins (1996) stresses. He argues that *stimuli can serve as stimulants*. Rather than just thinking of stimuli as something to be processed, the reception of stimuli can also set other forms of processing in motion depending on the context. If a tiger walks into your room you will not only process the stimulus information about the tiger but you will probably start thinking about how to escape. However, if you see a tiger walk into an empty room you may start thinking about how it was that a tiger came to be walking around the building in the first place.

Now many proponents of biased stimulus processing would accept the role that knowledge plays in cognition as a necessary complementary emphasis to their own work. Nevertheless, the example serves to illustrate the insufficiency of an approach to categorization based solely on stimulus processing. Obviously the psychological prepotence of the tiger as a stimulus does not depend solely on its novelty or complexity or the limitations of the perceiver's processing capacity in any way that has been discussed in this chapter so far. The tiger demands attention not because it is *seen* to be novel, but because it is *known* to be dangerous. Another equally novel stimulus, say an armadillo walking into the room, would also attract attention, but it would engage quite different processing on the part of the perceiver. The perceiver might wonder, for example, if an armadillo might turn nasty when cornered, or might damage the furniture, but the perceiver might be most likely to wonder how the armadillo came to be in the building, or even whether it really was an armadillo.

To take the example further, if the presence of dangerous tigers in our working environments were routine, but armadillos remained scarce (reflecting the armadillos' good judgement or bad luck in a tiger-rich environment) then we would still expect our knowledge of danger to control our psychological response to the tiger and not its (non-)distinctiveness. As Oakes and Turner (1986) argue in relation to social stereotyping, the *meaning* of a category in the context in which it is experienced determines the psychological prominence of that category, not the numerical distinctiveness of the category.

Researchers interested in knowledge activation and use have proposed a suite of distinctions which bear on the issues raised by this example (albeit, applied to more everyday occurrences). The distinctions on which Higgins (1996) focuses are between the concepts of availability, accessibility and **applicability** (or fit), **judged usability** and salience.

Availability refers to whether the knowledge is actually stored in memory. Obviously, knowledge cannot be activated unless it already exists, though new knowledge might be created at any time. If the constructs we are referring to are categories then the prior availability of the categories in question determines whether the process relates to category use or category formation.

Accessibility refers to the potential for activation of some available knowledge. It is not the actual *use* of that knowledge, or even the potential for the knowledge to be used, but the possibility of that knowledge being *activated*. The latter distinction is necessary because knowledge can be activated without being used – for example, where it is judged to be neither usable nor applicable. An important determinant of accessibility is recent activation. Knowledge that has been recently activated is more likely to be activated again and Higgins (1996) summarizes evidence for such effects lasting over periods of 24 hours or more. Knowledge that is *frequently* activated also has high levels of accessibility.

Applicability refers to the relation between the features of some stored knowledge and the attended (categorical) features of the stimulus. Where there is a high goodness of fit, or a high overlap between features of stored knowledge and features of the stimulus, the construct will be highly applicable. Higgins (1996) follows Medin and colleagues (1993; Murphy and Medin,

1985) in arguing that just as similarity defined in the abstract is not a sufficient principle to explain category formation, it is not a sufficient principle to explain applicability. This is because features vary in their relevance or importance. Thus overlap of features must be defined in terms of the features to which attention is paid. A construct which overlaps with a stimulus on irrelevant features will be less applicable than a concept that overlaps on relevant features.

Accessibility and fit (or applicability) are the basic variables that determine construct activation in Higgins's (1996) formulation and in Bruner's (1957) original formulation. Unfortunately in updating the definition of accessibility from Higgins and King's (1981) definition (accessible constructs are stored constructs which are readily usable) in order to develop a definition that is compatible with multiple models of accessibility, Higgins introduces circularity that was not obvious in Bruner's original formulation. If accessibility is defined as *potential for activation* then the statement that accessibility is a *determinant of activation* is a tautology. To say that the potential for rain determines actual rain (even if we qualify this statement as involving an interaction with other factors) begs a definition of potential for rain in terms of other constructs. Without such a definition the construct could be acceptable for predictive and descriptive purposes, but not for explanatory purposes, unless we go further and argue that accessibility is not an explanatory construct in itself but is a catch-all for non-applicability related influences on activation. That would make the definition of accessibility: 'the aspects of a construct that predispose it to be activated which are independent of the relationship between the stimulus and the construct'. In other words, definitions which *sound* incoherent can still be of practical use, but this discussion does demonstrate that it is essential for the notion of accessibility to exclude rigorously anything that relates to characteristics of the stimulus. Thus, as Higgins notes, accessibility is potential for activation in the absence of the stimulus or prior to the stimulus.

Judged usability must also be distinguished from accessibility. This is the judged appropriateness or relevance of some stored piece of knowledge. The variables which affect judged usability are (a) causal significance, (b) framing of the task or problem, (c) conversational norms and (d) perceived reliability and representativeness. With respect to categorization, judged usability relates to both using an activated exemplar as a standard of comparison and using an activated concept to categorize a stimulus.

Finally, for Higgins (1996) *salience* is a feature of a stimulus which draws or holds attention. It is thus something about the stimulus event that does not apply until exposure to the stimulus rather than something to do with stored knowledge. This means that considerations of statistical infrequency or novelty must be excluded from the concept as these can influence knowledge activation prior to, and independent of, stimulus exposure. Having said that, the comparative distinctiveness (properties in comparison with those of other stimuli) of stimuli can be considered to be part of salience. Another component of salience is natural prominence due to the absolute attention-grabbing features of a stimulus. Salience is a determinant of selective attention which influences applicability by focusing attention on particular features of the stimulus. It can be distinguished from instructional set, momentary goals and active expectancies which influence selective attention through accessibility.

A slight complication, however, emerges in relation to the ideas developed in the extended distinctiveness model of McConnell et al. (1994). The distinctiveness of individual stimuli may only become apparent when all members of a series have been presented. That is, stimulus distinctiveness may not be detected during the exposure of the stimulus, but involve reprocessing of the stimulus information (reactivation of the knowledge about the stimulus).

Higgins refers to activation and accessibility experiences. People can be aware both of knowledge being activated and of the ease or difficulty of that activation. These awarenesses are **metacognitions**. The ease with which it is believed some thought can be brought to mind can influence how knowledge is activated when it is used. For example, if someone believes that some thought is complex and difficult to access (say the solution to some mathematical problem or a memory from long ago) they may be less likely to think about it or to think about it in particular ways.

This discussion of accessibility experiences raises the more general question of whether knowledge activation is automatic or controlled. Bargh (1994; 1996) defines four criteria for distinguishing between **automatic** and **controlled processes**. Automatic processes are not governed by intention, occur outside conscious awareness, are uncontrollable (i.e., once started cannot be stopped), and are efficient (consume minimal resources and can occur in parallel). Few processes have all four characteristics and no social psychological information process has been shown to satisfy all. For example, there can be intentional automatic processes whereby an act of will is required to set a process in motion but it then continues automatically. An example would be deciding to reflect upon some past event or to pay attention to some current happening. Bargh (1996) suggests that, rather than treating each broad, complex process as being automatic or not, the broad process should be broken down into its component processes. The essence of automaticity for Bargh is **autonomy**: whether a process is capable of operating itself without need for conscious guidance once set in motion.

With respect to categorization processes, evidence assembled by Whitney et al. (1994) suggests that the process of behavioural classification may be relatively automatic but that *characterization* (or making dispositional inferences) as in impression formation may be more deliberative (and is more likely to occur in experiments) where participants are given impression formation instructions. The distinction between the classification of behavioural/trait information and categorizations based, for example, on social groups is also supported by the research of Andersen and Klatzky (1987), Ford et al. (1994) and Stapel et al. (1997).

A major theme in recent research on the activation of stereotypes and

social categories has been the importance of automatic and indeed unconscious processes in stereotyping. The thrust of this research has been that
stereotyping, and in particular prejudiced responses to members of particular categories, can occur on measures over which perceivers have limited
conscious control, but not on measures on which perceivers have conscious
control (such as trait ratings). Evidence of such unconscious prejudice, or at
least of unconscious social category activation, has been obtained by many
authors (Blair and Banaji, 1996; Devine, 1989; Lepore and Brown, 1997; see
Greenwald and Banaji, 1995, for an overview).

Models of priming effects

Two main types of model have been proposed to deal with priming effects in
knowledge activation. These include mechanistic models such as Wyer and
Srull's (1989) storage bin model and excitation transfer models such as
Higgins et al.'s (1985) synapse model.

The storage bin model maintains that all knowledge is stored in a 'bin'
with the recently activated units stored on top. Other things being equal, the
more recently activated of two constructs is more likely to be activated again.

The excitation transfer models postulate that the activation level of units
must exceed a threshold before they can be activated. The units, however,
retain a resting level of activation which keeps them going. Thus recently activated units will be closer to the threshold level that they need to reach to be
activated again.

In order to infer the category membership of a stimulus the storage bin
model suggests it is necessary to compute the likelihood that a category
member would have the features possessed by the stimulus. The features of
the stimulus that confirm or disconfirm this inference are taken into account.
The causal sequence therefore involves testing the applicability of constructs
(starting with the one at the top of the bin) to stimulus information. If the
match between the construct and the stimulus is insufficient (or the mis-
match too great) then the applicability of the next construct in the stack will
be addressed.

Essentially then, the storage bin model proposes a serial hypothesis-testing
approach to the applicability of categories. The clear implication of the serial
nature of the model is that frequent, recent activation of alternative concepts
should delay categorization (as the most accessible concepts are processed
first) and lead to categorization errors (as accessible but inappropriate categorizations are deployed).

The synapse model proposes quite a different account of applicability in
which the causal sequence runs from stimulus information to stored knowledge. A parallel process is envisaged whereby the stimulus serves as a
stimulant to activate all constructs which are related to that stimulus. The
interaction between accessibility and applicability takes the form that all
applicable constructs are considered and the one which maximizes accessibility and applicability is selected.

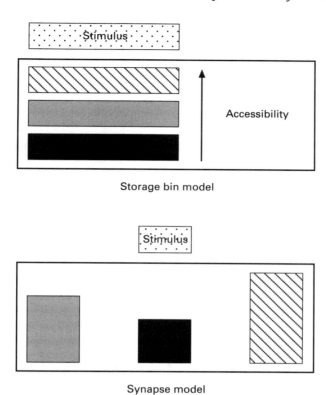

FIGURE 4.3   *Depiction of the differing structures of the storage bin and synapse models*

Thus the storage bin model suggests that all constructs including irrelevant ones are examined one after another until a sufficiently fitting construct is found. The synapse model suggests that all constructs which are similar to the target stimulus are tested in parallel.

In the depiction of the models in Figure 4.3, applicability is represented by the match between the patterns of the stimulus and the stored constructs.

Accessibility is represented in the storage bin model by the proximity of a construct to the top of the bin. The accessibility by applicability interaction is assessed for each stimulus sequentially until some criterion is reached.

For the synapse model the accessibility of the constructs is represented in the figure by the varying size of the rectangles so that the largest rectangle represents the most accessible construct. The accessibility by applicability interaction is assessed simultaneously for all applicable constructs.

Higgins argues that the two formulations make the same predictions in relation to the categorization of *ambiguous* stimulus information, that is, where two or more constructs have features which are strongly related to the stimulus. The storage bin model says that the construct closer to the top of the bin will be activated, the synapse model says that the construct with the higher excitation level will be activated.

However, the two models make different predictions for *vague* stimulus information (i.e., where the stimulus information is not clearly related to any construct). From the storage bin perspective, constructs which are high in accessibility will not be used to categorize unrelated stimuli. However, the synapse model allows extremely vague stimulus information to activate highly accessible constructs.

The differing predictions of the two formulations arise because of the serial–parallel divide. A highly accessible construct which has been rejected by the serial test applied by the storage bin model cannot appear again in the sequence. This linear restriction does not apply in the synapse model: a construct will be activated if it maximizes accessibility and applicability. Where applicability tends towards zero the differences in activation will depend upon accessibility. Higgins cites research by Higgins and Brendl (1995) as support for the synapse model in this regard.

To accommodate this finding the storage bin model only needs a small modification. If a random component to activation is included then this will have a disproportionately large effect when feature matching information is poor. If a linear sequence is tested in such a way that it terminates when a threshold is reached then the highly accessible concepts which are tested earlier in the sequence will be likely to reach the threshold owing to the contribution of the random component. That is, if the random component is sufficiently large it is highly unlikely that a run of non-activations of accessible constructs will occur.

This modification would work particularly well with Wyer and Srull's (1986; 1989) modification of the model which allows multiple representations of constructs. This means that highly accessible constructs would have multiple opportunities to be selected.

A more serious problem is whether the prediction that highly accessible constructs should be activated by vague stimulus information is sound for a wide range of conditions. Unexpected or novel information may be assimilated to the similar constructs that seem most relevant at the time (high accessibility) but this information can also play the role of logically negating those highly accessible constructs, that is, in demonstrating that existing constructs do not hold and new ones are needed. Thus rather than referring merely to stimuli which are related and unrelated to the constructs, we need to address the logical possibility that stimuli can both excite (validate) and inhibit (negate) constructs. In this vein, Macrae et al. (1995) have assembled evidence of inhibitory processes in stereotyping: that is, processes which suppress stereotypic thoughts or reduce stereotypic beliefs (see also Macrae et al., 1994; 1997; 1998; Wegner and Erber, 1992). That is, some constructs may have low levels of activation because they are suppressed (parallel constraint satisfaction models such as that of Kunda and Thagard, 1996, contain both excitatory and inhibitory inputs: see Chapter 10). These and other issues suggest that much more work needs to be done to separate the storage bin from the synapse model empirically (despite their clearly different structures).

Bodenhausen and Macrae's (1998b) model of stereotype activation and inhibition combines important concerns dealt with so far in this chapter. These authors emphasize, correctly in my view (and certainly in line with a developing emphasis in social cognition), that there are inhibitory and excitatory factors in the use of categories and the activation of stereotypes. In constraint relations terms these can be thought of as positive or negative constraints on category use. Where categorization does occur, however, it leads to biased interpretation and subsequently to discrimination. However, once the stereotype has been activated the subsequent stage of biased interpretation is constrained by personal endorsement/rejection of the stereotype and the final stage of discrimination is constrained by social normative factors which are pro- or anti-discrimination.

This model could be seen as a very pure social cognitive model of categorization, stressing as it does many of the traditional concerns of social cognitive approaches. Categorization is seen to lead to inevitable error and aspects of the person are seen to be separate from or even opposed to social factors. Thus, categorizations and stereotypes are mistakes that people make unless they personally reject these views, or where the concern to be egalitarian leads to the concealment of the stereotype. These errors can also be exacerbated by personal endorsement (leading to motivated reasoning which supports the stereotype) or by social norms which support discrimination.

The problem with the assumption of an opposition between personal control and social control arises fairly immediately in the model. The experimental manipulations that Bodenhausen, Macrae and colleagues use to achieve personal control are instructions from the experimenter. That is, participants are asked to try not to stereotype (e.g., in the study by Macrae et al., 1994, where participants were instructed not to stereotype skinheads).

My interpretation of these instructions is that they strongly engage what Bodenhausen and Macrae call social control: telling participants that they should not stereotype implies that the experimenter thinks that stereotyping is wrong. In other words, it seems wrong to attempt to distinguish social and personal factors as relating to different processes (see Abrams and Masser, 1998, for a much more detailed critique).

The more general issue of whether stereotypes and categories should be thought of as distorting processes is one we shall return to. Bodenhausen and Macrae maintain that they are agnostic on this point. I think we have to trust the details of their model, however, which strongly suggests that stereotypes and categories are distortions (see Kobrynowicz and Biernat's, 1998 comment). This suggests that categorization and stereotyping are processes that lead to distortion unless other processes are engaged to prevent those representations from being expressed. As we will see in the next few chapters this view is keenly contested by self-categorization theorists and others.

applicability The match between stored knowledge and the attended (categorical) features of a stimulus. Applicability is another term for Bruner's notion of fit.

automatic process Such processes tend to have four characteristics: (a) they are not intentional, (b) they are not conscious, (c) they are not controllable once started, and (d) they are efficient and can operate easily in parallel with other processes.

autonomy A characteristic of processes whereby they do not need conscious control once set in motion.

controlled process A process which tends not to have the hallmarks of automatic processes and is under conscious control.

judged usability The judged relevance or appropriateness of applying some knowledge to a stimulus.

metacognitions Subjective beliefs or understandings about the operations of cognitive processes.

C. Affective, evaluative and motivational influences on categorization

A variety of approaches to the influence of affect and evaluation on categorization have been developed over the last 20 years. In this section I merely wish to signpost some major approaches so that readers can follow up this material in more detail.

Attempts to articulate the role of affect on categorization or categorization-like processes occur in the work of authors such as Brewer (1988), Fiske and Pavelchak (1986; Fiske and Neuberg, 1990) and Forgas (1994). An approach that combines both extensive empirical investigation and a detailed application to the categorization is found in the work of Isen and colleagues and I will focus on that here.

One underpinning principle of recent research on affect and cognition is that people make judgements congruent with their mood (the mood-congruency effect). We expect people to react more favourably to others when they are in a good mood and more negatively when they are in a bad mood. How might this effect impact on the categorization process? One possibility is that people will be more likely to judge neutral or ambiguous stimuli to belong to desirable categories when they are in a good mood. This seems highly plausible: if you were about to ask a favour of somebody who did not know you very well you would definitely want to ensure that they were in a good mood when you asked. That is, you would want them to assign you (a neutral or ambiguous stimulus) to a desirable category.

The work of Isen and colleagues explains how this process could function. Isen (1987) argued that positive affect increases the accessibility of cognitive information. One effect of this should be increased category breadth for positive or neutral stimuli. That is, neutral stimuli should be assigned to positive categories and not to negative categories, and this is what Isen et al. (1992) found with respect to social categories. The process which could be involved here was articulated further by Isen (1993) who argued that positive affect leads people to focus on the positive aspects of the stimulus, making it appear more similar to the positive category that is primed in that context. An equivalent process does not occur for negative categories: that is, neutral stimuli are not more likely to be assigned to negative categories. This is because positive affect is only held to increase the accessibility of positive knowledge, and thus there is no basis for more connections between the neutral stimuli and the negative categories.

To these priming differences must be added several other effects on categorization-like processes detailed by Forgas (1994). He argues that affect may induce motivated processing to achieve mood repair (negative moods) or mood maintenance (positive moods). He also argues that there is evidence of different processing styles. In particular, positive moods may induce simplified, heuristic processing strategies and sad moods may trigger careful and substantive processing (related ideas can be derived from the work of Fiske and Pavelchak, 1986). Bodenhausen et al. (1994) argue, however, that anger produces simplified, heuristic processing which is similar to the effects of happiness. The measure of simplified, heuristic processing was the effect of an activated stereotype on judgements. As we will see in the next two chapters there is substantial disagreement about whether it is sensible to equate stereotyping with simplified processing.

On the whole, research on the effects of affect on categorization/processing appears to be highly congruent with the biased processing and knowledge activation approaches. There are varying amounts of emphasis on whether affect has a direct effect on processing or whether affect is effective on processing through the information it conveys to the perceiver about external events and the appropriate response to it. Having said that, there appears to be a strong consensus that affect is an important moderating or qualifying variable for the categorization process in terms of both the effects of cognitive load and the priming of activated constructs. That is, despite its enormous breadth research on affect sits comfortably across the perspectives introduced earlier in this chapter rather than being a separate substantive approach.

In recent years the reintegration of motivational processes with cognitive processes has become important in social psychology. In summarizing the evidence Kruglanski (1996) suggests that beyond mere knowledge activation most cognition is goal-dependent. That is, it involves a discrepancy between an actual and a desired state (regardless of whether that goal is consciously recognized).

Kruglanski shows that motivation has been suggested to be involved in categorization-based processes in a number of ways. A very important set of processes relate to the distinction between motivational and cognitive capacity explanations of the effects of cognitive load on processing. Kruglanski distinguishes a strong and a weak version of the capacity limitation thesis. The strong version is that the exhaustion of cognitive capacity *prevents* processing whereas the weak version is that it *restricts* processing.

The strong version is inconsistent with a motivational account because it does not allow for the possibility of perceivers increasing their effort. Kahneman's (1973) argument was that attention is a pool of resources that can be augmented by increased effort (Norman and Bobrow, 1975, make it clear though that the potential for increases in performance can be strictly limited by task conditions). The weak version is compatible with a motivational account. Kruglanski argues further that the strong version of the cognitive capacity argument would need to have additional principles added to it to explain variations in evaluations and preference that occur when restrictions are placed on information processing by time pressure and so on. These additional principles are necessarily motivational constructs. One possible motivational principle is need for closure: that is, the need to achieve some outcome or solution. For example, Kruglanski and Webster (1991) found that group members tended to reject opinion deviates more when they were under time pressure. They explained this effect in terms of the increased threat to closure that the deviates represented in the time pressure condition.

More generally, Kruglanski suggests that there are two main ways in which motivational constructs can influence cognition (cf. Kunda, 1990): motivation may initiate or terminate cognitive activity. People should begin a sequence of categorizing when a discrepancy between a desired and an actual state is established and cease categorizing when that goal is achieved or replaced with another goal.

Kruglanski casts some doubts over the prospect of unmotivated cognitive processing. A considerable amount of research suggests that categories can be activated automatically by mere exposure to the category member. For example, the impression formation models of Fiske and Neuberg (1990) and Brewer (1988) both assume automatic, primary categorizations are applied immediately to individuals encountered. However, a wide range of research cited by Kruglanski (1996) suggests that even seemingly spontaneous, automatic cognition is goal-dependent because changes in instructions in experimental tasks can have profound and immediate effects.

In concluding this section it is pertinent to note that there has been a resurgence of interest in individual differences and their effects on categorization. For example, people high in need for structure were found by Moskowitz (1993) to show stronger degrees of social categorization. Other studies have found prejudiced persons to categorize in particular ways (e.g., Schaller et al., 1995), and Huber and Sorrentino (1996) discuss the implications of individual differences in uncertainty orientation on categorization phenomena. As yet though it is difficult to see which findings on individual differences are essential to aiding our understanding of the categorization process in general. A great deal of this individual differences work relates to individual differences in motivation, and the chapter by Fiske et al. (in press) includes a very useful review of some of this material.

Combining contemporary views: selective attention drives categorization and cognition

Taking elements from the biased stimulus processing approach together with the knowledge activation tradition it is possible to abstract a view of the categorization process in social cognition that draws on many disparate elements. Obviously not all the ideas contained within this view would be accepted by all theorists. It is even possible that all theorists would disown some aspects of the view that I am now about to articulate (though it is often best to judge theorists by what they do rather than what they say). Nevertheless I will make the claim that the view represents the weight of opinion in the field of social cognition.

The central precept of contemporary social cognitive approaches to categorization is also the central precept of the field as a whole. Categorization is an application of the more general phenomenon of selective attention to stimulus events and to stored constructs.

Categorization occurs because of the need to selectively attend to stimuli and its operations are determined by the need to be selective. Categorization is a goal-directed process of explanation that is motivated by a need to make capacity-overwhelming, diffuse stimulus information coherent. Categories imply hypotheses or enable inferences. Information which is inconsistent with hypotheses and/or expectancies is attended to when there are sufficient resources/motivation to individuate, or when knowledge about the individual is activated. Category-consistent information will be attended to when categories are activated. Which categories are activated is driven by the interaction between accessibility and fit (applicability).

Thus the causal sequence in judgement is that perception proceeds from the retrieval of exemplars which closely match a target. Similarity is determined by the dimensions that are attended to, and attention is determined by context. Some aspects of categorization are automatic but categorization is also affected by insight and experience. The process of individuation appears to rely heavily on control.

The flavour of much of this research is changing rapidly, with a renewed emphasis on motivational and evaluative/affective factors in cognition and a new emphasis on inhibitory as well as excitatory influences. Some of this work is considered in more detail in Chapter 6.

5 Categorization as Meaning Creation I: Self-Categorization Theory and some Other Developments

A. The social categorization tradition

The tradition of work that follows from the insights of Tajfel and others can be referred to as the social categorization tradition, the social identity approach, or the European intergroup perspective. I have referred to this body of research on a number of occasions throughout the previous chapters. What I want to do briefly in this chapter is address some common misconceptions about this line of research.

Tajfel argued that categorization was a sense-making process which allowed perceivers to derive meaning by making different classes coherent, separable and clear. The accentuation processes by which this coherent, separable nature was achieved were discussed in Chapter 3. These are held to apply equally to the perception of social and non-social stimuli.

Tajfel and Turner's (1979; 1986) social identity theory added two more principles to the categorization process in an attempt to provide a theory of the social psychological processes involved in intergroup relations. These principles were *identification* and *comparison*. Social comparison was derived from the earlier work of Festinger (1954) and relied on the idea that people derived positive self-esteem by comparing themselves favourably with relevant other people. Tajfel and Turner extended this to social comparison by members of social groups. That is, people could derive self-esteem from seeing their own group as being relatively better than relevant other groups. The two processes of social categorization and social comparison cannot be understood, however, without the idea of social identification. That is, that people are deriving a sense of *who they are* from their membership in social groups.

The terms 'identity' and 'identification' therefore have two technical meanings. An identity is the nature or essence of some thing, but two things are *identical* if they share that nature or essence. For social identity theorists the statement that 'Person X identifies with group Y' means both that 'Person X sees group Y as an aspect of his or her self' and 'Person X sees themselves as being relatively similar to other people who belong to group Y (and different from people who are not in group Y).'

In terms of the constraint relations model of categorization that I have been using here we can see the prospects for confusion from these related uses. The idea of social identity cuts across two important ideas involved in categorization: categorization involves working out what something is, and to do that one must work out what that thing is similar to and different from. Does this then mean that identification is the same as categorization? As it turns out, it does not. Identification is best understood as a set of constraints on the categorization process, but it is easier to see this in the context of self-categorization theory in the next section, and I will return to this point in Chapter 9.

The social identity tradition has, however, led to a vast amount of research on social categorization. A great deal of this research repeats a popular misconception of the original implications of social identity theory. This misconceived idea is that social identification automatically creates intergroup discrimination and prejudice. To select an example on the basis of its currency, Schaller et al. (1998) review theoretical development intergroup processes and schematize the social categorization approach as the idea that:

social identity → prejudice → stereotypes and discrimination

Although the causal mechanisms outlined above do hold under some conditions they represent a dramatic oversimplification of the original social identity ideas (having said that, I think Schaller et al.'s characterization correctly describes much of the work in the social identification tradition which has made the same oversimplifications). Social identity theory does not maintain that a positive evaluation of the ingroup relative to the outgroup (what Schaller et al. refer to as prejudice) is an inevitable consequence of social identification, nor are stereotypes and discrimination inevitable consequences of ingroup favouritism.

Contrary to a widely received view, social identity theory specifies precise condition where social identification will produce discrimination (Bourhis et al., 1997; Turner and Bourhis, 1996). The actual relations anticipated by Tajfel and Turner (1979) are that motivation for a positive self-concept produces positive distinctiveness which will be expressed in the attempt to achieve superiority over relevant outgroups on relevant dimensions. A football team is likely to attempt to achieve superiority over other football teams on dimensions of sporting success but not on cultural, aesthetic or intellectual dimensions. However, the members of a football team might devalue the importance of cultural or aesthetic dimensions when comparing themselves with a ballet troupe. Similarly, charity workers may see their own organization to be more charitable than other charities, but their competition will be expressed not by allocating resources to their own group but by contributing to the welfare of the needy. Charity may begin at home, but all legitimate charities judge their success by their generosity to those less fortunate than themselves rather than to *themselves.*

There is another important sense in which I must disagree with Schaller et al.'s (1998) equation of prejudice with a favourable view of the ingroup.

Prejudice implies a prior judgement or view. The favourable judgements that are created through processes of social categorization need not have any existence prior to the formation of those categories. In the famous example of the minimal group paradigm (Tajfel et al., 1971) there is no prior interaction or history between the members. It is at best misleading to call these immediate reactions prejudice.

We (McGarty and Grace, 1996; see also Chapter 9) have argued that it is also a mistake to assume that so-called ingroup bias is any more a bias than any disagreement that occurs between people. When members of one group judge their own efforts or views as being superior to those of other groups this is often interpreted as a distortion, error or bias. However, exactly the same process can be seen when individuals judge their own efforts or views. That is, individuals see their own views as being superior to the alternative views of other people. This is not surprising because when two people disagree, at least one of them must be wrong (see McGarty et al., 1993b). If we believe that our own views are correct then it must also be true that the alternative view is wrong. The belief that our own views are superior to the conflicting views of other people need reflect nothing more than disagreement. Of course, this effect can be augmented by the process of social validation that occurs within groups because we are more likely to believe our own views are correct when they are endorsed by ingroup members (McGarty et al., 1993b; Turner, 1991) but these and other related issues are discussed in Chapter 9.

Such arguments aside, the social categorization tradition over the last 30 years has generated an extensive body of research on a variety of topics. The principal implication of this work is that it has followed the original social identity idea that social categorization has consequences for the treatment of group members, even though the nature of those consequences can be substantially qualified, for example, by whether the action has positive or negative consequences (Mummendey and Schreiber, 1983; Mummendey and Simon, 1989) or whether the ingroup and outgroup members are seen to be typical members of the group (Marques et al., 1988). Three research areas are considered here.

First, a continuing tradition addresses the consequences of crossed categorization (for a review and meta-analysis see Urban and Miller, 1998). This work examines the effects of overlapping social categorizations on judgements. A major impetus for this line of work was established by Deschamps and Doise (1978) when they showed that people who were members of overlapping categories showed reduced intergroup discrimination. As Miller et al. (1998) note, however, there are at least six different patterns of results that have been found in this area.

Secondly, another tradition of research focuses on stereotyping change and the effects of intergroup contact. The three key variants of research can be summarized as stressing the importance of *decategorization, recategorization* or categorization for creating positive intergroup contact and stereotype change.

The common theme in all of these approaches is that the way that groups interact will be affected by the ways in which people construe intergroup relations. Thus Brewer and Miller (1984) argue that intergroup contact will involve more positive relations when people decategorize, that is, when they see themselves and others as unique individuals rather than group members. Essentially, this argument is that positive relations are created by eliminating intergroup contact. Gaertner et al. (1989) argue that what is important for successful intergroup contact is recategorization (this idea is clearly prefigured in self-categorization theory), that is, positive relations are achieved by members of different groups who are able to see themselves as one group.

There is considerable merit in each of these ideas. However, it could be argued that both approaches involve removing the groups from consideration. Hewstone and Brown (1986) argue that if an improvement in intergroup relations is not to be ephemeral, it must rely on favourable contact where people are thinking of themselves as members of the relevant social groups. This is consistent with a cognitive analysis of intergroup contact that follows from the work of Rothbart and John (1985) and is pursued by Hewstone and Lord (1998). A key idea is that unless perceivers construe people they are judging in group terms they will be able to explain away evidence that is inconsistent with their stereotypes by assuming that the counter-stereotypic behaviour actually has nothing to do with the target's group membership. If I have a negative stereotype of the Ku Klux Klan then my stereotype is unlikely to change when I see Klan members doing positive things unless I am thinking of those Klan members as Klan members. Technically, Hewstone and colleagues have argued that their research shows that the perceived typicality of disconfirming instances mediates the process of stereotyping change: perceivers will change their stereotypes to the degree that they perceive people who act inconsistently with the outgroup stereotype to nevertheless be members of that outgroup.

Thirdly, a number of writers have emphasized the consequences of the effects of social categorization for the perceptions of social groups. An important figure in this line of research has been Wilder (e.g., 1978; 1986) who has shown that the level of perceived homogeneity within a group can have consequences for the treatment of that group. For example, groups which were perceived to be homogeneous were more likely to be the targets of intergroup bias. More recently, Vanbesalaere (1996) has shown that homogeneous ingroups are treated in the same way as heterogeneous outgroups.

Group memberships can also have consequences for social categorization. This point was also made clearly by Schaller and Maass (1989) who showed that the illusory correlation effect (see Chapters 4 and 8 of this volume) was eliminated when participants belonged to the minority group (and Spears et al., 1985, had earlier found that the salience of own position may weaken the effect). That is, the conventional effect was qualified under these conditions. Branscombe, Doosje, Ellemers, Spears and others have made an extensive study of the interrelations between social categorization and social identification. We will return to key concerns in these areas in Chapter 9, but let us first consider self-categorization theory in more detail.

B. Self-categorization and categorization

Self-categorization theory is a theory of self-perception which anticipates that aspects of social behaviour, especially group behaviour, can be explained by variations in self-perception. That is, the way people act in social situations depends on the way that they perceive themselves in those situations, and in particular, the way in which people perceive themselves to be similar to or different from other people. The theory contains a small number of principles that describe the process of categorization in general, and other principles which relate specifically to social categorization. Some of the social categorization principles can easily be generalized to non-social categorization, others cannot be so easily generalized. When we discuss self-categorization theory as a theory of categorization (as is the interest here) it is important to bear the scope of the principles in mind.

The first statement of self-categorization theory (SCT) was the chapter by Turner (1985; several of the ideas are anticipated in Turner's earlier work). A more comprehensive source is the book by Turner et al. (1987), but a number of ideas in this work are modified in subsequent writings (Oakes et al., 1994; Turner and Oakes, 1989; Turner et al., 1994; Turner and Onorato, in press). In some cases these are changes in terminology (reflecting changes in emphasis and understanding) and in other cases they are more detailed changes in thinking. For the purposes of elucidation (and to avoid the definitional problems that have arisen with social identity theory) I will assume that what self-categorization theory currently *is* is whatever Turner maintains it to be in his most recent writings on the topic. For maximum clarity I will use the more recent versions of terminology where a choice is available.

Before we go further it is probably helpful to differentiate between the terms used by knowledge activation theorists such as Higgins and by self-categorization theorists. The purpose of Table 5.1 is not to equate the knowledge activation and self-categorization concepts: the concepts on the left and right hand sides are not identical. Rather, the concepts serve equivalent roles in the two formulations. The point of the table is to demonstrate that there is almost no overlap in the language used and that anyone sampling both literatures risks confusion.

TABLE 5.1 *Equivalent concepts in knowledge activation (Higgins, 1996) and self-categorization theory (e.g. Oakes et al., 1994)*

Knowledge activation	Self-categorization
Activation	Salience
Accessibility	Perceiver readiness (formerly relative accessibility)
Applicability	Fit
Salience	—[1]

[1]Formally there is no equivalent concept, but the terms 'stimulus distinctiveness' or 'perceptual prominence' might be used by self-categorization theorists.

The key concept of self-categorization theory is that self-perception is hierarchically organized. That is, at different times, people see themselves as being members of categories that vary in inclusiveness. At some times people see themselves as unique individuals in comparison with other individuals, and at other times they see themselves as members of groups in comparison with members of other groups. At still other times they may see themselves as members of the human race, that is, as a person in contrast to non-human organisms.

These variations in self-perceptions reflect true changes in reality as it is understood or experienced from the point of view of the perceiver. That is, perceiving self as a group member is as valid a self-perception as perceiving self as a unique individual, the principal difference being that in the former case the self is seen to be interchangeable in relevant ways with those other people. In linguistic terms, the transition in self-perception can be seen as the change from saying 'I think X' to 'We think X.'

Comparison between stimuli under SCT therefore rests on a higher-order equivalence in a hierarchy. That is, in order for two stimuli to be compared they must be identical in terms of some more abstract or more inclusive category which entirely contains that subordinate category. More inclusive categories cannot be included within less inclusive categories and the position of the category in the hierarchy, and not specific features of the category, establish its inclusiveness.

SCT is a highly developed constraint relations model. The theory maintains that cognitive activity in the form of pre-existing knowledge and perceived similarities and differences constrains category use: the extent to which a categorization is psychologically prepotent, switched on or activated. As we will see, for self-categorization theorists this usually means that new categories are formed and not that pre-existing categories are retrieved from some knowledge store. The term used for the psychological prepotence of some categorization is salience.

The constraint relations involved are shown in Figure 5.1. Perceived similarities and difference constrain category use, but using categories also

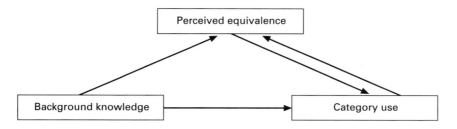

FIGURE 5.1   *Principal constraint relations envisaged in self-categorization theory*

constrains perceived similarities and difference. At the same time the range of categories that can be used is constrained by the active body of knowledge, and the perception of similarity and difference is constrained by the knowledge about the social meaning of categories.

SCT at this stage has less to say about the storage of long-term knowledge or the constraints of perceived equivalence on background knowledge, but long-term knowledge is constrained by category use in the sense that the knowledge which is relevant in some situation depends on the categories used.

The constraint relations between category use and perceived equivalence can be considered under the heading of the **meta-contrast principle** and **comparative fit** (which Oakes, 1987, originally called 'structural fit'):

> Category formation (categorization) depends upon the comparison of stimuli and follows the *principle of meta-contrast*: that is, within any given **frame of reference** (in any situation comprising some definite pool of psychologically significant stimuli), any collection of stimuli is more likely to be categorized as an entity (i.e., grouped as identical) to the degree that the differences between those stimuli on relevant dimensions of comparison (intraclass differences) are perceived as less than the differences between that collection and other stimuli (interclass differences). (Turner et al., 1987: 47)

The meta-contrast ratio (MCR) is defined as the ratio of average interclass differences to average intraclass differences. The formula for the meta-contrast ratio is shown in Equation (5.1) which converts the text in the quote above to algebraic form:

$$\frac{\sum\limits_{d=1}^{n_d} \sum\limits_{i=1}^{n_x} \sum\limits_{j=1}^{n_y} \left| x_{di} - y_{dj} \right| / (n_d n_x n_y)}{\sum\limits_{d=1}^{n_d} \sum\limits_{l=1}^{n_x} \sum\limits_{m=1}^{n_x} \left| x_{dlm} - y_{dml} \right| / ((n_d n_x)(n_x - 1)) \text{ for dlm} \neq \text{dml}} \tag{5.1}$$

where n_d is the number of relevant dimensions; n_x is the number of members of some category X; n_y is the number of members outside category X; and the x and y values are the positions of a member of one or the other category on a particular dimension. When the value of this ratio is greater than 1 then category X will be perceived to be an entitative category.

In practice, equation (5.1) is rarely operationalized empirically by self-categorization theory researchers. What is more commonly done is to use the idea of *meta-contrast ratio of a stimulus* to define its *prototypicality* (Rosch, 1978); that is, the extent to which the stimulus is representative of the category as a whole. The average meta-contrast ratio of all of the category members can be used to estimate the homogeneity of a set of stimuli with respect to a frame of reference. Thus:

$$\mathrm{MCR} = \frac{\left(\displaystyle\sum_{b=1}^{n_b}\left|x_s - x_b\right|\right)/n_b}{\left(\displaystyle\sum_{a=1}^{n_a}\left|x_s - x_a\right|\right)/n_a} \tag{5.2}$$

where x_s is the position of the stimulus S on the dimension under judgement; x_a is the position of another member of the same category A of which S is a member; x_b is the position of a member in category B; n_a is the number of other members in category A (e.g., the ingroup); and n_b is the number of members in another category B (e.g., an outgroup).

Equation (5.2) defines the use of MCR as a specific measure of prototypicality of a stimulus (e.g. Haslam and Turner, 1992; 1995; McGarty et al., 1992; Turner et al., 1987; variants on the equation have been used by Berndsen et al., 1998; McGarty et al., 1993a). The equations are considered further in the appendix to this chapter.

The constraints of prior knowledge on perceived similarities and differences can be considered under the heading of **normative fit**. The normative component is based on the social meanings of behaviours and attributes which vary with the type of social self-categorization made. For example, being intelligent may be normatively relevant to a racist when comparing whites with blacks, but it is less likely to be highly related to the differences between supporters of two football teams. The football supporter might believe that supporters of his team are more intelligent, but this feature is likely to be less important than in the racial context where beliefs about intelligence pervade the social meaning of some racial categorizations.

More technically, Oakes et al. (1994) use the term *normative fit* to refer to the match between category and reality in terms of content and not just the comparative fit of the dimension. Oakes et al. (1991) conducted an experiment which illustrates the difference between these concepts (experiment 2). They had participants rate groups under conditions of varying normative and comparative fit. Four of the six cells in the design are sufficient to illustrate how this works. Comparative fit was manipulated so that there was either conflict or consensus between the groups. Normative fit related to whether the direction of that conflict or consensus was consistent with conflict and consensus of the groups in reality. In the experiment the groups were arts and science students and the attributes were whether the students emphasized enjoying the social life (arts stereotype consistent:AC) or hard work (science stereotype consistent:SC) at university.

The design is shown in Table 5.2 (with the deviance condition included in parentheses). The meta-contrast ratios as calculated following equation (5.1) are shown for each group. To calculate the MCRs I have assumed that the average differences between members holding the same attitudes are small (represented by a value ε which is close to zero) relative to the differences between the attitudes.

TABLE 5.2 *Normative and comparative fit in arts/science experiment*

| | Category | | | | | | | |
| | Science | | | | Arts | | | |
				MCR				MCR
Consistent/ consensus	AC	AC	AC	$\varepsilon_1/\varepsilon_2$	AC	AC	AC	$\varepsilon_1/\varepsilon_2$
Consistent/ conflict	SC	SC	SC	$1/\varepsilon$	AC	AC	AC	$1/\varepsilon$
(Consistent/ deviance)	SC	SC	SC	$0.33/\varepsilon$	AC	SC	SC	0.5
Inconsistent/ consensus	SC	SC	SC	$\varepsilon_1/\varepsilon_2$	SC	SC	SC	$\varepsilon_1/\varepsilon_2$
Inconsistent/ conflict	AC	AC	AC	$1/\varepsilon$	SC	SC	SC	$1/\varepsilon$
(Inconsistent/ deviance)	AC	AC	AC	$0.33/\varepsilon$	SC	AC	AC	0.5

ε is a very small number.

As ε is a very small number, $1/\varepsilon$ will be a very large number; this means that there will be a large difference in the degree of comparative fit between the consensus and conflict conditions. Normative fit is introduced into the design by the consistency factor. Normative fit should be high when the positions espoused by the targets match the stereotypical position of their groups, that is, when arts students express an arts-consistent position and science students express a science-consistent position. Normative fit is thus clearly higher in the consistent than the inconsistent conditions.

Unfortunately, normative fit is also higher in the consistent/conflict than in the consistent/consensus condition because the position espoused by the science students in the consensus condition is actually inconsistent with their stereotypical position. That is, the distribution in that cell does not match the participants' knowledge of the differences between arts and science students.

Thus, the clear test of the normative fit hypothesis applies in the comparison of the consistent/conflict with the inconsistent/conflict condition. On the judgement of the similarity of an arts student to other members of her group there was perceived to be significantly more similarity in the consistent/conflict than in the inconsistent/conflict condition ($p < .05$ by planned comparison). The Oakes et al. (1991) design does not allow a clear test of conditions with differing comparative fit and similar normative fit (but this hypothesis has received support in many other studies, e.g., Haslam and Turner, 1992; 1995; Haslam et al., 1995b). Although this lack of orthogonality in the design does not really imperil the conclusions drawn from the data by Oakes et al. (1991), it does point to the difficulty of manipulating normative fit and comparative fit orthogonally.

In summary, normative fit constrains the dimensions on which groups can be seen as similar and different, which in turn constrains category use. It serves the same functions in the theory as those posited for thematic integration and structural alignment by Bassok and Medin (1997; see Chapter 3).

Constraints of prior knowledge on category use can be discussed under the heading of **perceiver readiness** (which was originally called 'relative accessibility' by Turner et al., 1987). This idea refers to the way in which perception is constrained by the perceiver to reflect the perceiver's vantage point at a particular time. This is what Turner et al. refer to using the term 'cognitive choice': it is the 'selective representation of phenomena from the vantage point of the perceiver' (1994: 462). The formation of these categories follows principles of comparative fit and normative fit which have been outlined above.

Oakes et al. make four points about perceiver readiness of which they suggest the last two are more difficult to understand:

1 Through the influence of perceiver readiness stimuli are *elaborated* in terms of categories provided by one's own past experience and the body of ideas, theories and knowledge acquired from one's culture (a perceiver not primed in this way is one who has literally learnt nothing and categorizes in ignorance).
2 Perceiver readiness leads to the *selective* categorization of the world in a way that is *meaningful, relevant and useful* in terms of the needs, goals and purposes of the perceiver.
3 It ensures that the categories used by the perceiver *evaluate* reality from the perspective of his or her own standards, norms and values.
4 It represents and judges reality *from the vantage point of one's own place in it*, from the perspective provided by one's own particular position. (1994: 201, emphasis in the original)

Considering these in a slightly different order, point 2 is essentially a statement of the constraining effect of prior knowledge on the categories used. Forming categories by relying on the pool of previous knowledge ensures that the categories are meaningful; forming categories on the basis of that part of previous knowledge which corresponds to current needs ensures that the categories are relevant and useful to the perceiver's current needs and goals. It can be *meaningful* to think that a coffee mug is like a Ming Dynasty vase providing we *know* something about coffee mugs and Ming Dynasty vases; it will probably not be relevant or useful to do so unless our knowledge of the Ming Dynasty is currently activated or can be made relevant.

Point 1 suggests that the constraining effect of perceiver readiness on category use is not just a direct link but is mediated by experience of the stimuli. When Oakes et al. (1994) refer to the elaboration of stimuli in terms of categories provided by past experience they are referring to ways of reconciling the infinite number of potential similarities and differences amongst stimuli. For example, the Ming vase and the coffee mug are both fragile and can both contain liquid, but they differ in value and composition.

Point 3, however, relates to the evaluative nature of perceiver readiness. Not only do we choose categories that describe reality in terms of available and accessible knowledge, but relations between categories enable us to determine whether some statement about category membership is not merely meaningful and useful, but is correct from the point of view of the perceiver.

When we decide not to water the pot plants with the priceless vase, even though we know it belongs to the category 'water container', we have made that decision because the categorization is incorrect from our point of view: a point of view which places a value on the vase as a work of art and/or as a rare object. This leads us to look for some more suitable container. All of this depends on the interplay of current goals and the possible category memberships of the vase. We might make no objection to assigning the vase to the category 'water container' if we needed to extinguish a dangerous fire.

Oakes et al.'s (1994) thesis is that the consideration of the validity of social stereotyping rests on these possibilities. The categories used or formed are unerringly meaningful, useful and relevant from the point of view of the perceiver because categorization is a valid and adaptive process of deciding what some thing is from *the point of view of the perceiver*. It can be no more or less error-prone than categorization-free processes because, for SCT, *there are no such categorization-free processes* (following Bruner, 1957: 123: 'Perception involves an act of categorization'; see Oakes, in press, for a detailed treatment).

Imagine that we saw a house guest use a priceless vase to water the pot plants. According to SCT we can disagree with the content of their categorization from our *own point of view* but we cannot contest the guest's categorization from their point of view. That is, we cannot impose some other standard that leads us to say 'Person X has miscategorized that priceless vase as a water vessel from his or her own point of view' because their own psychological activity guarantees subjectively valid experience. We cannot contest that they do think something is X. We can contest that thing is X: that is, we can disagree with the appropriateness of their categorization without it necessarily being the case that their psychological processes are deficient. Oakes et al. (1994) take the example of contesting political stereotypes. Fascists are wrong because we and they have different values which lead us to disagree with them. Neither we nor they are wrong because our psychological processes are deficient, nor are we or they wrong because our opinions are value-laden. If perception reflects reality from the point of view of the perceiver then, if our (or their) values are part of the perceiver (and hence part of reality), perception would fail to reflect reality if it did not reflect those values. As Oakes et al. ask, what would be the point of holding political views, for example, that did not reflect one's own values?

To return to the vase example: the guest is right from their point of view when they perceive the vase to be a water container. We nevertheless disagree with and object to the categorization that they have chosen for the object, preferring instead some other categorization that is meaningful, relevant and useful for our own goals, needs and purposes.

Oakes et al. (1994) have made a number of important and challenging contributions in the treatment of the relationship between categorization and reality. My reservations about some of their ideas are presented in the chapters to come (see especially Chapters 7 and 11).

In the discussion of perceiver readiness I referred to a case where some categorization differed from our own categorization because it was not meaningful, useful or relevant. It should be obvious from the preceding discussion that what can be defined as one's *own* categorization, purpose or goal varies with the level of abstraction of self-perception. When we think of ourselves as group members our goals and values shift from being the goals and values that we espouse as a unique individual in some setting to the goals, values and categorizations that we share with other people who we perceive to be interchangeable with ourselves (or to share a social identity with ourselves). The transition in self-perception is referred to as **depersonalization**. The choice of terminology is unfortunate because it does not describe a loss of identity but refers to a transition in identity from the personal to the social.

Depersonalization is held to underlie group phenomena but it is variable and continuous. Depersonalization is not an all-or-none process. In almost no circumstance do we respond to the world solely in terms of personal or social identity. On the contrary, self-categorization operates continually at different points between those extremes. However, it is important to remember that personal identity and any particular social identity exist in a **functional antagonism**. This does not mean that the content of beliefs associated with personal and social identity must be inconsistent, or that several social categorizations could not be salient at a given time.

To make some of these points clearer it is useful to consider a statement attributed to Einstein:

> If my theory of relativity is proven successful, Germany will claim me as a German and France will declare that I am a citizen of the world. Should my theory prove untrue France will say I am a German and Germany will declare that I am a Jew.

Einstein's statement is a convenient illustration of how self-categories can be used flexibly (assuming, for the sake of argument that Einstein was correctly describing the self-perception of French and German people). When Einstein is positively valued he is assigned to the least abstract self-category that is relevant for the perceiver (German or citizen of the world). When Einstein is negatively valued though he is assigned to a relevant outgroup category (German or Jew) that enables the perceiver to differentiate self from Einstein (Table 5.3).

TABLE 5.3 *Categorization of Einstein*

Perceiver	Work	Einstein assigned to category
German	Success	German
German	Failure	Jew
French	Success	Citizen of the world
French	Failure	German

For Germans and French the least abstract category that includes all relevant stimuli is different. Germans can compare themselves with Einstein as Germans, but the French need to use some more inclusive category: Einstein uses the term 'citizen of the world'. If both groups wish to perceive themselves and Einstein to share a positive self-category in the light of his success, they need to use such abstract categories. If they wish to differentiate themselves from Einstein in view of his failure, they need to use a sub-category that they do not share with Einstein which invokes an intergroup distinction. For the French that sub-category is *German*, for the Germans it is *Jew*. I will consider the point that *Jew* and *German* can be seen as equally abstract in general (comprising overlapping sub-categories of the global 'citizen of the world' category) in Chapter 10.

Having introduced the key concepts of the theory it is useful to dwell upon the way in which the processes have interrelated effects. Generally speaking, SCT argues that category salience is the product of the interaction between perceiver readiness and fit. In practical terms it is difficult to define normative fit, perceiver readiness and comparative fit in probabilistically independent terms. This is illustrated by the discussion of perceiver readiness, where Oakes et al.'s (1994) arguments suggest that perceiver readiness has a direct effect on category use and that through perceiver readiness prior knowledge elaborates stimuli (assuming that stimulus elaboration refers to detecting similarities and differences). Given these mutual dependencies it is sensible to consider the constructs as constraint relations rather than as isolated entities.

The issue of which dimensions are used to make intercategory differentiations has also been explored in the work of Reynolds (e.g., 1996). Her work on impression formation showed that the dimensions used in comparisons between stimulus individuals were determined by the higher-level category that was made salient. That is, different dimensions were used for comparing the *same* two female science students when they were categorized as women than when they were categorized as science students, and the dimensions chosen were those which were relevant to the higher-order category. Essentially, Reynolds's results suggest the important role played by structural alignment and thematic integration as per Bassok and Medin's (1997) analysis.

In constraint relations terms, Reynolds's results can be put in the form shown in Figure 5.2. Initial category use involves a question: 'Are stimuli X and Y members of category A?' Asking such a question activates knowledge about the dimensions that distinguish within the categories and also the dimensions that distinguish between the categories. In Gentner's (1983) terms this is structural alignment (but I argue it is accompanied by ubiquitous thematic integration). Where there are no activated dimensions that distinguish X from Y, or the dimensions that distinguish X from Y are not those that distinguish A from not-A, the perceived equivalence of X and Y is increased and the use of the category is confirmed. Note that in Figure 5.2 the self-categorization theory constructs are represented as constraint relations. There is no

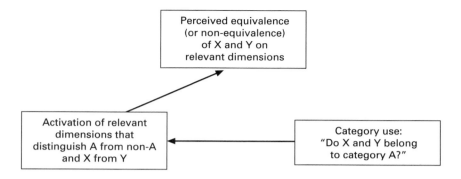

FIGURE 5.2   *Constraint relations shown in Reynolds's study*

box in the figure that can be called 'normative fit' or 'perceiver readiness' but these constructs are implicit. For example, the actual phrasing of the question in the category use box assumes that the perceiver is ready to use category A. The activation of dimensions for differentiation is dependent on the congruence between the meaning of A and not-A.

The dimensions which enable the perceiver to distinguish between A and non-A and between X and Y enable the derivation of what McGarty and Turner (1992) call *differentiated meaning*. This is meaning which makes concepts separable and clear. To say what something is, we need to be able to say what it is not and why it is not some other thing. These ideas have been applied to a number of domains, particularly the outgroup homogeneity effect and the illusory correlation effect, which will be discussed in much more detail in Chapter 8. The easiest way to explain the effects in terms of a limited number of principles is that the use of categories involves answering questions about the identity and nature of stimuli and categories by comparing stimuli and by comparing categories. The nature of the question addressed determines which dimensions are seen as relevant to the particular judgement and this in turn constrains the perceived equivalence of the entities being compared (for much more detailed elaborations and evidence see Haslam et al., 1996c; McGarty and de la Haye, 1997; Oakes et al., 1994). In each of the following examples the constraint relations take a form similar to that shown in Figure 5.2.

Thus when judging two members of an ingroup perceivers are engaged in answering questions of the form 'Are these two people different from each other?' The knowledge that will be activated in response to that particular goal or purpose will reflect knowledge about the dimensions that help us to distinguish between members of that group. No dimensions that help to distinguish *between groups* need be activated because intergroup comparison is not necessarily relevant to the task at hand. This will in turn increase the perceived non-equivalence of members of the group (ingroup heterogeneity) because differentiations between persons are being made. Of course, should intergroup differentiation become relevant then dimensions that discriminate between groups will become relevant, leading to increased perceived equivalence of the ingroup members. That is, the two people will be similar to the degree that they are not like the members of the outgroup.

When judging two members of an outgroup perceivers are engaged in answering not only a question of the form 'Are these two people different from each other?' but also a question of the form 'Are these two people different from *us*?' Dimensions which distinguish between members of the outgroup and dimensions that distinguish between the ingroup and outgroup are immediately relevant for answering these questions. However different members of the outgroup may be from each other on dimensions which distinguish between outgroup members they will be similar to each other, and different from the ingroup, in that they belong to the outgroup. This enhanced perceived equivalence creates the conditions for the outgroup homogeneity effect.

Imagine the situation where an Australian considers whether two other Australians are similar to each other and where the same Australian considers whether two Americans are similar to each other. In answering the first question the consideration that the two Australians are similar in that they are not American is relatively unlikely to affect judgement unless the perceiver is primed to contrast Australians and Americans (perhaps by experimental instructions). When answering the second question such a contrast *is* primed by the question and this puts the perceiver in an intergroup context.

Finally, when judging two groups of differing size perceivers are engaged in answering the question 'Are the members of group A different from the members of group B?' Those dimensions that distinguish between groups A and B and between their members become relevant. To the extent that variations on the dimensions reveal the nature of one group more clearly (owing to the greater amount of information available about the larger group) than the other group, the perceived non-equivalence of the two groups and the perceived equivalence of the members of each group will be enhanced (the illusory correlation effect). This example introduces an additional principle, *diagnosticity*, that will be discussed in Chapter 8.

However, there is some slipperiness in the SCT terms 'interpersonal' and 'intergroup'. This occurs for a number of reasons. A conversation between a man and a woman could be an interpersonal interaction in SCT terms or it could be an intergroup interaction (e.g., as it could be in a debate about feminism). Moreover, it could be an intergroup encounter for one participant and an interpersonal encounter for the other. Worse still, the extent to which it is an intergroup or interpersonal encounter will almost certainly vary across the course of interaction as changes in salience occur. This suggests that SCT must reject diagnostic categories that are readily accepted in everyday language and by most social psychologists. Two people having a casual conversation would almost invariably be perceived by most observers to be engaged in interpersonal interaction. Under SCT it is only unambiguously an interpersonal interaction from the point of view of either perceiver when he or she conceives self and other to share some higher-level group membership.

This terminology becomes strained when the 'groups' comprise single members. The protagonists in a boxing match or a street robbery will in some cases be acting as representatives of competing social groups, but in others they may be engaged in a contest for individual gain or expressing personal enmity that does not rest on a shared group membership. Thus it does not make sense to call this an intragroup encounter because the processes of cooperation and mutual social influence that would be engaged in a genuine intragroup encounter are not involved, even though the processes of competition and differentiation that would be engaged in any other intergroup encounter may be. At the same time each protagonist may be seeing self as relatively unique. We must therefore distinguish a genuine intragroup encounter, as might occur when two boxers compete for the right to represent their nation, from an encounter between two persons who are not acting as representatives of some group and either do not perceive, or only weakly perceive, themselves to share a group membership.

There are several solutions that could be consistent with SCT, but the analytic solution involves three steps for SCT researchers: they should (a) always specify the group memberships in a putative intergroup relationship, (b) avoid the term *interpersonal* where possible, and (c) avoid equating personalized self-perception with intragroup interactions. A boxer competing with an opponent, or a deviate being expelled from a group, may be engaged in what is best termed an intergroup encounter, but self-perception for the boxer or deviate might be highly personalized.

Another abiding concern in self-categorization theory research is the flexibility of cognitive constructs. Turner et al. (1994) suggest that stability in self-perception is afforded by constancy in relations between social groups (and other features of reality) and by relatively enduring higher-level knowledge frameworks (what Oakes et al., 1994: 192, refer to as 'the body of social knowledge and theory the perceiver brings to interpretation'). The process of category use, however, is entirely fluid and involves the formation of new categories for particular purposes.

Turner and Onorato (in press) do address alternatives to the flexible categorization model. One alternative is that relevant self-categories are stored prior to activation. Turner and Onorato consider this proposal implausible for reasons of cognitive economy, in that it is unlikely that so many self-categories would be retained. I would note that this is a highly idiosyncratic invocation of principles of cognitive economy as nobody has established that long-term memory capacity is *limited*. Network models such as the autoassociator (see Smith and de Coster, 1998; and Chapter 10 here) allow massive amounts of information to be 'stored' (or more correctly retrieved) by means of a relatively small number of connections. More critically, in my view, Turner and Onorato also argue that the proposal is deficient because it does not provide an account of the formation of new categories.

The views developed by Turner et al. (1994), Oakes et al. (1994) and Turner and Onorato (in press) represent a significant departure from the original assumptions of self-categorization theory. Turner and Onorato (in press) interpret Turner et al. (1994) to have suggested that the self-concept is not a cognitive structure in the information processing system. Assumption 1 of SCT states:

> A.1 That the self-concept is the cognitive component of the psychological system or process referred to as the self. *The self may be understood at least in part as a cognitive structure, a cognitive element in the information-processing system.* The self-concept may be defined as the set of cognitive representations of self available to a person. (Turner et al., 1987: 44, emphasis added)

This represents a substantial shift in position. My own reading of Turner et al. (1994) suggests no need for a dramatic revision to the original theory if we allow that the *self* cannot be understood as a cognitive structure but that the self-concept is open to this interpretation. I would therefore recommend retaining the term *self* for the process of generating spontaneous self-depictions (what Turner et al., 1987: 44, refer to as 'self-images', but 'self-categories' could be an equally good term) and retaining the term *self-concept* for long-term knowledge about the particular biological-psychological entity which is generating the categories. I presume this knowledge is implicated in determining the readiness of perceivers to use certain categorizations.

The ideas of higher-level knowledge and theory await further developments in self-categorization theory writings. In part, SCT writers have been influenced by the work of Medin, Murphy, Barsalou and colleagues on the role of theories in constraining categories (e.g., Barsalou and Medin, 1986; Medin and Wattenmaker, 1987; Murphy and Medin, 1985). As we have seen, these authors advocate a change from a view of concepts as static, neatly organized packets of knowledge to the idea that the representation of categories varies dynamically with experience and current **comparative context**, and that they serve to generate useful expectations, regardless of whether these have a high probability of being true, or have other criteria which suggest conventional logical adequacy. The example considered in Chapter 3 was that it is vitally important to remember that snakes *can* be poisonous when we encounter a snake, even though *most* snakes are not poisonous. Context specificity improves prediction but it also represents an argument against static representations, and suggests that we need to understand relations between concepts (cf. Thagard, 1989; 1992).

In this vein Brown (1999; Brown and Turner, 1998) has explored the form that these theories take in providing content for stereotypical beliefs (an issue closely related to the concept of normative fit). Theories, like context (see the discussion of Reynolds's work above), can constrain and guide perceptions of consistency/similarity within groups, the meaning of categories, and the dimensions used to differentiate between social groups.

Brown and Turner (1998) manipulated the explanation of unemployment that participants endorsed by presenting them with an extreme individual responsibility or social deterministic theory and asking them how much they agreed with it. Brown and Turner reasoned (correctly as their results indicate) that rejecting an extreme view would be associated with adopting the opposite view. They found that stereotyping increased so that there was more stereotyping of a stereotype-consistent unemployed person when an individual responsibility stereotype was used and less when they endorsed a social responsibility stereotype.

In analysing stereotype and category content Brown develops the following points. First, regardless of what else it might be, part of stereotype content must be the comparative relations involved. That is, stereotype content is not so much based on an appreciation of the differences between and similarities within groups, but *is* those differences between groups and similarities within groups. Necessarily these similarities and differences change as the frame of reference changes because similarities and differences cannot be defined without reference to contrasting categories. These aspects of stereotype content can therefore be expected to be inherently fluid and subject to contextual variation, and Brown has assembled an impressive amount of evidence of this fluidity (building also on the work of Haslam and colleagues: see Haslam et al., 1995b; 1996c).

Most of Brown's work focuses on the theories or explanatory ideas that people hold in relation to stereotypes. A very important point in this regard is that the labelling system used to distinguish between groups can itself be understood to be a type of theory. That is, labels like group A or group B as might be used in experiments are useful to the extent to which they serve to explain some situation. As McGarty et al. (1993a) argue, this can even apply in the illusory correlation paradigm where there are minimal conditions for differentiating between groups but the existence of the differing group labels leads people to expect differences between groups. This motivates them to find ways in which the groups differ.

Self-categorization theorists such as Oakes et al. (1994) and Turner and Onorato (in press) have claimed that categories are not stored but are constructed on the spot to take account of the current context. Although this idea is well worth investigating it does beg the question demanded by the preceding analysis of what form longer-term enduring knowledge takes. If we accept that there is such a thing as long-term knowledge, and that we can have long-term knowledge about groups, then it follows that long-term knowledge must also be relative, comparative and, most importantly, categorical. We cannot know, for example, that some piece of information is normatively consistent with the stereotype of some group unless we also know of the existence of that group, and in particular we must know that such groups are distinct or at least potentially distinct from other groups.

These are difficult points and I shall certainly return to them. For the moment though I wish to suggest that it seems that the sort of long-term knowledge which is anticipated by self-categorization theory requires categorical ideas and this must be reconciled with the proposal that categories are created on the spot for the current purposes. The solution that I will pursue in the chapters to come is to argue for a distinction between the *category* as the immediate usable representation of some group or set of objects which is created on-line, and *categorization schemes* which represent longer-term knowledge structures and explanatory processes which need not have a rational representation that appears in consciousness.

In summary, SCT is a well-developed constraint model that avoids some of the pitfalls that exist in the categorization literature. The theory also makes a number of hard choices on controversial issues about categorization. Some of these choices will be investigated further in Chapter 7, but before we do that I will review several more sense-making approaches in Chapter 6.

---

comparative context The stimuli taken into account by the perceiver in some setting (see *frame of reference*).

comparative fit The perception of similarities and differences amongst stimuli on relevant dimensions which provide a basis for categorizing. It is instantiated in the meta-contrast principle.

depersonalization A shift in self-perception so that the self is seen as interchangeable with other members of a given social category (self-stereotyping). This is not a loss of personal identity but a change in identity. The opposite process is called personalization.

frame of reference Formally in SCT the pool of psychologically relevant stimuli, but the term is also used to refer to the range of psychologically relevant stimulus positions.

functional antagonism The tendency for the salience of different levels of categorization to be inversely related.

meta-contrast principle The idea that category formation proceeds on the basis of the detection and maximization of the ratio of relevant differences and similarities.

normative fit The match between a categorization and the social meaning of the stimuli.

perceiver readiness The preparedness to perceive some set of stimuli to share a category membership. The term was preferred by Oakes et al. (1994) to relative accessibility.

Appendix: other equations for meta-contrast

It is worth noting that the equation for meta-contrast retains a problem in that it is unconstrained when the differences between members of the group on the bottom line of the equation approach zero. As the denominator approaches zero the ratio becomes a large positive number, and it becomes undefined when there are no differences. In the example above drawn from the study by Oakes et al. (1991) I have assumed that there are differences, but that these are very small so that the meta-contrast ratios for the conflict conditions are $1/\varepsilon$ (a very large number) rather than infinity. The problem with using this equation for comparative quantitative purposes is that we have to estimate the value of ε. For example, if ε_1 on the top line of the equation is 0.01 and ε_2 on the bottom line of the equation is 0.004 then we obtain an MCR of 2.5 for the consensus condition. If we reverse these assignments we obtain an MCR of 0.4. This is clearly fanciful arithmetic for two reasons. First, the meta-contrast ratios of two categories which do not differ in any relevant way should both be defined to be 1.0 with respect to each other – regardless of the amount of similarity within the categories. Secondly, the MCR should not be sensitive to variations which are much smaller than the degree of discriminability of the stimuli in the current context. To address this problem I recommend adding a constant to both lines of the equation, so that equation (5.1) becomes

$$\frac{1 + \sum\limits_{d=1}^{n_d} \sum\limits_{i=1}^{n_x} \sum\limits_{j=1}^{n_y} \left| x_{di} - y_{dj} \right| /(n_d n_x n_y)}{1 + \sum\limits_{d=1}^{n_d} \sum\limits_{l=1}^{n_x} \sum\limits_{m=1}^{n_x} \left| x_{dlm} - y_{dml} \right| /((n_d n_x)(n n_x - 1))} \tag{5.3}$$

and equation (5.2) becomes

$$\mathrm{MCR} = \frac{1 + \left(\sum\limits_{b=1}^{n_b} \left| x_s - x_b \right| \right) / n_b}{1 + \left(\sum\limits_{a=1}^{n_a} \left| x_s - x_a \right| \right) / n_a} \tag{5.4}$$

These changes deal with the problem of MCR approaching infinity, but the choice of 1 as a constant to be added to each line is arbitrary. A superior solution would be to choose a constant that was related to the degree of discriminability of the stimuli on the scale of measurement used. Thus when comparing stimuli on a seven-point scale, adding a constant of 1 might suffice; but with a 100-point scale a constant of 10 might serve better. Yet another alternative would be to constrain the ratio to a set range (such as –1 to +1 or 0 to 1) which *might* allow comparability across circumstances (note that such a metric would be quite different from the biserial correlation between category membership and position of the stimulus on the dimension).

A cautionary note is necessary in relation to all these points though. The instantiation of self-categorization theory ideas in numerical form can be helpful but it can also lead to certain problems. This is because the equations are not much use without a measurement theory that tells us how to assign magnitudes on the dimensions that are presumed to be of interest. Self-categorization theory implies that the task of deriving such a measurement theory should be very difficult. Self-categorization theory suggests that judgements are not unalterable, fixed properties of stimuli or even of differences amongst stimuli, but that they vary with the context. Hence the appropriateness of measurement theories will vary with that context.

6 Categorization as Meaning Creation II: Other Sense-Making Approaches

In this chapter I propose to address a range of approaches to social categorization and related phenomena which adopt what could be termed a sense-making approach. These approaches overlap considerably with each other, and with the approaches presented in the previous two chapters. For the purpose of this chapter I have classified the approaches on the basis of the key constructs emphasized in each formulation. These constructs are really derived from the various ancestries of the approach. Those which descend most directly from social categorization research tend to stress coherence, those which descend from work on person perception stress explanation, and those which descend from social judgement stress assimilation and contrast.

A. Coherence-based approaches

A prominent recent approach is the optimal distinctiveness theory of Brewer (1991; 1993a; 1993b). This theory represents an amalgamation of self-categorization theory and uniqueness theory (Snyder and Fromkin, 1980). The central postulate is that both differentiation of the self from others and inclusion of the self into larger social collectives are powerful motives which function as opposed processes. Social identities are self-categorizations which encompass both of these motives. The optimal social identity (a point of equilibrium in some social setting) is that which best satisfies the need for distinctiveness and for inclusion.

The two drives define a dimension of inclusiveness of the self-concept, and threats to self-integrity exist at both extremes (thereby creating pressures for moderate inclusiveness). Being too distinctive allows social isolation and stigmatization; being immersed in a highly inclusive group provides an insufficient basis for comparative appraisal or self-definition (there is a tension between this idea and Festinger's, 1954, suggestion that we seek similar others for comparison purposes).

For Brewer, the particular mechanism which defines the level of inclusiveness of some social category is the number or variety of people that can be classified to share a category. Thus, other things being equal, identifying with a larger group will be associated with a more extended self-concept.

Although no equivalent drives for uniqueness and differentiation can readily be identified for non-self stimuli there are some ideas that are directly relevant to an analysis of general categorization processes. Brewer suggests that identification with larger or more diverse (greater variety of persons) groups leads to a loss of individual distinctiveness. However, there is a conflict between this idea and the work discussed previously by Mullen (1991) and others (e.g., Brewer and Harasty, 1996; Brewer et al., 1995) suggesting that minorities are more entitative than majorities. Thus, minorities are held to be entitative and majorities are less so, but associating oneself with a larger group and (one would think from these arguments) less entitative group is held to threaten personal distinctiveness. Clearly, at least one set of these ideas must be wrong, and in Chapter 8 I discuss the suggestion by McGarty et al. (1995) that there is no simple relationship between entitativity and relative group size (where the work of B. Simon, e.g., Simon, 1993; Simon and Hamilton, 1994; Simon et al., 1997, and others is considered) and that the relationships between diversity, variability and group size must be considered further.

A number of writers who adopt a social cognitive perspective have argued that categorization processes represent a search for coherence. Much of this work is a variation on the selective attention approach that was discussed in Chapter 4.

The proposal of an exemplar theory of social judgement by Smith and Zárate (1992) that we discussed in Chapter 2 is an example of such a contribution. Indeed a great deal of work by Smith and colleagues stresses the search for coherence (Carlston and Smith, 1996; E. R. Smith and Mackie, 1995; 1997).

Another general approach which is structurally quite different but which shares some concerns with Smith's approach stems from an associational model whereby stereotypes are seen as mental representations based on associations in memory between category labels and attributes. When a category label is activated this activation spreads from the category to the connected attributes. In the terms used by Stangor and Lange (1994) an example of the model can be presented in Figure 6.1 (the lines of varying thickness represent the strength of the links).

With respect to social categories the attributes linked to the category nodes are normally trait terms but can be other types of characteristic. The associated characteristics are those which are most typically associated with the category. The strength of the associations reflects the degree of the typicality whereby new inputs are interpreted on the basis of prior knowledge. It follows that associations which are consistent with prior expectations will be more highly activated because of their high links with the category label. If we encounter a concert violinist the category will activate the attributes such as *cultured* and *highly trained* rather than *violent* and *generous* even though such new associations could be learned over time.

Stangor and colleagues have conducted extensive research on the rela-
ıship between stereotype/expectancy-consistent and -inconsistent
·mation. The consensus is that people have better memories for

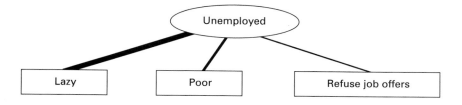

FIGURE 6.1   *Example of a stereotype structure in Stangor and Lange's associational model*

expectancy-inconsistent information except when stereotypes are activated (Stangor and McMillan, 1992). Under these conditions people start to ignore inconsistent information and look for stereotype-consistent information. The implication is that stimuli which are congruent with expectations will tend to be overrepresented in memory (Fyock and Stangor, 1994).

An important idea that emerges from the work of Stangor and Ford (1992) is that the development of these strong expectancies, and motivation to find stereotype-consistent information, derives from a desire to arrive at a simple coherent impression of the groups (Brewer's optimal distinctiveness theory stresses similar features).

This point illustrates why the approach of Stangor et al. can be characterized as taking a middle road. The account stresses coherence and sense-making but it is sense-making with a cost, that cost being error. For the sense-making account envisaged by SCT the cost is in the effort after meaning: if people really were mental sluggards they would not categorize under certain conditions, because as Spears and Haslam (1997) suggest, categorization can be effortful.

This associational model does not encompass links between the attributes or activation of the higher-level category node by the activation of lower-level nodes. A model of impression formation which allows reciprocal activation has been proposed by Kunda and Thagard (1996).

B. Explanation-based approaches

The pragmatic approach championed by Leyens et al. (1992; 1994) has been represented as an alternative to the conventional social cognitive stance. The pragmatic approach is expressed most clearly in social judgeability theory. These authors argue that perception, including categorical perception, is governed not only by what it is appropriate to believe/perceive because it is true, but by what it is appropriate to believe/perceive because it serves the interests of the perceiver, that is, it is useful.

Leyens et al. (1994) see their vantage point as being from the bridge between a social cognitive approach and what they term a social identity approach (I would describe this as a *self-categorization theory* approach as most of the issues they discuss are well beyond the scope of social identity theory). They consider the social cognitive approach with its focus on the distortion of reality produced by social perception to have been carried too far by its proponents, but at the same time they see the idea of self-categorization theorists that social perception serves to produce a greater match between perception and reality to have gone too far as well. The core of the objection is that the entirely fluid, context-dependent perception that SCT advocates, whereby any and all stimulus information can be reinterpreted by the perceiver, is too unconstrained. Fiske and Leyens elaborate this point:

> Does that mean that our perception of people varies constantly with context? To a Belgian, Americans, for instance, are in-groupers if compared to Iraqis, but out-groupers if compared to Belgians. Without denying the role of context, the shortcoming of SIT/SCT is that it does not make sense that we are forever fluctuating in our perception of ourselves and of others. To the same extent that, in adaptation-level experiments, a croquet ball may seem lighter after lifting a bowling ball but is not confused with a ping-pong ball, people's perceptions may be somewhat altered by the context, but they will rarely be turned upside down. (1997: 99)

I am not aware of self-categorization theorists predicting that such perceptions would be turned upside down (arguing as they do that enduring aspects of reality provide constraints on perception), but straw men aside, the arguments derived from the pragmatic approach demand close attention. Essentially, the work centres on the *adequacy* of perception as the overarching concept rather than alternatives such as accuracy or efficiency that follow from social cognitive work. They argue for a multiple-level approach where the levels relate to differing concerns about the adequacy of judgement. These concerns stem from differing conceptions of the world and also, importantly, from the conception of the judgement situation. In this sense the work of Leyens et al. has some affinities with that of Bless et al. (1993) and Schwarz et al. (1991) on the role of conversational logic in structuring perceptions and also the work of Kunda and colleagues (Kunda, 1990; Kunda and Sherman-Williams, 1993; Kunda et al., 1997) on motivated reasoning.

The problem that the social judgeability theory addresses then is: given the infinite number of possible categories that people have available to them, how do they arrive at adequate judgements? At the level of objective reality, judgements are adequate if they can be seen to provide a match to the data; thus in order for a category to be applied it must provide some fit to reality. This idea cuts across the SCT concepts of comparative and normative fit.

However, given the vast number of categories that can be applied to what is a relatively stable and enduring reality, reality itself cannot arbitrate which categories will be deployed. The other criteria for adequacy of judgements that can be deployed are the *cultural*, *integrity* and *theoretical* levels.

The aim in using each of these levels is to provide a useful fit with reality rather than an exact match with reality, and in particular, to allow people to interact with other people. In constraint relations terms each of the levels of adequacy reflects the constraints of particular types of knowledge on category use. The cultural level of adequacy reflects people's propensity to follow the social rules within a particular culture at a particular time. An example of such a social rule that is immediately relevant to this discussion (and is introduced by Leyens et al., 1994: 5–6) is that in many Western societies it is seen as wrong to treat people at the categorical level (i.e., to stereotype them) without paying attention to individuating information.

The integrity level relates to the personal and social integrity of the judge. The suggestion is therefore that people avoid applying categorizations which would threaten the identity of themselves as individuals or of groups to which they belong. Thus, a supporter of a political party may resist forming an impression of their leader as corrupt, despite evidence of dubious deals, because that impression would have negative consequences for the party, the supporter's self-esteem and so on.

The theoretical level of integrity relates to the degree to which the judgement explains the relationships between the information that is to be integrated. Under this view a judgement should comprise an *enlightening Gestalt* that gives meaning to the world and allows communication. These ideas closely correspond to the ideas of Medin, Murphy and colleagues on the naive theories that underpin categorization behaviour, and the particular idea of psychological essentialism (Medin, 1989; and as applied to social categories by Rothbart and Taylor, 1992). Put simply, theoretical integrity refers to the perceived correspondence between a judgement and some theory of the world.

Social judgeability theory thus emphasizes the importance of *social validity* in judgements. That is, in order for judgements to be useful in social interaction it is necessary for them to be true in some sense, and truth is a complex construct with many levels. Judgements are made in the context of the effort after meaning, to make sense of the world and to make sense of the situation the judge finds themselves in. Importantly 'situation' here includes the judgement situation. Where people feel that they have an adequate basis for judgement at the relevant levels they develop a sense of social judgeability and make the judgement in line with their concerns: otherwise they refuse to judge.

Leyens et al. (1994) note that a consideration of different levels of adequacy already occurs implicitly in a lot of the contemporary research. In that respect, the social judgeability approach can be seen as formalizing and teasing out a perspective that exists in implicit form in the literature. Leyens et al. (1994: 127) argue that both social cognitive and social identity approaches pay a great deal of attention to the reality level, where the social cognitivists argue that perceivers fail to grasp reality adequately, and the social identity theorists stress the complexities of reality and the necessity of being selective. Both approaches are said to be silent about the cultural level of adequacy in relation to commonly studied stereotyping phenomena. They argue that the social part of the integrity level had attracted some interest from social identity theorists and that the theoretical level is attracting increasing attention.

To illustrate the social judgeability approach an experiment by Yzerbyt et al. (1994) serves well in relation to the use of categorical and individuating information in impression formation. These authors reasoned, following the social judgeability approach, that people would avoid making a categorical judgement (stereotyping) if they felt that their judgement was ill informed (because they had insufficient information about the individual). This is because making categorical judgements under such conditions violated a social rule in the Western society the participants belonged to. The question was how to release that categorical judgement. This is problematic because providing people with detailed information may lead them to use this information as the basis of their judgement. In order to release the categorical judgement the experimenters therefore had to create the illusion for the participants that they were well informed.

The illusion was created by means of a dichotic listening task where participants were asked to pay attention to information in one ear while text was read to the other non-attending ear. Half of the participants were told that this text (which was actually unrelated to the message) was really information about the target individual. Thus an illusion of knowledge was created. These participants were more likely to make a categorical judgement than were people who did not have this knowledge.

In a not unrelated vein, Wittenbrink and colleagues (1997; 1998) have developed the view that stereotypes provide background knowledge which allows perceivers to form coherent impressions of people. Their approach is inspired by work by such authors as Asch and Zukier (1984). Asch and Zukier (1984) emphasized that impressions of persons often involved reconciling apparently conflicting traits through interpretation of the interrelations between attributes. These interpretations can be understood to be based on mental models which relate observations to the world. For Wittenbrink et al. (1998) one function served by stereotypes is that they serve as a source of such integrating knowledge (Wittenbrink et al. draw on the concept of mental models for this purpose).

To take an example, if a perceiver sees an unemployed person refuse a job offer then stereotypes of the form 'unemployed people are often lazy' and 'unemployed people are often offered jobs for which they are highly over-qualified' would serve to inform the impressions formed of the interaction in quite different ways. The target might be expected to be perceived more negatively in the first case and to be expected to refuse other job offers in the future. If the second stereotype was active then there is no reason to expect that a negative impression will be formed or that future job offers will be refused unless the job is for a position the target is over-qualified for. It is worth noting that the two stereotypes perform differing cognitive functions. The first stereotype can also provide an explanation of unemployment, whereas the second one must be linked to some other principle (the state of the job market). This mirrors the fact that the first stereotype involves dispositional attribution (laziness is a characteristic internal to the person) and the second is situational (external).

This is an unusual set of circumstances though. It is unlikely that a single attribution (laziness) would be able to explain the nature of some person and other relevant states of affairs in the world. It may be the parsimony of this explanation (along with the justification it provides for the maintenance of less than generous treatment of the unemployed in many societies) that makes it so pervasive.

Returning to Wittenbrink et al.'s (1998) work, these authors reiterate the points about flexibility of categorizing that follow from the work of Barsalou, Medin, Murphy and others. They therefore suggest that stereotypic knowledge should be considered as a diffuse set of constraints on categorizing. Their views on these points are thus very similar to those of Turner et al. (1994) considered in the previous chapter.

C. Assimilation and contrast approaches

The final tradition that I wish to address in this chapter is one which has a long and continuing heritage in social psychology. It is a tradition that has clear links to ideas discussed in Chapter 3 in relation to categorization effects, and is also intimately related to the tradition of research on construct activation that was discussed in Chapter 4.

This tradition could be referred to as the assimilation-contrast approach. The core idea is that perceivers form judgemental standards and that either they assimilate stimuli to these judgemental standards or they contrast stimuli away from them. All of these approaches trace their heritage from theorists such as Helson (1964), Sherif and Hovland (1961) and Upshaw (1965). The approaches differ in (a) the extent to which they endorse a perceptual or semantic view of judgemental shift (see Chapter 3), (b) the manner in which the judgemental standards are computed, and (c) the predictions for assimilation and contrast.

Sherif and Hovland's view (see also Sherif et al., 1965) was that the range of possible positions could be classified into three regions: the latitude of acceptance, the latitude of rejection and the latitude of non-commitment. Opinions which fell into the latitude of acceptance would be assimilated to own position, opinions which fell into the latitude of rejection would be contrasted away from own position, and opinions which fell into the latitude of non-commitment would be neither assimilated nor contrasted. Thus for Sherif and Hovland (1961) own position defined the standards and determined whether there would be assimilation or contrast: own position enabled specification of a set of categories into which other positions could be interpreted.

Other writers have defined other methods for defining standards. For example, Biernat et al. (1998) have presented a shifting standards model (based on a tradition of research by Manis and colleagues) which establishes similar categories to stereotypic perception. The core of their model is that seeing a person with relevant stereotypic cues leads to the activation of a stereotype. This stereotype allows the activation of judgemental standards (what Biernat et al., 1998, describe as a triggering of the comparative context) against which that person can be judged. Where the target's characteristics are consistent with the stereotype or ambiguous with respect to the stereotype the target will be subjectively assimilated to the judgemental standards. Where the target's characteristics are inconsistent with the stereotype the perceiver will be subjectively contrasted from the standards.

Up to that point the model is a straightforward extension of Sherif and Hovland's (1961) ideas. Biernat et al. (1998) suggest, however, that while assimilation and contrast will occur on subjectively anchored dimensions, quite different effects will be observed on objective or externally anchored dimensions. The latter are dimensions which are measured on dimensions that do not change despite the target's category membership. On such dimensions they expect assimilation to group stereotypes. They give examples of such units with constant meaning as units of distance, time and wealth as well as standardized test scores and rank orderings of stimuli. These are understood to provide a basis for absolute judgement because they are held to be invariant attributes of the object. Thus, if the maximum speed of a car is 200 km/h then that speed can be considered to be slow or fast (a subjective standard) depending on whether it is a racing car or a street vehicle, but it cannot be considered to be 150 km/h or 250 km/h because maximum speed is understood to be an invariant property.

The assumption that some dimensions contain units which do not vary in their meaning is tenuous but it is less contestable that certain properties of objects and people are seen to be variably variable. We expect people to vary from context to context in the extent to which they are perceived to be short or tall, but we do not expect their height to vary from context to context. In other words, although there is variability *between* adults in height there is not much variability within adults. Biernat et al.'s argument is thus that objective dimensions are not context specific (see Chapter 7 for a further discussion of related points).

The final extension of the model is that zero-sum behaviours are predicted to follow from the objective judgement. Zero-sum behaviours are those which restrict the behavioural options of other people. This could involve the allocation of limited or valuable resources. For example, targets could be positively or negatively evaluated on subjective dimensions which reflected their position with respect to other dimensions, but still be allocated resources on the basis of their category membership. Thus a female applicant for a male-stereotypic job might be regarded as an 'excellent applicant, *for a woman*' but still be unlikely to be awarded the job.

Still another view is contained within Schwarz and Bless's (1992) inclusion–exclusion model. Their argument is similar to that contained in Kahneman and Miller's (1986) norm theory that contrast/assimilation results from a process of comparison of reality with some of its alternatives. In particular, information that is categorized as belonging to the same category is assimilated and information that is categorized differently will be contrasted.

In empirical studies of this model Bless and Schwarz (1998) showed that when a respected person's political party membership was primed, the evaluation of the party was assimilated to the favourable impression of that respected person (the exemplar). When, however, features which differentiated the exemplar from the social category were primed the party was contrasted away from the exemplar. That is, participants saw the political party less positively.

Bless and Schwarz (1998) argue that the inclusion-exclusion model provides a coherent and unifying explanation of this phenomenon. Many other formulations would appear, however, to predict identical results. While the model and its empirical investigation appear sound, more distinctive evidence of the utility of their formulation is required to justify the claims made. In short these authors appear to be approaching the same phenomena as authors such as Haslam and Turner (1992; 1995) and Wilder and Thompson (1988) and indeed Biernat et al. (1998).

Finally, Martin et al. (1990) have argued that different standards of comparisons are developed when a category label is primed than when a category label and traits are primed. The effect of priming the category label plus the associated traits should be to produce contrast of an ambiguous new target individual whereas priming the category label on its own is less likely to produce contrast. This is because priming a label and traits should create a more explicit or overt standard against which to compare the target.

These ideas were examined further by Ford et al. (1994) who argue that it is important to distinguish between priming social categories and behavioural traits. They argue that the effects shown by Martin et al. (1990) and their own research point to the adaptability and context-dependent nature of social judgements in that they show clearly how the same perceiver can perceive the same person in different ways. Their own research shows that a person with dual category membership (two-major student) was contrasted away from a single-major prime when the traits associated with that single major were primed. In other words, an interpersonal distinction was made. In experiment 2 they found that when a category label was primed the judged likelihood of the target belonging to that group was lower when associated traits were also primed.

A continuing topic of interest in this area is the effect of awareness of the events that produced the priming on assimilation and contrast. Moskowitz and Roman (1992) found that when participants memorized trait-implying sentences they appeared to generate unconscious primes which led to an assimilation effect in subsequent judgements. However, when participants were given explicit impression formation instructions there was a contrast effect (Higgins, 1996, points out that such contrast effects due to awareness of priming events are not inevitable and the results obtained by Stapel et al., 1996, concur with this).

On balance there is a high level of agreement between assimilation and contrast formulations as well as considerable overlap between the predictions of these approaches and self-categorization theory. Some differences are more apparent when we consider some branch points in the social categorization literature in the next chapter (but for the application of self-categorization theory to social judgement see Haslam and Turner, 1992; 1995; Oakes et al., 1994).

7 Contrasting Perspectives on Motivated Relative Perception

In the previous three chapters I have contrasted approaches based on the principles of selective attention and of sense-making or knowledge creation. As a structure on which to hang a treatment of divergent perspectives on categorization, however, this starts to look somewhat shaky. Although the principles of selective attention and of knowledge creation provide a contrast there is also overlap on these dimensions.

For example, few if any social cognitive theorists would disagree that the function of categorization is sense-making. Does this mean that there is no fundamental disagreement in social psychology over categorization?

I think the easiest way to make the oppositions clear is to examine the questions that are sensible to ask from the mainstream social cognitive point of view and then to consider the type of competing questions that are implied by SCT and some related sense-making approaches.

A. How do limits on capacity affect categorization?
versus
Do limits on capacity have any effect on categorization?

Despite the importance of the idea of capacity limitations for social cognitive approaches to categorization, Spears and Haslam (1997) observe that the relationship between cognitive load and categorization/stereotyping remains underexplored. To consider this relationship, it is probably helpful to start by identifying what form limits on capacity might take and then to examine how they could be related to the categorization process. A common assumption seems to be that capacity limitations are much like the processing capacity of the CPU of a computer. That is, processing capacity provides a continuous absolute limit on the performance of the system. Another way to conceive of capacity limits though would be to think of a water tank connected to a tap. The tank has a profound effect on the operation of the tap only when the absolute limit is reached (it is empty). The implication of this metaphor would be that just as the tank sets no limit on the water supply to a tap until it is empty, so capacity limits may have a critical but occasional effect on human information processing (see also Kruglanski, 1996).

The fact that we may have varying success in applying either of these metaphors implies they may not be particularly apt for cognitive processes. Short-term memory (STM) is seen as having a small finite capacity (the magic number seven plus or minus two items: G. A. Miller, 1956) which can be continuously challenged by externally imposed demands. This seems close to the CPU analogy. Long-term memory, however, is routinely seen to be unlimited in terms of the total number of items which can be stored, that is, neither metaphor seems appropriate.

A common explicit assumption is that load affects the effective performance of cognitive tasks. Traditionally, this has been determined by the accuracy of recall or recognition memory, speed of processing (often priming in a reaction time task), or accuracy of judgement. The implicit assumption therefore is that stable standards of accuracy or effectiveness exist against which performance can be assessed. As we will see, the existence of stable standards of accuracy has been challenged by the self-categorization theorists (Oakes et al., 1994; Oakes and Reynolds, 1997). It is more difficult to direct the same challenge at measures of speed of processing. However, accuracy remains an issue because the speed of response is meaningless without a consideration of the accuracy of response.

A wide variety of processes might be seen to be affected by capacity limits. For example, although the capacity of long-term memory is effectively unlimited, the process of storing that information is by no means perfect. Memory is a probabilistic process whereby only some of the stimuli we encounter are encoded with any detectable trace. This is particularly true where the perceiver pays little attention to the stimuli. This implies that there may be limits on the capacity of the *process of storing* information. A variety of other claims can be made about other phases. The list in Table 7.1 is by no means exhaustive, and it is certainly not uncontested.

TABLE 7.1　*Processes affected by capacity limits*

Process	Hindered by	Implies limits on
Detection of stimuli	Distractor stimuli	Attention
Storage of perceived stimuli	Low attention	Encoding capacity
Interpretation	Distractor tasks	Interpretive capacity
Category/rule learning	Disconfirming instances	Attention or STM
Retrieval	Competing cues	Decoding capacity
Exception learning	Categorization	Attention or STM

The short list in Table 7.1 suggests that different limitations may apply to some stages of information processing. The question I want to turn to immediately is how categorization could relate to capacity limits for some of these stages of processing.

Categorization should aid attempts to learn rules and perceive covariation. That is, a perceiver should be better able to learn relations if they treat stimuli in categorical terms than when they do not. This in itself is fairly obviously true given that category formation is, in part at least, the process of learning equivalence relations. The advantages of categorization, however, will only be obvious where the categorization is appropriate to the situation (bearing in mind, though, that there are difficulties in defining exactly what an appropriate categorization might be).

The process of categorization could be expected to work against exception learning because a focus on category-level information might lead perceivers to ignore individuating, disconfirming or expectancy-incongruent information. Thus categorization should lead, for example, to perceivers being slower to recognize differences between stimuli belonging to the same category than to recognize differences between stimuli belonging to different categories.

On these two points there is reasonably strong agreement between perspectives based on self-categorization theory and perspectives drawn from mainstream social cognitive work. Where the approaches diverge sharply is in relation to the implications of evidence of the effects of capacity limitations.

The dispute between perspectives can be reduced to the following set of principles. Let us take the selective attention stance first (these points are a recapitulation of ideas discussed previously):

1   Stimuli have invariant features, distinguishing them from other stimuli which can be discovered by the allocation of attention. These features represent aspects of objective reality.
2   Processes such as categorization lead people to ignore the invariant, objective aspects of stimuli and thus cause errors.
3   Categorization is an energy-saving process. Categorizing involves an automatic tradeoff between accurately picking up the stimulus information and reducing the total amount of effort.

In contrast, the alternative meaning-seeking view is based on the following set of ideas (e.g., as developed by Spears and Haslam, 1997, building on the work of writers such as Oakes et al., 1994; Oakes and Turner, 1990):

1   Stimulus features do not provide an invariant set of differences which can be detected by appropriate allocation of attention. Rather stimuli are seen to be similar or different depending on whether they are categorized as belonging to the same or different categories (Turner et al., 1987; see Medin et al., 1993, for a related view).
2   The process of categorization does not lead to errors or distortion but instead provides a framework for deciding which similarities and differences are currently relevant to the comparison involved.
3   The process of categorization is an interpretive process which can be effortful and thus can consume rather than save cognitive resources.
4   Being an interpretive process, categorization is shaped by the understandings that the perceiver brings to the stimulus situation. A change to cognitive load may also change the meaning of the situation, leading to changes in categorization which are independent of the changes to cognitive load.

5   There are many possible relationships between cognitive load and categorization.

Point 4 is in some ways the most fundamental and is highlighted in work on illusory correlation (Berndsen et al., 1998; Haslam et al., 1996a; McGarty and de la Haye, 1997; McGarty et al., 1993a) and outgroup homogeneity (Haslam et al., 1995b, 1996c). If we ask participants to perform additional tasks which increase cognitive load we may at the same time give them cues about the relative importance of the focal task. If, for example, we ask participants to remember an eight-digit number at the same time as receiving individuating and categorical information about some stimulus person we not only increase cognitive load but may also persuade participants that their *real* task is to remember the number and not to learn about the stimulus person. This is the substance of Spears and Haslam's (1997) criticism of the study by Macrae et al. (1993) and a body of related work. Nobody disputes that people will perform differently when they do not pay attention to the stimulus information; the question boils down to an examination of the reasons why perceivers do not pay attention to the stimulus information in the high-cognitive-load condition. Is it because they do not have the resources to pay attention and therefore *cannot* pay attention, or is it because they *chose* not to pay attention when they had the opportunity, because they thought they were supposed to pay attention to something else?

To take an equivalent example. If I ask you to monitor how many times the letter 'e' occurs in a string of text and then actually ask you to nominate the number of times that the letter 'u' occurred in the text we would expect your performance to be worse than that of a perceiver who had not been misled in this way by the experimenter (see McMullen et al., 1997, for a related comment). Does this tell us anything about the limits that cognitive economy places on performance? Probably not. What researchers would have to do to examine cognitive economy in this case would be to compare the performance on 'e' monitoring of perceivers who had been asked to monitor 'e' only with those who had been asked to monitor 'e' and 'u' (and for good measure compare them with the performance of people who had been given no such instructions).

Point 5 follows from Spears and Haslam's (1997) curvilinear hypothesis. Their meaning-seeking approach to cognitive load suggests that there is an inverted U-shaped relationship between cognitive load and stereotyping. Stereotyping will be greatest under conditions of moderate load. Under conditions of low load there may be no gain from treating the individual stimuli in categorical terms and under conditions of high load it may be very difficult to do the interpretive work necessary to form the categories. A categorical representation of the situation may therefore be most useful and applicable under conditions where there is a moderate load: that is, where there is both time to perceive the stimuli and time to interpret them in categorical terms.

Spears and Haslam are therefore recommending a functional approach to categorization in order to understand what the effects of cognitive load are.

In order to understand how people categorize we need to understand what they do with categories. In a context defined by only a few stimuli where there is (a) little prospect of encountering future exemplars of that category, (b) no good reason to treat subsets of stimuli as equivalent, and (c) no reason to believe that the individuating information that differentiates stimuli is irrelevant, there is little point in developing categorizations to imbue the stimuli with meaning in order to make sense of the situation. The very judgement that individuating information is relevant or irrelevant in some context is categorical and suggests a particular way of making sense of the situation. Presenting participants in an experiment with many stimuli may increase cognitive load but it may also provide cues to participants that it is inappropriate or unnecessary to remember the characteristics that differentiate between individual stimuli and that instead it is appropriate to look for the characteristics that differentiate between the groups.

Consider, for example, cognitive load in the illusory correlation paradigm (as per Spears and van Knippenberg, 1997). On the basis of previous research we could expect illusory correlation with a set of 36 stimulus statements, but we might not with four stimuli or with 400. With four stimuli there would be no information loss because the capacity of short-term memory to transfer the information to long-term memory and to retrieve that information would be close to perfect. As we know from Fiedler's (1991) work (see Chapter 8) there can be no illusory correlation effect on the standard measures without at least some information loss.

With 400 stimuli, however, the task may be so difficult that it is impossible to encode the stimulus information in the form of a stereotype. In other words, limits on encoding capacity may be reached with such a large stimulus set and consequently no stereotype is formed.

I think Spears and Haslam (1997) are on much weaker ground when they maintain that categorization *should* be no more effortful than individuation because both involve the same process of categorization. Obviously the same process could be more effortful at one time or another: memorizing an entire page or a single line from the phone book might involve the same processes but obviously the former will require more effort. These authors' general point, that the level of categorization is determined not so much by how much effort can be saved but by how the target of perception is best understood from the perspective of the perceiver, is well taken though.

At times it appears, however, that research on cognitive load may not be sufficiently well developed to sustain a useful debate about categorization. The competing views on categorization make the research priorities from the competing perspectives mutually unintelligible. Opposed views on the functions and effects of categorization mean that it is difficult to use the same terms to refer to similar concepts. This is most notable in relation to such concepts as *accuracy*, *distortion* and *veridical perception*: the meaning and nature of all of these concepts is hotly contested.

In order for work on cognitive load to repay the interest that scholars of social categorization have paid to it I believe the following two conditions need to be met:

1   Empirical investigations should not rely exclusively on measures of accuracy of judgement. Given that there is considerable controversy in the field over the status of accuracy (see next section) then measures such as reaction times are more likely to provide data that will be genuinely useful for all scholars. If we observe a person say 'X is Y' then we can debate whether 'X is really Y'. If we observe a person respond faster to stimulus X than stimulus Y then the debate about the accuracy of the response is more circumscribed. Having said that, reaction time measures are susceptible to changes in attention owing to variations in perceived meaning of the kind that I discussed above (see Spears and Haslam, 1997, for a more detailed discussion).
2   Researchers need to specify the process or sub-process under consideration before invoking the concept of capacity limits. Capacity limits will affect different processes in different ways and the implications for categorization may be multi-faceted (Gilbert and Hixon, 1991).

Although much of the research in the 1990s has been sensitive to these considerations, the second point requires further illustration. The clearest illustration of the existence of a process with a limited capacity is short-term memory. We are able to remember around seven items. Where short-term memory capacity is threatened then one obvious strategy is 'chunking', combining smaller elements into large chunks (H. A. Simon, 1974). For example, if we need to remember the 14 letters

C   A   T   D   O   T   H   E   A   T   B   O   A   T

we will do better at remembering them if we break them into syllabic chunks such as 'cat', 'dot', 'heat' and 'boat' (of course, the same advantage might not be achieved if the entities were not meaningful words which could be differentiated from other meaningful words).

Chunking, in this case, leads to conclusions quite different from those which would be expected if we believe that categorization should distract perceivers from the individual stimulus information, leading to a reduction in accuracy as they focus on the categories and not the specific stimulus information. Chunking here can be conceived of as a categorical sense-making process whereby perceivers establish that the series of stimuli can be understood in terms of some grouping scheme such as words or syllables. Remembering such higher-order elements does not prejudice the retention of the lower-order elements because rather than trying to remember the individual elements in isolation it is far easier to remember the word, the representation of which is associated with the scheme for spelling the word.

The chunks in this example are based on what could be called expectancy-congruent information (they are all based on regular English words). If the chunks involved expectancy-inconsistent information then we might expect the effects to take a different form. This, however, is consistent with the more general claim to be made here that there are many different relations between cognitive load and categorization.

Finally, the idea of a fixed capacity is itself highly questionable. As I have mentioned previously, cognitive research (e.g., Kahneman, 1973; see also Kruglanski, 1996) suggests that attentional capacity is modified by effort. That is, there is not a fixed pool of resources but a pool that varies in size depending upon how hard we are trying. The variation in capacity is interesting because it suggests that there will be different **speed–accuracy tradeoffs** between performance and effort for different situations. Unfortunately, this means that it will be very difficult to draw simple conclusions about the relations between categorization, accuracy and load. In particular relationships between performance and effort will vary for different tasks.

The implications of this point can be seen in Figure 7.1 which illustrates performance increasing with effort up to a point (point B for both curves in the figure for ease of presentation only). This is said to be *resource-limited performance* (Norman and Bobrow, 1975). Beyond point B it does not matter how much effort increases, performance will not improve because performance is limited by the quality of the stimulus data (*data-limited performance*). Data limitations can exist for very easy tasks or for very difficult tasks (for which the acceleration of the function between A and B and the level of performance before reaching the plateaus will differ). Serious attempts to study the relationship between cognitive load and categorization need to vary multiple levels of task difficulty and effort and must avoid assuming that cognitive resources such as attention are fixed.

The final way I wish to address this issue is to imagine, as a thought exper-

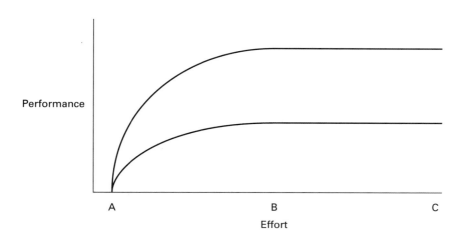

FIGURE 7.1   *Some tradeoffs between performance and effort*

iment, alien beings visiting earth with unlimited information processing capacity. Would these extraterrestrials stereotype?

What would be the implications of not stereotyping or stereotyping for the aliens? A being with unlimited capacity which did not form stereotypes would have difficulty making predictions based on relations between objects. That is, although they should be able to form predictions about one human based on prior examination of the specimen, they would have no way of deciding whether two humans would react in the same way because they would be unable to decide whether humans were *similar* in relevant ways. On the other hand, beings with unlimited capacity would presumably retain information about individuals that humans would dispense with and which might later become relevant. Unlimited processing capacity therefore could actually serve to increase the prospects for categorization by providing additional possible categorizations: it is impossible to use some feature as a basis for categorization if we have forgotten, ignored or otherwise failed to encode that feature.

When I set this question as a third-year exam in my social psychology course the answers I received tended to fall into two groups. One reflected the work of Bruner in that students argued that regardless of how much information processing capacity the aliens had they would still need to stereotype to increase the stock of knowledge. The other trend to the answers was clearly influenced by the work of Asch: these students argued that regardless of the aliens' information processing capacity, and regardless of their own social organization, the aliens would need to stereotype if they were to be successful in understanding *us* (a species with an organized social structure and collective behaviour).

A fairer answer would probably be that if the aliens were similar to humans in every other respect except their processing capacity they would show stereotyping effects on some measures and not on others. This is because the phenomenon that we call stereotyping is actually a complex array of sub-processes, some of which can be expected to be affected by capacity limitations and others which will not be (see also Chapter 11).

Our discussion of cognitive load has been punctuated by considerations of the accuracy of perception. Perhaps one way of deciding whether categorization is driven by overload is to ask whether the accuracy of perception depends upon its categorical nature. It is to this issue that we now turn.

---

speed–accuracy tradeoffs In a recognition or identification task, the decrease in accuracy that occurs as the observer attempts to perform the task faster.

B. Does categorization lead to error and biases?
versus
Do the notions of error and bias have any role to play in understanding cognition?

Again the first question is framed from the point of view of the social cognitive selective attentional model and the second question is framed from the point of view of the meaning-seeking perspective. A useful place to commence this discussion is Judd and Park's (1993) analysis of the issue of stereotype accuracy. They point out that researchers have long attempted to establish the accuracy of stereotypes by comparing the content of those stereotypes with the actual characteristics of the members of the groups in question. Judd and Park acknowledge that this enterprise has proved difficult in the past, but they suggest that improvements in methodological and theoretical sophistication mean that this long-anticipated goal for the science of social psychology may be achieved.

One way of setting out the alternative models is to detail the hypothesized relations between subjective and objective reality that are envisaged as being brought about by categorization/stereotyping.

The selective attention model normally assumes that there is an underlying objective reality to be perceived but that social perceptual processes intervene so that subjective reality is a distortion of underlying reality. For authors like Judd and Park (1993) the objective reality in relation to group judgements is provided by the individual characteristics of the people who make up those groups. Thus for Judd and Park the characteristics of the individual (as might be gleaned from a reliable and valid personality test) provide the standards of objective reality. Thus if we say that 73 per cent of Germans are efficient and in truth only 54 per cent are efficient then the discrepancy between reality and the stereotype is 19 per cent. This discrepancy implies that the stereotype is a degraded representation of reality. The mediating role that categorization plays between perception and reality is shown in Figure 7.2. Without categorization the representation closely matches reality. Categorization, however, serves a distorting role leading to a less accurate view (depicted by the lower-case letter 'r'). The constraint relations envisaged here are that category use

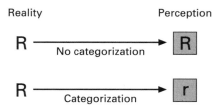

FIGURE 7.2 *The distorting effects of categorization envisaged by Judd and Park and others*

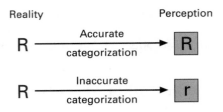

FIGURE 7.3   *The beneficial effects of accurate categorization (as per Jussim)*

produces increased equivalence which in turn results in (degraded) knowledge of reality to at least the same degree.

For Lee et al. (1993), however, stereotypes are based on objective features of social groups. Jussim (1991) has provided the clearest detailed statement of the relationship between belief and reality that is consistent with this approach. His reflection-construction model anticipates tight links between perceptions and reality because perception is based on cues which are probabilistically related to objective reality (Figure 7.3).

The relations envisaged in this model are much more complex than those encompassed by the Judd and Park (1993) approach. For Jussim (1991) there is a two-way influence of belief upon reality because beliefs potentially determine both the target's behaviour/attributes and judgements of those behaviours/attributes. In addition to this, background information determines target behaviour and social beliefs. This implies that there should be a correspondence between beliefs and perception, partly because the beliefs reflect reality, partly because beliefs modify reality (as reflected in the target's behaviour), and partly because beliefs influence the construction of that reality.

Applying this model to historical perceptions of group differences in intelligence it might be argued that blacks were perceived to be less intelligent than whites because they were expected to be less intelligent, but that these expectations could have influenced the behaviour of blacks so that they acted in line with expectations, thereby appearing to be less intelligent than they would otherwise be. The model leaves open the possibility (and I have chosen this controversial example quite deliberately to show the tricky terrain that researchers on this topic must negotiate) that there could be *real* differences in intelligence between blacks and whites. Where there were real differences (in line with the perceived differences) the stereotype would serve to enhance the accuracy of perception. Where there were no such differences the stereotype would serve to reduce the accuracy of perception. Thus, if the stereotype, or other cateogorization, is itself accurate there will be a closer match between perception and reality, otherwise there will be a distortion.

Oakes and Reynolds (1997) suggest an alternative accuracy-oriented approach to stereotyping. In this respect they follow Oakes et al. (1994) and

Oakes and Turner (1990). From this point of view, stereotyping and categorization are seen as allowing selective representation from the vantage point of the perceiver.

Their argument is that all perception is categorical and that categorization involves finding some way to represent reality from the point of view of the perceiver. Rather than being a source of distortion, categorization is actually a way in which perception can be brought into line with reality. This means taking selective slices of reality that reflect real similarities and differences and crystallize them.

Such categorization processes are necessarily selective and necessarily based on the point of view of some perceiver. As Oakes et al. (1994) ask: why would a perceiver seek to represent reality from a point of view other than their own? Perceivers may imagine the world from another's point of view but they can hardly see it from another's point of view without that point of view becoming their own (see also Turner and Onorato's, in press, critique of the utility of the concept of a *looking glass self*).

Perception is therefore held to be selective and context-dependent. Is it possible nevertheless to define the accuracy of such perceptions? The answer adopted by Oakes and her colleagues is that the perceptions are psychologically valid from the point of view of the perceiver. That is, they are perceived to be accurate from the current point of view of that perceiver, and they are meaningful, relevant and useful for the perceiver, but beyond that the accuracy of perception can only be established with respect to social validity, the degree to which some relevant ingroup shares the perception.

In this respect, Oakes et al. (1994; Oakes and Reynolds, 1997) closely follow earlier self-categorization writings (e.g., Turner, 1987) which have in turn been influenced by Moscovici (e.g., 1976). The starting point is that the correspondence between reality and experience is never itself directly given in experience. That is, although we can be sure of what we see, we can never be sure that what we see is present in reality. To overcome this deficiency we must instead rely on perceived correspondences and divergences between our own behaviour and that of relevant others. Importantly, such consensus and dissensus is informative chiefly because it is diagnostic of reality. If people with whom we expect to agree act in the same way and people with whom we expect to disagree act in another way then this provides the basis for deciding when our own perceptions are right and wrong (perceptions which will be allied to experiences of certainty and uncertainty). In this way, perceptions are brought into line with reality. Note that Oakes, Turner and colleagues adopt a materialist perspective in that they accept the existence of a physical substrate to reality, but in contrast to a long line of realist thinkers they reject the possibility that appeal to this physical substrate can serve as an arbiter in disputes over truth (except through social processes of agreement and disagreement).

Applying this idea to stereotyping, the only test that can appropriately be applied to the accuracy of a stereotype is its social validity: the extent that a relevant ingroup would agree. Thus the characteristics of individuals do not provide the standards against which the accuracy of stereotypes or group behaviour can be judged. Rather truth can only be judged in relation to group norms.

Does this mean that all stereotypes are equally valid and equally deserving of respect? Oakes et al. (1994) argue that it is possible to go beyond irreconcilable disagreements and a *laissez-faire* relativism by seeking higher-level agreements: that is, by seeking consensuses which are reflective of norms shared by all people and not just by some group.

If we accept this argument, however, we must be aware that the scope of these claims cannot be limited to stereotypes (broad as this class of beliefs is). The same claim can be developed for any statement: for example, the statement that develops from Oakes and Reynolds's (1997) view that Judd and Park's (1993) analysis is wrong. From Oakes and Reynolds's point of view Judd and Park are wrong because they violate some ingroup consensus which is diagnostic of underlying reality, but not because their views are *demonstrably* at variance with underlying reality.

That is, statements about truth are statements about reality but they cannot be resolved by appeal to arbitration by reality because (a) we do not have direct access to that reality and (b) reality tends to be complex and variable and defies attempts to establish univocal correspondence with perception.

Oakes et al. apply their analysis of stereotype accuracy to categorical perception in the Tajfel and Wilkes (1963) paradigm:

> Instead, we believe that even where the stimulus is incapable of effecting change itself (as in most judgemental studies), veridical perception will still involve accentuation (at some level of categorization).
>
> This point applies to the results of Tajfel and Wilkes (1963) where . . . subjects are typically understood to have distorted reality by, amongst other things, representing the difference between the longest of the four short lines and the shortest of the four long lines as 1.9 cm when the 'actual' difference was 0.9 cm . . . We would argue that judgements of lines made in isolation using a metric ruler are not inherently more valid, accurate or useful than judgements which reflect the category memberships of those lines. This is because the ruler itself must be understood simply as a classification device which is consensually employed to make judgements at a particular level of abstraction. As it is, subjects' responses served to reflect the fact that there were *important and meaningful* differences between the two categories of lines (A and B), a significant higher level structural property of the stimulus situation that *cannot be conveyed* by use of a ruler. (1994: 156–7, emphasis in the original)

These are challenging and, presumably, controversial ideas. Oakes et al. establish a dichotomy between judgements made in isolation (though they would accept the reasoning of Turner, 1987, and Moscovici, 1976, that the person is acting as a representative of society in accepting the ruler as an embodiment of social norms about distance) with the aid of a ruler and categorical judgements which reflect other truths.

Consider the statements 'Men are taller than women' and 'Men are more intelligent than women.' Both are statements that could reflect some stereotype but for Oakes et al. (1994) the accuracy of either statement can only be established through social validity. An attempt to establish the accuracy or inaccuracy of either statement following the logic of Judd and Park (1993) by seeking to establish the objective differences between men and women on either variable would be bound to failure. Accuracy in both cases could be established by a political act and would not be resolvable by recourse to the methods of psychological science (Oakes and Reynolds, 1997).

While the metaphysics of this argument are interesting (see Chapter 11) they do serve to obscure an important distinction. If we follow Oakes et al.'s metaphysical argument then Judd and Park are no more wrong than anyone else who attempts to make a statement about reality. In that sense Oakes et al.'s arguments may have very little to do with stereotype accuracy or the distorting effects of categorization. However, Judd and Park may be wrong in the sense that they apply inappropriate standards as a baseline for deciding what is accurate. It is on this point that Oakes et al. appear to be on much stronger ground.

It is useful to articulate the constraint relation between categorization and reality that is anticipated by Oakes et al. (1994) (Figure 7.4). This view is endorsed by Kobrynowicz and Biernat (1998) in contrast to the views implied by Bodenhausen and Macrae's (1998b) model (see Chapter 4). That is, where an appropriate categorization (e.g., one which is consistent with relevant group norms) is applied to the situation there will be a better match between reality and perception than when the categorization is inappropriate. Thus, error is present in categorization not in terms of whether the category is accurate or whether the category produces distortion but in terms of whether the appropriate categorization (the categorization that is relevant, useful and meaningful from the current point of view) is activated. Put in these terms the gap between this perspective and certain ideas drawn from social judgeability theory narrows.

I will close this section by reiterating that there is some tension in the work of Oakes et al.: they note that 'Given that groups are real, not to represent them would be inaccurate' (1994: 189). The logical status of such

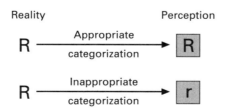

FIGURE 7.4 *The consequences of appropriate categorization on veridical perception*

inaccuracies is difficult to establish on the basis of the writings of Oakes and colleagues. If a perceiver were to fail to perceive the existence of a group, would they be making a mistake? In one sense this may be a moot point. Oakes et al. (1994: 195) claim that the available data from Haslam and Turner (1992) show no evidence of distortion. They could also point to the evidence obtained by McMullen et al. (1997) that apparent error (e.g., base-rate neglect) arises because participants have been misled by experimenters to focus on appropriate dimensions (thereby leading them to misconstrue the sample space they have been presented with). Similarly, Cheng and Novick (1990) have shown that attributional 'biases' can be understood as variations produced by the different understandings that participants and experimenters have of social psychological experiments.

More importantly, there is still some sense in which the perceiver would be engaged in a psychologically valid perception of the group members as individuals, even though that perception may fail to explain the collective action of the group being perceived. It is possible for a soldier in a war to see the enemy as individuals, but clearly it is wrong to interpret the collective action the enemy take against that perceiver as personally motivated. What this example seems to imply is that the psychological validity of categorizations depends to a large extent on what the perceiver is going to do with the categorization. Perceiving the enemy as individuals may accurately describe the perceiver's psychological orientation to the enemy and be helpful for predicting and explaining the perceiver's behaviour. However, the same categorization is far less helpful when it comes to *explaining and predicting* the enemy's behaviour. These are points which we will consider further.

C. How are previously stored categories activated?
versus
Are there such things as stored categories?

The third branch point between the selective attention models and the sense-making model relates to the question of whether categories actually have a prior existence which allows them to be activated. The resolution to this question is rather important for the knowledge activation approach: if constructs do not already exist they can hardly be activated but rather must be formed anew. The debate therefore hinges on the issue of whether categories have an enduring existence in which they slip in and out of psychological prominence, or whether they are constructed on a case-by-case basis to meet current circumstances (as would also be anticipated by the exemplar model of social judgement: Smith and Zárate, 1992).

The self-categorization theory version of the sense-making account and a variety of parallel-distributed processing accounts of categorization tend to assume that categories are constructed afresh for each processing situation. That is, there are no stored categories which can be activated to allow us to categorize in some particular setting. What is relatively stable on the other hand is a set of background knowledge about the world and 'higher-order knowledge frameworks used to give coherence to varying instances of group behaviour' (Oakes et al., 1994: 199). More generally in relation to self-categories, Turner et al. observe:

> We doubt whether the idea of self as a relatively fixed mental structure is meaningful or necessary. If self-categories are contextual definitions of the individual, how can they be stored prior to their use? How can they be stored as pre-formed givens independent of the context in which they are used? Social contexts are infinitely variable, as are our relationships to them, yet we are never at a loss for an appropriate self-definition. If a stored set of self-concepts is adjusted in some way for new contexts, then theoretically what is needed is an explanation of how the adjustment occurs, a principle of the *generation* of the concepts used, and once we have one (as in the fit hypothesis, for example), it is not clear that the notion of prior-concepts-waiting-to-be-activated plays any further useful explanatory role. (1994: 458-9)

The principles embodied here are readily generalized to categories other than self-categories and indeed Turner et al. (1994) hold that their ideas are similar to those of Barsalou (1987), who argues that categories are generated on the spot as a function of an interaction between long-term, higher-order, 'continuous' knowledge and the specific set of instances being represented.

Without some further specification of what this long-term knowledge might be, and how it can be distinguished from categories in terms of a construct other than the brevity of existence, not much progress can be expected in elaborating these points. Self-categorization theorists refer to these issues under the general heading of normative fit but efforts to differentiate normative fit from other constructs in empirically realizable terms have been relatively slow.

I must also reiterate the point I made in the previous chapter in relation to work by Brown and Turner that even if categories are constructed on the spot a great deal of long-term knowledge must be categorical in that it relates to differences between groups. Long-term knowledge must include knowledge that groups are different.

The question posed by Turner et al. (1994) as to what further explanatory role is played by a principle of adjustment of existing concepts over and above a principle of generation of concepts demands attention. Obviously categories can be generated otherwise we could not form new categories. It is also obvious that we can remember aspects of our own categorizing behaviour and we can also store knowledge which takes a categorical form. The question is whether the retrieval of these categories is the same as remembering the process of categorizing. Does remembering the use of a category on a previous occasion, for example, increase the perceiver's readiness to use a similar categorization again? Clearly, Higgins (e.g., 1996) would argue strongly for this position.

An adjustment principle would more readily explain the existence of memory for previously used categories and the effects that this memory has. For example, if 'old' categories which currently have low accessibility are activated/generated more rapidly or more easily than 'new' categories with similar accessibility then this would suggest that there is something to be explained by the adjustment principle. Some development of a generation principle such as the fit hypothesis would need to occur before it could explain such a memory advantage.

The question can be addressed in part by examining evidence of priming effects in social categorization. In two experiments Stangor et al. (1992) failed to obtain categorization effects of priming. That is, when participants were given two overlapping categorizations (sex and race) of a set of stimulus individuals they were no more likely to use the one that was primed than the one that was not. Stangor et al. (1992) argue though that sex and race are such chronically accessible categories that it may be difficult to increase their accessibility through short-term contextual manipulations such as priming.

In order to address this problem van Twuyer and van Knippenberg (1995) used other overlapping categorizations (university major and university town) which they believed to be less chronically accessible (and on which they found weaker categorization effects than on sex). They found that priming one or the other led to a greater use of that categorization (as shown by an increase in the relative number of confusions of members of the same category). From van Twuyer and van Knippenberg's results it appears that there is evidence of priming effects for social categorizations. This certainly suggests the possibility of an explanatory role for an activation-based approach or adjustment principle and demands an account in self-categorization theory terms. Subsequently there have been many other studies demonstrating the priming of social categories, some of which were considered in Chapter 4.

The adjustment/activation principle also avoids a difficulty that occurs in the self-categorization theory discussion of perceiver readiness. It is easier in logical terms to discuss the 'accessibility of' or 'readiness to use' something which already exists than something that is yet to be formed. This problem was not present in earlier versions of SCT:

> An individual who defines him- or herself as an 'Australian', for example, may never think about nationality for days at a time, yet if that self-definition did not exist as a latent identity, it could hardly become salient in relevant settings. (Turner et al., 1987: 54)

Turner et al. also refer to group formation occurring on the basis of the '*internalization* of some *preformed*, culturally available classification such as in terms of sex, nationality, class, occupation, religion, or race' (1987: 51, emphasis in the original). This is a clear acknowledgement of the need for enduring constructs which are categorical and relational in nature.

Even from this short discussion it is apparent that an appropriate conclusion for this section is that although there are problems in establishing how pre-existing concepts are activated or adjusted there are also non-trivial obstacles in the path of the spontaneous generation principle. The obvious response from a revised self-categorization theory standpoint is to argue that priming social categories really involves priming knowledge about such categories rather than the categories themselves. This would appear to be consistent with the results of Smith et al. (1996) who show that priming attitudes which are relevant to a categorization leads to increased activation of that categorization. Generally though, the empirical challenge for the field is to show whether priming a category and priming knowledge which increases perceivers' readiness to use a category exist as distinct and separable phenomena. Given that it seems difficult to avoid the conclusion that long-term knowledge is itself categorical, then this would seem to be a very onerous task.

Conclusion: the relativity of perception

To summarize the key points from this chapter:

1   Limits on capacity have been underexplored, and where they have been explored the process which is involved has rarely been specified in sufficient detail for the relations between capacity and performance to be understood.
2   There is no straightforward reason to assume that capacity limitations create the conditions for categorization.
3   Even if all forms of information processing were unlimited in capacity, categorization could still be expected.
4   Three different models of the relationship between perception and reality anticipate that categorization can serve to improve or debilitate the quality of representation. One class of model (Judd and Park, 1993) argues that categorization distorts reality. A second model (Jussim, 1991) holds that categorization can increase or decrease the match between perception and reality. A third class of model derived from SCT holds that appropriately categorizing always serves to increase the match between perception and reality.
5   Categorization can be understood in terms of a principle of activation of stored knowledge or of a principle of generation of spontaneous categories. The key advantage of the latter approach is that it is not necessary to assume the existence of an infinite number of prior categorizations stored to suit every possible context. An apparent advantage of the activation approach is in accounting for memory and priming effects. We thus need to know whether remembering a category is, or can be, the same as reusing that category.

The arguments in this chapter establish some vantage points for considering the consequences of relative perception for categorization. I think that they clearly illustrate that there are sharply divergent approaches to social categorization. As I have implied throughout this chapter there is still considerable work to be done in answering these questions. I will provide my own preferred answers in the final chapter, but before we get there I wish to look at some more specific developments in the study of social categorization.

PART II

SOME EXPLORATIONS IN SOCIAL CATEGORIZATION

8 Group Variability and Consistency

Whereas Part I was a wide-ranging coverage of the field of categorization, this chapter and the next two have a more modest aim. I propose to address a series of scientific problems in the social categorization literature and suggest some steps towards solutions. The selection of the topics is driven by my own interests, certainly, but also by my judgement that these are the areas which are ripe for advances. Having said that, the ideas addressed are generally more complex than those in Part I.

In this chapter I look at an interrelated set of issues to do with perceptions of the coherence of social groups. By coherence I am referring to both the variability of social groups and the 'groupiness' of those groups. Obviously the tradition of research on differentiation between social groups is important here. Recently, however, there has been renewed interest in the entitativity of social groups (see Chapter 5). Entitativity is the degree to which the group is seen as a real *entity* or thing. Much of the interest in entitativity stems from the work of Campbell (1958) and the suggestion of Rothbart and Taylor (1992) that Medin's (1989) idea of *psychological essentialism* applies strongly to social categories.

I suggest that entitativity and another principle which I will term *diagnosticity* enable us to see links between a number of phenomena that are often treated separately. The search for this commonality is the core of this chapter. I believe that judgements of groups are powerfully constrained by attempts to understand their nature and to use that derived knowledge to understand aspects of society including the behaviour of those groups. Having said that, I am certainly not trying to account for everything associated with the vast literature on each of these topics: each individual phenomenon can be expected to be controlled by a host of moderating variables. My goal here is thus to show that the phenomena are part of the same forest and not to map the individual trees.

To do this I start with the idea that categorizations are explanations. I assume that when people make judgements of themselves and others in categorical terms they are attempting to explain the relations between persons and groups and/or between groups. The perceiver's ability to articulate an explanation rests upon their ability to understand the phenomenon. Thus, factors which impede understanding should affect the nature and scope of the explanation. In this chapter I discuss the importance of these precursors to explanation in terms of the principle of *diagnosticity*. My central claim is that the relative perception of groups and individuals rests on the ability of the perceiver to draw a clear impression of those groups, and that key phenomena in group perception rest on the relative diagnosticity of those targets.

A. Group variability judgements

Many of the central ideas in the application of the categorization process to group variability judgements have already been discussed in previous chapters so I will only reiterate these ideas briefly here. The central finding in research on group variability judgements has been the evidence for the outgroup homogeneity effect. That is, people have often been found to judge greater similarity between members of outgroups than ingroups. These effects have been found on a wide variety of measures (for reviews and/or meta-analyses see Haslam et al., 1996c; Mullen and Hu, 1989; Ostrom and Sedikides, 1992).

For example, Quattrone and Jones (1980) found Princeton University students predicted that more people at Rutgers University would have the same musical preference than Princeton students. Thus, 55 per cent of Princeton students were predicted to choose to listen to rock music compared with 75 per cent of Rutgers students.

Linville et al. (1989) discuss how the effect can be demonstrated on two key variables. The first is perceived variability which relates closely to conventional measures of dispersion such as range and variance. The second is attribute differentiation. Linville et al. (1989) recommend measuring this in terms of the construct probability for differentiation (P_d). This construct is the probability of distinguishing between two group members in terms of a given dimension. It is given by:

$$P_d = 1 - \sum_{i=1}^{m} p_i^2$$

where p_i is the subjectively perceived proportion of members of a group who share a feature or the level of the attribute in question.

Although perceived variability and probability of differentiation are correlated they are not identical. P_d is maximized by a flat rectangular distribution whereas variability is maximized by a bimodal distribution where all members are maximally distant from the mean (variability corresponds to the sum of squares of differences between scores and the mean).

Park and Judd (1990) suggest that the general distinction to be made amongst measures in this area is between measures of dispersion and measures of stereotypicality. A group can be seen to be homogeneous if all of its members are similar on some dimension (low dispersion) or if the members tend to adopt a few positions or to share the same characteristic (high stereotypicality).

The conventional effect has been explained in terms of processes which relate closely to models of the categorization process which were current in the 1980s. Linville et al. (1986; 1989) argued that the outgroup homogeneity effect could be explained in terms of an exemplar model based on differential familiarity for members of the two groups.

There are two ways in which this exemplar-based model predicts greater homogeneity from increased familiarity. The first and explicit argument is that varying homogeneity is due to biased statistics that are used to compute sample variability. The other implicit implication rests on the varying sizes of the population of exemplars stored for familiar and unfamiliar groups.

Linville and Fischer (1998: 128) make the misleading assertion that the model's prediction of outgroup homogeneity rests on statistical principles which guarantee that the larger the size of a random sample the larger the variability of the sample. Statistical principles guarantee instead that both large and small random samples from a population will be estimates of the same population variance. All that larger sample size guarantees is that the error involved in estimating this population variance will be smaller. However, the sample variance is a biased estimate of the population variance and the size of this bias is relatively larger for small sample sizes than large sample sizes (the bias is corrected by changing the divisor from N to N-1). For large sample sizes like 100, the choice of divisor makes very little difference; for small sample sizes like five, the divisor makes a big difference to the size of the variance.

Linville et al.'s PDIST formulation rests on the assumption that estimates of variance computed from memory are biased in the same way that sample variance is a biased estimate when the N divisor is used. That is, the mind is like a scientific calculator in statistical mode. However, it uses the N button and not the N-1 button for computing variability. These points were made clearly by Linville et al. (1989) but they cannot be ignored without misrepresenting the true situation. Park et al. (1991) argue that the equation of number of exemplars with familiarity is problematic because the statistics used to measure attribute differentiation and perceived variability are biased (see above). This is problematic for small sample sizes because the predicted relationship between heterogeneity and familiarity could be an artefact of this bias.

The validation of Linville et al.'s idea rests on demonstrating that estimates of perceived group variability show the same form of sample size bias as PDIST. The PDIST formulation should predict not only an outgroup homogeneity effect but relatively more homogeneity for small ingroups and for large outgroups. Simon and Brown (1987), however, found no difference in perceived homogeneity between a majority and a minority when participants were not members of either group.

The simple exemplar model above is a simplification of Linville et al.'s (1989) views. They actually (1989: 177) anticipated a mixed model which allows exemplars to be both instances and abstractions about the category (or sub-groups of the category). In practice, though, the principles for generalization and forming abstractions are given very little consideration in their discussion of the PDIST model.

The second (implicit) implication of the model is that perceptions of variability should be affected by bias owing to the varying size of the population of exemplars stored in the mind about different groups. Thus the model implies that for ingroups there will be many exemplars stored in memory and for the outgroup there will only be a few exemplars. This means that there is a lower probability that any two exemplars retrieved from memory will be different for an outgroup sample than for an ingroup sample. If perceived similarity is computed from a process of retrieving exemplars from memory then this similarity will be greater for outgroups than for ingroups.

An analogy can be made to sampling (with replacement) marbles from a bag of 100 marbles (the ingroup) and a bag of five marbles (the outgroup). The probability of drawing the same marble twice in the small bag is much greater with the smaller bag than the larger bag: thus the average similarity of marbles drawn from the small bag would be greater than the average similarity of marbles drawn from the large bag. Familiarity under this view depends on the number of exemplars encountered that belong to the category. The more exemplars encountered, the richer and more differentiated will be the view of the groups.

Thus, outgroup homogeneity might rest on what could be termed 'spurious sameness': similar recollections are spuriously similar if they are actually recollections of the same person (sampled with replacement). Similarity is not spurious if two recollections of two different persons are the same. Note that this bias is due to the small size of the populations sampled relative to the sample size under conditions of sampling with replacement, rather than being due to the small sample size *per se*.

Linville et al. (1989) obtained an outgroup homogeneity effect in perceptions of young and old people and different nationalities (Irish and Americans) but not different sexes (who have roughly equivalent levels of contact). However, other studies (Judd and Park, 1988) have found asymmetries in men's and women's perceptions of group homogeneity. Lorenzi-Cioldi (1993; Lorenzi-Cioldi et al., 1995) has found that the outgroup homogeneity effect is more common for males perceiving females than for females perceiving males. The differential effects were explained in terms of the differing status and power of men and women.

Following similar work by Wilder (1984) and Simon and Brown (1987), research by Judd and Park (1988) found the outgroup homogeneity effect in minimal group studies. Obviously there can be no prior contact or greater familiarity with members of minimal groups. Linville et al. (1989) therefore argue that differential familiarity was sufficient but not necessary for the out-group homogeneity effect and that plausible alternatives included differential motivation to process ingroup and outgroup exemplars and differing representations of ingroups and outgroups. Subsequently, Oakes et al. (1995) found in a field study that perceived homogeneity of an ingroup on group-defining dimensions increased with familiarity while Lord et al. (1991) found more knowledgeable members were *more* likely to display a typicality effect, that is, they tended to treat different members of the same group in the same way.

The arguments of Goldstone (1998) in relation to the role of familiarity in perceptual learning are intriguing. Caucasian participants in the United States are generally better able to identify Caucasian than African-American faces, but people in general are faster at categorizing faces that are difficult to identify. However, research by O'Toole et al. cited by Goldstone suggests that people are better able to apply a male–female categorization to members of their own race. This evidence would seem to suggest that familiarity with a perceptual category enables people to learn important features for distinguishing between that category and other categories and for differentiating between members of that category. This would seem to imply that familiarity increases intergroup and intragroup distinctions implying that there should be no main effect for familiarity. This is what the available data appear to show.

Other exemplar-based approaches have been proposed by Kashima and Kashima (1993) and by Smith and Zárate (1992). The latter's exemplar account differs from that of Linville et al. (1989) in some ways (and is based on a modification of Nosofsky's, 1984, 1986, generalized context model) in that it depends not so much on the number of exemplars encountered but on the number of dimensions that are attended to for the purposes of differentiating between stimuli (a point similar to the initial insight of Linville and Jones, 1980). The exemplar theory of social judgement holds that both ingroups and outgroups have an exemplar-based representation but that the exemplars of the outgroup appear more similar to each other because they have fewer attributes to be used as a basis for differentiation between them. Let us again conceive of the store of exemplars as a set of marbles in a bag, but this time they differ in size as well as colour. The perceived differences between the marbles will be greater if we attend to differences on both dimensions as opposed to just one dimension. That is, two red marbles of differing size can be seen to be very similar if we are only interested in colour; they will be less similar if we take into account size as well. If people pay more attention to the individuating attributes of the self and fellow ingroup members then they will perceive ingroups to be more variable than outgroups.

A later development on the Linville et al. exemplar model is the perceived covariation model of Linville et al. (1996). This model suggests that mental representations of groups require knowledge of covariations of features. They suggest therefore that impressions of groups can be based on overestimations and underestimations of the covariation between attributes of the groups. In particular, Linville and Fischer (1998) argue that perceived covariation between attributes should be greater for outgroups than ingroups because of the greater familiarity perceivers have with ingroups. They cite three reasons for this effect:

1   Illusory correlation research shows that people can perceive a correlation even when one is not present.
2   High covariation under conditions of low familiarity is consistent with sampling theory in that the sample covariation should be a biased (over-) estimate of the population covariation.
3   Covariation under conditions of low familiarity should be based on knowledge of second-hand exemplars learned from other people rather than direct experience. These second-hand exemplars should be strongly stereotypic.

The shift in interest to covariation is interesting because, as Linville and Fischer note, covariation has also been implicated in analyses of causal attribution – the process by which reasoners develop explanations for behaviour and other events (see e.g., Hewstone, 1989; Kelley, 1967). Given the existence of repeated claims in the literature about links between categorization and explanation (sense making) this would appear to be a promising emphasis (see also Chapter 10).

However, these authors repeat some previous imprecisions. Linville and Fischer fail to acknowledge that aligning their theory with sampling theory rests upon the assumption that the process of information aggregation used by perceivers is biased in the same way as certain sample statistics are biased (ignoring the criticism of Park et al., 1991). The value of the claim that the model is consistent with sampling theory is therefore highly questionable.

The other surprising omission from the model is a consideration of the constraining effect of background knowledge (other than in the form of familiarity with exemplars) on perceived correlation. As we saw in Chapter 3 a major emphasis in the cognitive literature on categorization in the last 15 years has been to show that background knowledge serves to constrain covariation (using processes of structural alignment, e.g., Gentner, 1983, or other mechanisms). While Linville et al. (1996) may have found evidence of differences in covariation, the experience in the cognitive literature indicates that a featural-similarity-based approach is unlikely to be able to explain why it is that some features come to be correlated and others are not. Put simply, Linville and Fischer's account suggests that all unfamiliar categories will be subject to an overestimation of covariation effect on all dimensions. It seems more plausible, however, that the overestimation would be stronger on relevant dimensions (see the next section).

As an alternative to the exemplar models, Judd and Park (1988; Park and Judd, 1990; Park et al., 1991; but originally Park and Rothbart, 1982) proposed a dual-process model. Under this model group representations are based on both (a) individual-level knowledge (i.e., knowledge about specific group members, exemplars) and (b) group-level knowledge including group-level knowledge about central tendency and perceived variability in the group.

The outgroup homogeneity effect arises because, in the case of representations of the ingroup, group-level knowledge was likely to be supplemented by a great deal of individual-level knowledge, but for outgroup members there would be little supplementary information and perceivers would be forced to rely on abstraction-level information. In either case estimates of perceived variability and central tendency are formed spontaneously on-line as instances of categories are encountered and these estimates are stored in memory.

This situation is analogous to trying to draw a conclusion about the contents of bags of marbles about which you already have some general information (like 40 per cent of the marbles are red) and varying amounts of specific information about individual marbles in each bag. The general information should be more important where we have limited information about individuals. There is more reason to rely on the abstraction-level information and less reason to reject this information in favour of the individuating information where perceivers have a great deal of information. In particular, groups with which we are familiar, or are motivated to pay attention to, will have abstraction-based representations. Interestingly, this implies that abstraction-based information is presumed to be used more for groups which we have less information about. This would seem to be inconsistent with the idea that abstraction-level information is used as a short-cut or summary for an overload of exemplar-level information.

Evidence consistent with this approach shows that people can identify more ingroup sub-groups and that, when they do identify these sub-groups, group homogeneity is reduced (Park et al., 1991). This knowledge of sub-groups is an example of more specific information that can be used instead of abstract information. Kraus et al. (1993) showed that more sub-groups were spontaneously generated when judging an ingroup than an outgroup. They interpreted their findings as support for a model in which groups are represented by frequency distributions with fewer categories for outgroups than ingroups.

A rather different note was sounded in work by Simon and Brown (1987) which showed that members of minorities (minimal or real) are likely to see their group as more homogeneous than relevant outgroups. This was explained in terms of an effort by minority members to deal with their numerical inferiority by perceiving more ingroup homogeneity than outgroup homogeneity. Indeed Simon (1992) argues that all ingroups perceive themselves to be more homogeneous than outgroups on group-defining dimensions. In this vein, Kelly (1989) has found that members of political parties perceived more homogeneity within ingroup than outgroup political attitudes. This finding in particular is consistent with the rallying call that 'United we stand, divided we fall.' That is, there are occasionally good reasons to value and expect more consistency within an ingroup than an outgroup. An orchestra, for example, would pride itself on its discipline and responsiveness to the conductor and not on the capriciousness of individual members.

This work (and some supporting data by Doosje et al., 1998) underscores the importance of *valence* (evaluative positivity or negativity) in group variability judgements. Group members tend to perceive outgroup members to be more similar to each other because they share characteristics which are stereotypical of the outgroup. Not coincidentally those characteristics are often ones which are viewed negatively by the ingroup (and sometimes by both groups). Indeed perceiving outgroup members to share stereotypically unfavourable characteristics and ingroup members to share stereotypically favourable characteristics is a very direct way in which the evaluative processes of differentiation that are anticipated by social identity and self-categorization theories can apply.

Simon's (1993) model of egocentric social categorization (ESC) maintains that the cognitive construal of ingroups and outgroups is different owing to the presence of the self as a member of the ingroup. The distinction between 'me' and 'not-me' is blurred for ingroups because at some times ingroup members are considered to be interchangeable or identical with self and at other times ingroup members are considered to be distinct from self. On the other hand, the distinction between 'me' and 'not-me' facilitates the distinction between ingroups and outgroups, but more importantly, it does not facilitate or create distinctions within outgroups. Thus, the special role of the self in categorization creates or augments differentiations within ingroups, but because the personal self is not a part of outgroups, it does not provide a basis for differentiation between outgroup members.

By highlighting the special role of the personal self in social categorization, Simon has made an important contribution which is extended in a series of more recent publications (Simon, 1997; Simon et al., 1995; 1997). The particular importance of this contribution is that it suggests the categorization process works in different ways for social categories because of the role of the self as category member.

Self-categorization theory was applied to the outgroup homogeneity effect by Haslam et al. (1995b; 1996c; see Chapter 5 in this volume). SCT proposes that under conditions of high social category salience both ingroups and outgroups should be perceived to be homogeneous. However, contextual changes can lead to variations in salience so that ingroups and outgroups are actually being perceived in different circumstances. This leads to asymmetries in the perception of ingroups and outgroups.

As discussed in Chapter 5, when a person makes a comparison between themselves and other members of an ingroup it is an intragroup encounter. The differentiation is between 'I am like this' and 'You, he or she is like that.' On the other hand, when making a comparison between self and members of an outgroup it is an intergroup encounter that involves differentiations of the form 'We are like this' and 'They are like that.' Thus the outgroup homogeneity effect arises because of different categorical realities – namely the fact that in experiments outgroups are typically judged in an intergroup context and ingroups are typically judged in an intragroup context. In responding to these different contexts participants attend to intragroup differences when judging the ingroup (and thereby perceive heterogeneity) and attend to intergroup differences when judging outgroups (and thereby perceive homogeneity). The differing levels of homogeneity therefore reflect different selective perceptions in the different contexts.

The SCT analysis of outgroup homogeneity was tested by Haslam et al. (1995b; 1996c). Haslam et al. (1995b, experiment 1) found that when Australians were judged alone, ingroup stereotypic traits were seen to apply to 57 per cent of that ingroup. When Americans were judged alone, outgroup stereotypic traits were applied to 75 per cent of that outgroup (i.e., evidence of an outgroup homogeneity effect). However, if Australians were judged at the same time as Americans, Australian stereotypic traits were seen to apply to 74 per cent of Australians and American stereotypic traits were seen to apply to 74 per cent of Americans. Clearly, the outgroup homogeneity effect had been eliminated.

The implications of the SCT account for the representation and processing of group variability are extensive. There is no need to posit a special form of representation for ingroups as opposed to outgroups. This means that the relative merits of exemplar and prototype representations (a distinction that has declined in importance in cognitive approaches to categorization) is not important. Indeed Haslam et al. (1995a) argue that there is no sense in which individual exemplars have a fixed and invariant weight in determining category representation. There is no need to posit differential encoding or retrieval of prior experiences about ingroups and outgroups. This means that the theory accounts for homogeneity effects in minimal groups with which the perceiver has no prior experience. Although no specific exemplar traces need be encountered, the idea that outgroup homogeneity depends upon the dimensions selected for comparison (as per Smith and Zárate, 1992) remains critically important. Finally, there is no need to posit a special psychological role for the personal self to explain outgroup homogeneity.

Thus, outgroup homogeneity derives from a motivated effort on the part of the perceiver to make sense of reality by focusing on dimensions which are currently relevant. Under different conditions, features which stress the cohesion or the lack thereof within social groups will determine the perceived variability of the group.

To understand these pressures it is useful to return to the concept of valence. The broad conditions are mapped out in Table 8.1 (which captures the spirit of views of authors such as Haslam et al., 1995b, 1996c, and Spears and Manstead, 1990). The table is an attempt to clarify answers to the question: when will outgroup homogeneity or ingroup homogeneity occur owing to the accentuation of the perceived prevalence of some characteristic? I have cast the hypotheses in the form of perceived prevalence on the assumption that estimated prevalence of some characteristic reflects the way in which judges communicate the relative stereotypicality of some characteristic where judgements are not heavily constrained by other knowledge of the prevalence of the characteristic. Where some characteristic was known to be stereotypical but rare (e.g., winning the Nobel Prize might be seen as a representative characteristic of a university but the number of winners might be known to be a small integer), the accentuation effects would instead take the form of accentuating the representativeness or strength of ingroup characteristics. That is, where variation is constrained by knowledge on one dimension, other dimensions will be chosen for the comparison.

The answers given in the table invariably take the form: it depends on the valence of the characteristic in the perceiver's group. That is, homogeneity involves a stereotypicality × valence interaction. The comparisons assume that a comparative context is established by having people make judgements of both ingroup and outgroup on some dimension. In this way the meaning and desirability of some characteristic become relatively fixed when compared with the full range of possibilities. For a white racist sunbather, darker skin tone might be a desirable characteristic in an intraracial context but an undesirable one in an interracial context. A characteristic can be seen to be stereotypical of one group (A), of the other group (B), or of neither group. A characteristic can also be seen to be desirable or undesirable by one or both groups. I assume that there is consensus across both groups on the stereotypicality of the characteristic, but obviously this need not be the case.

TABLE 8.1   *Group homogeneity and perceived prevalence*

Characteristic	Stereotypical of	Evaluation by group		Perceived prevalence	
		A	B	Perceiver A	Perceiver B
I	Group A	+	−	A >> B	A >> B
II	Group B	−	+	A << B	A << B
III	Group A	+	+	A >> B	A > B
IV	Group B	+	+	A < B	A << B
V	Group A	−	−	A > B	A >> B
VI	Group B	−	−	A << B	A < B
VII	Neither	+	+	A > B	A < B
VIII	Neither	−	−	A < B	A > B
IX	Neither	+	−	A > B	A > B
X	Neither	−	+	A < B	A > B

Evaluation by = viewed positively or negatively by the group.
A < B = characteristic perceived to be less prevalent in group A than in group B.
A << B = characteristic perceived to be much less prevalent in group A than in group B.

As an example consider the first line in Table 8.1. Characteristic I is stereotypical of group A and is perceived favourably by group A and unfavourably by group B. Both groups are expected to accentuate the perceived prevalence of characteristic I in group A relative to group B. If we measured only group A's judgements of both groups our results would appear to show ingroup homogeneity, and if we measured only group B's judgements of both groups our results would appear to show outgroup homogeneity.

The outcomes in the table reflect the prevalence of the perceived characteristic by members of one group relative to its perceived prevalence in the other group. No statement can be made about absolute prevalence as stereotypical characteristics of a group can have a low absolute but high relative prevalence. These comparisons are not intended to be meaningful across characteristics and they assume that both ingroup and outgroup are judged in an intergroup context.

There are several interesting features of this table. For example, intergroup agreement is expected under some conditions. Where one group sees a characteristic as desirable and the other group sees it as undesirable this conflicting view of reality can give rise to disagreement or to agreement. This might occur where an adolescent gang saw law-breaking as a virtue, a view which might be contested by another group in society, but both groups might agree that law-breaking was prevalent in the gang. Note that this table assumes that the processes of group variability judgement and social projection (see third section) are strongly related. Ryan and Judd (1992) argue, and de la Haye (1998) demonstrates, that self-ascription of characteristics is an important variable in its own right and that false consensus produces predictions that conflict with the outgroup homogeneity effect under some circumstances.

What the table does not show, however, is that the valence × stereotypicality interaction is not a sufficient principle to account for group homogeneity in general. This is because no predictions emerge for neutral non-group-defining traits (i.e., perceived neither positively nor negatively). Returning to the study by Quattrone and Jones (1980), why should greater outgroup homogeneity be seen amongst Princeton students on an ostensibly neutral trait such as 'likes rock music'? However, homogeneity on neutral traits might itself be seen as a negative outgroup characteristic. More parsimoniously though, the self-categorization theory account suggests that the different comparative contexts invoked by a two-group comparison and a single-group comparison produce relative outgroup homogeneity because the two-group case enables differentiation between groups (the caveat being that judging a single outgroup is an implicit two-group judgement).

The predictions in Table 8.1 can be put into constraint relations terms in the following manner. Relative group homogeneity is constrained by the process of comparing the ingroup favourably with the outgroup. Knowledge which achieves those favourable comparisons is activated and interpreted to constrain the perceived equivalence of ingroup members, outgroup members and the ingroup and outgroup in a variety of ways. Note that in the constraint diagrams in Figure 8.1 the definition of positive and negative dimensions is from the point of view of the perceiver in the comparative context provided by the task of judging two different groups. Note also that in Chapter 10, the same ideas are presented in terms of the support theory (Tversky and Koehler, 1994) concept of categorical unpacking.

Imagine a group of Australian students judging Australians and

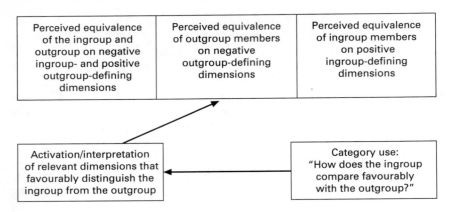

FIGURE 8.1   *The constraint relations involved in relative group homogeneity effects*

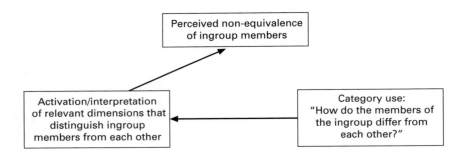

FIGURE 8.2   *Constraint relations involved in intragroup differentiation*

Americans (as per Haslam et al., 1995b). They are expected to seek to distinguish between Australians and Americans on dimensions where the end which they perceive to be positive is stereotypical of Australians and dimensions where the end which they perceive to be negative is stereotypical of Americans. They are also expected to de-emphasize dimensions on which the groups do not differ. The overall effect is for the groups to be seen to be different from each other. This pattern is fully consistent with Goldstone's (1998) arguments in relation to category effects in perceptual learning (see above).

Under conditions where only an ingroup comparison is invoked by the comparative context a simpler set of relations hold as discussed in Chapter 5. Under such circumstances only dimensions which allow perceivers to distinguish between ingroup members are activated and relative heterogeneity should be obtained (Figure 8.2).

In summary, contextually variable judgements of relative homogeneity are obtained because the task and the perceiver's orientation make different categorizations salient and activate different types of knowledge and expectations and create different interpretations of the same information. The general principle here is that variations in group homogeneity judgements arise from motivated attempts to interpret the relations between persons in terms of their group memberships. This is a reasonably comprehensive account of relative group homogeneity judgements under conditions of at least moderate social category salience. Moderating principles derived from other perspectives can be readily incorporated into this approach (e.g., Smith and Zárate's, 1992, unbiased exemplar formulation). I would anticipate that the effects of these moderating variables would be weakest under conditions of high salience. However, the ability of perceivers to gain a clear impression of groups can be moderated by the quality and quantity of the information that the perceiver has to work with. The *diagnosticity* of the stimulus information qualifies the picture obtained here for some other judgement phenomena that I discuss next. That is, under some circumstances the ease with which the stimulus information can be used to form a clear impression of one or another of two groups can vary. This is most obvious in relation to the illusory correlation effect.

B. Illusory correlation

The illusory correlation effect has attracted considerable interest from students of social categorization owing to the possibility that the formation of social stereotypes could be explained by the biased encoding of stimulus information. The robustness of the effects in laboratory explanations suggested the provocative possibility that a cognitive account which did not rely on the role of the social context or concepts such as shared social norms or even ingroups and outgroups could provide a satisfactory explanation of stereotype formation.

The initial distinctiveness-based explanation posited that novel or infrequent behaviours by novel or infrequent people (minority group members) were doubly distinctive and were likely to be overrepresented in memory and would therefore dominate impressions.

In addition to Hamilton and Gifford's (1976) distinctiveness-based explanation a range of other explanations based on the stimulus information have been proposed. These include the extended distinctiveness-based explanation of McConnell et al. (1994) which was discussed in Chapter 4 and the memory-based explanations of Fiedler (1991) and Smith (1991).

Fiedler's and Smith's explanations invoke different principles but Fiedler (1996) has argued that they explain the illusory correlation effect in the same way. Smith's account follows from Hintzman's MINERVA2 multiple-trace exemplar model. Smith posits that the judgement is computed by an aggregation of information. This judgement is sensitive to the difference in positive and negative items rather than the proportion of positive and negative items.

Empirical support for their models was provided by Fiedler et al. (1993) who showed that the effect was associated with impaired memory rather than enhanced memory for distinctive stimuli.

The aggregation principle is a powerful idea that makes good statistical sense. To illustrate, imagine some social psychologists are interested in establishing the prevalence of some phenomenon and conduct two surveys: study 1 with 12 participants and study 2 with 24 participants (perhaps run after a suggestion by an journal editor to replicate the phenomenon with a larger sample). Eight participants show the effect in study 1. Sixteen participants show the effect in study 2. From a statistical point of view there are two readily apparent truths. Based on the law of large numbers we should be more confident of the effect in study 2 than study 1, but we have no reason to believe that the effect is stronger or more prevalent in study 2 than study 1.

The relevance for the illusory correlation effect is when these two ideas become conflated. Imagine that we ask the researchers to summarize what they found. Their summary might very well take the form that 'Study 1 was ambiguous, however, study 2 showed clear evidence of the effect.' This statement is perfectly analogous to saying 'Group B is neither clearly positive nor negative, and group A has a clear majority of positive behaviours.'

Thus the illusory correlation effect can be seen as analogous to the issue of researchers equating effect size with statistical significance. The problem becomes apparent in the illusory correlation paradigm because of the relation between judgements of group A and group B. Developing a more favourable impression of group A than group B is much like saying that study 1 shows the effect and study 2 does not.

For Fiedler (1991; 1996) the statistical basis of this argument emerges from the principle of information loss. Owing to random processes of forgetting and poor retrieval, information is lost about both large and small groups. In statistical terms the 'sample' here is that subset which is retained in memory from the total stimulus set (population). The effect of this information loss is disproportionately larger for the small group which will tend to be more different from the overall positive impression provided by the stimulus data.

Thus the larger group will provide a relatively stronger impression of positivity than the small group. There is a major problem with this analysis though. As with all of the applications of Fiedler's (1996) BIAS model, the way in which large samples differ from small samples is that the larger sample is a closer approximation to the representation of some prevailing tendency in the stimulus data. Thus here the 'general' tendency reflected in both groups is that a majority of behaviours are positive (the model works equally well for a majority of negative behaviours) and the aggregation of a large number of pieces of information is more likely to provide a close approximation than an aggregation of a small number of pieces of information. This occurs for exactly the same reason (the law of large numbers) that, other things being equal, a large sample will be a better estimate of some characteristic than a small sample (readers may wish to consult a treatment of the law of large numbers, e.g., Haslam and McGarty, 1998: Chapter 7).

The implications of this postulate are (a) tentatively, that the strength of the illusory correlation effect should increase with the square root of the number of statements; (b) more certainly that the actual level of relative positivity within the distributions provides a ceiling on the effect, and (c) that the presence of two or more groups in the comparative context is not essential for the phenomenon to occur.

The first two points await empirical investigation. The last point, however, is particularly important.

The aggregation principle implies that if participants were exposed to a sample of positive and negative behaviours about a large group in isolation they should form a more positive impression of that group than of a small group. This is because the aggregation principles suggest that perceivers develop independent judgements of group A and group B and the difference in these judgements depends solely on size.

Thus if we were to give different groups of participants just the group A stimuli or just the group B stimuli we should obtain a more positive impression of group A than group B. In other words, the illusory correlation effect should be equally strong for a within-subjects paradigm where participants judge both group A and group B as for a between-subjects paradigm where participants judge either group A or group B.

Some supportive evidence for this idea was provided by Berndsen (1997: studies 3.2 and 3.3) who found that the illusory correlation effect occurred in what she termed 'group-constrained' conditions where participants were only provided with statements about group A (the majority). However, Berndsen's participants were told to judge both group A and group B (the minority) and were told that there was more information about group A. In other words, there was an explicit intergroup contrast. In research currently in progress I have found so far that presenting group A or group B alone without contrastive information produces no differences. This would suggest that the aggregation principle on its own is an unsatisfactory explanation of the illusory correlation effect.

The idea that a comparative context which involves differentiating between social groups may be critical for the phenomenon provides the starting point for the analysis of illusory correlation (IC) that originated at ANU and has been developed by researchers at Amsterdam and Louvain-la-Neuve (Berndsen et al., 1996; 1998; Haslam et al., 1996a; McGarty et al., 1993a; Yzerbyt et al., 1998a). The approach is also very similar to that developed independently by Anne-Marie de la Haye and colleagues. The core of the idea is that although stimulus conditions such as distinctiveness and information loss can contribute to the illusory correlation effect, these phenomena do not lead to stereotype formation. Rather stereotypes result from expectancies of differences between groups.

Thus illusory correlation is a multiply-determined phenomenon, but some of these determining processes are also the processes that produce stereotypes. That is, stereotypes form because people expect differences between groups, and also illusory correlations are perceived because people expect

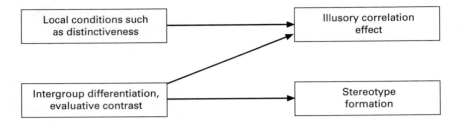

FIGURE 8.3 *Determinants of illusory correlation and stereotype formation according to McGarty and de la Haye*

differences between groups, but stereotypes do not form because people perceive illusory correlations. Schematically, the argument developed by McGarty and de la Haye (1995; 1997) looks like that in Figure 8.3.

McGarty and de la Haye (1997) review the strong evidence that differentiation between social groups or evaluative contrast is a pervasive feature of the illusory correlation paradigm. When people are given two groups they can expect, owing to the conversational logic of the experiment (Bless et al., 1993), that there should be some difference between the groups: why else would the experimenter have asked what the difference was? As Alloy and Tabachnick (1984) suggest, it is also more difficult not to perceive covariation than to perceive covariation.

Research by de la Haye and colleagues (see McGarty and de la Haye, 1997) shows that there is considerable evidence of intergroup differentiation or evaluative contrast when people are asked to judge two groups about which they receive equal amounts of information. That is, people always seem to favour one or the other group and therefore absolute differentiation is a consistent phenomenon. Why is it then that people come to favour the larger of the two groups when the majority of statements are about group A and a majority of statements describe desirable behaviours?

The answer that we came up with (McGarty et al., 1993a) was based on an analogy. Imagine that I show you three marbles, one of which is red and two of which are blue. I also tell you that one of the marbles was made in France and two were made in Germany, and then ask: what colour is the French marble? On the basis of the information given the 'rational' response is 'red', but the structure of the question can lead us to entertain the possibility that there is an association between nation of manufacture and the colour of marbles. Why else would I give you the information about nation of manufacture if it was not relevant to the question? The answer is that I would only give you irrelevant information if I were trying to trick you. Our analysis of the illusory correlation paradigm therefore is that participants are being tricked. That is, participants are given information about the desirability of behaviours of members of two groups and then asked if groups differ on this dimension (on memory and judgement measures). They therefore *expect* that there should be differences and examine the stimulus information to see, not so much whether there are differences between the groups, but what form these differences take.

A number of related reasons can be proposed for participants to expect and entertain the possibility that the larger group is associated with the majority tendency. One of these is that there is an implicit fit between group size and the prevailing tendency for the behaviours to be positive and therefore participants assume that any differences reflect this fit.

More specifically, an examination of the actual information does allow an interpretation that suggests that the majority is more positive than the minority. In particular if we allow the possibility that participants approach the situation with a view to testing hypotheses that the groups are different then the standard stimulus information can actually provide support for such hypotheses.

If we assume that participants wish to make sense of the situation by determining in what ways the groups are different then one possible way of construing the information is to consider the possibilities that group A is good and group B is bad and the possibility that group A is bad and group B is good. The information to test these possibilities is found by comparing the frequencies on the main diagonal with the other diagonal. Of 39 pieces of information in the standard paradigm, (Hamilton and Gifford, 1976), 22 support the possibility that group A is good and group B is bad and only 17 support the possibility that group A is bad and group B is good.

	Desirable behaviours	Undesirable behaviours
Group A	18	8
Group B	9	4

Yet another way of construing the situation is to imagine that participants conduct evaluations of group A and group B to determine whether each group is more positive than negative. The evidence that group A is positive is much clearer (18 pieces of evidence for, 8 pieces against) than the evidence that group B is positive (9 pieces of evidence for, and 4 against). This is entirely consistent with the aggregation principle (and hence the accounts of E. R. Smith, 1991, and Fiedler, 1991) that participants' responses can be sensitive to the absolute difference in the number of positive and negative statements rather than the ratio.

The implication is that expectations of differences between groups lead participants to construe the information in ways which favour the majority over the minority, and when they have detected such differences they accentuate the differences between groups in order to develop clear, separable and coherent impressions of the groups. That is, the key ideas that distinguish this self-categorization theory account from the aggregation account are that the SCT account assumes that the process of forming impressions of groups is motivated by a contrastive approach of deriving differentiated meaning, and that this is supplemented by processes of accentuation whereby perceived differences become magnified. Thus the process of accentuation serves the same purpose as a magnifying glass, in that it enables things to be seen more clearly (but see Chapter 11).

Quite a few studies have tested different aspects of this account. For example, McGarty et al. (1993a) removed the identifying group information from the stimuli and gave standard measures of the phenomenon to participants. In this way the stimulus information which is central to the accounts of Hamilton and Gifford (1976), Fiedler (1991), McConnell et al. (1994) and Smith (1991) was removed. We found extraordinarily strong evidence of illusory correlation. This was consistent with the differentiation-based account.

Haslam et al. (1996a) showed that the illusory correlation effect was removed, however, when expectancies of intergroup differentiation were reduced. This was achieved by telling participants in one condition that the minority group comprised left-handed people and that the majority group comprised right-handed people. We reasoned that people would expect there to be no differences in the desirability of behaviours in those groups.

In a related vein Yzerbyt et al. (1998a) showed that manipulating the validity of the classification affected the strength of the stereotypical impressions formed. We reasoned that psychology students would perceive a computer program as an invalid mechanism for classifying people and would expect no real differences between the groups, but they would expect differences when the people had been classified by an expert in human behaviour. Thus when participants were told that the behavioural statements had been classified by a computer program they perceived weaker illusory correlations than the standard condition and when the statements had been classified by a clinical psychologist they perceived more illusory correlation than in a standard control condition.

Berndsen (1997, study 2.2) also showed that the IC effect was attenuated when participants were told that the majority and minority were classes in different years at their own university (1993 and 1994). She reasoned that participants would have no expectation of differences between those years and her results are thus consistent with the idea that expectation of differences between groups is a necessary precondition for stereotype formation. Berndsen's results and those of Yzerbyt et al. (1998a) rule out the objection that can be made of Haslam et al.'s (1996a) study that participants have pre-existing stereotypes of left-handers and right-handers so that the study does not address stereotype formation.

Berndsen (1997) reports a wealth of other relevant studies on these issues. For example, she showed (study 2.1) that increasing the prominence of the group dimension (by accentuating the minority status of group B) led to an increased level of intercategory differentiation and that this variable mediated differences in the illusory correlation effect produced by these variations in prominence. Berndsen (study 2.3) also found that perceived coherence of the groups was a mediator of the effects.

In studies of process using think-aloud techniques Berndsen (study 2.4) found that most participants in the paradigm reported that they engaged in the processes that were hypothesized by McGarty et al. (1993a). That is, participants engaged in a general search for ways in which groups could differ and they actively tested hypotheses about differences between groups.

In a second series of studies Berndsen (1997) found that the stimuli perceived by participants in the illusory correlation paradigm were reinterpreted over the course of the experiment. That is, participants came to see desirable behaviours performed by the minority as less positive and undesirable behaviours performed by the majority as more positive. This suggests that the stimulus information is not fixed but undergoes reinterpretations which are expected from the differentiated meaning or evaluative contrast approach. Supportive evidence was also obtained on think-aloud measures.

Finally, Berndsen found very specific evidence in favour of the categorization-based approach of McGarty et al. (1993a). In this study (see Berndsen et al., 1998) she manipulated the scope for reinterpretation of the stimuli, the expected coherence of the stimuli and the amount of intragroup differences within the stimuli.

The rationale for this study was that the process of differentiation between groups is dynamic and that it involves both the perception of similarities as a precursor to the categorization process and the accentuation of such similarities following categorization.

Berndsen et al. (1998) observe that groups can be coherent in terms of expectations about consistency within groups or in terms of the demonstrated level of similarity (Ford and Stangor, 1992, provide evidence for the role of the latter data-based coherence in the formation of group stereotypes). This is essentially the process envisaged by the tradition of research on categorization effects (Tajfel and Wilkes, 1963) and by cognitive researchers such as Medin et al. (1993). Put another way, similarity provides the basis for categorization but it is also increased or solidified by perceptions of shared category membership.

Given its dynamic nature the process of reinterpretation provides an important but complex basis for the categorization process. In order for the illusory correlation effect to be maximized there must be expectations that the groups are separable and coherent, and there must be a basis for perceiving similarity (relatively small differences between the stimuli in the groups). Even when these conditions are present, however, there must also be scope for reinterpreting the stimulus information in a way that accentuates or magnifies those differences.

Berndsen et al. (1998) found very strong support for this analysis on a variety of measures. This work suggests quite a complex account of stereotype formation in the illusory correlation paradigm. This does not rule out the role of distinctiveness or aggregation principles as an explanation of the laboratory phenomenon of illusory correlation but suggests that the wider phenomenon of stereotype formation and the specific phenomenon of illusory correlation can both be explained in terms of the principles of intergroup differentiation. I will attempt to provide a reconciliation of these ideas at the conclusion of this chapter.

C. Entitativity and relative group size

In Chapter 4 the idea of the importance of relative group size for social perception was introduced. A large number of authors have suggested that the
particular importance of minority groups is that smaller groups are perceived
to be more entitative (Campbell, 1958) than other groups. Over and above the
discussion of the special role of minorities there has been a burgeoning of
new interest in the concept of entitativity.

Empirical evidence aside there are two main reasons for researchers to be
interested in the distinctive perceptual role of minorities as coherent. The first
is that minority influence theorists have posited that minorities are more persuasive than majorities by virtue of the coherence of minorities and the
consistent style of behaviour used by minorities to achieve successful influence (Moscovici, 1980; 1985). The second aspect that makes the idea of
entitative minorities interesting is the idea of a special role of distinctiveness
as an attention-grabbing process (Mullen, 1991).

As I discussed in Chapter 4 the justification in terms of the distinctiveness
account is difficult to sustain. Increased attention to the minority should
have the effect of individuating the members, thereby making them more
likely to be perceived as individuals rather than as an entitative group. Mullen
(1991) begins to address this concern under the heading of the 'paradox of
prototype representation of the ingroup' where he suggests that the problem
is apparent rather than real because most studies which have examined
ingroup members' perceptions have studied ingroups which are of equal size
or larger than outgroups. In other words, there has been a confound in the
previous research such that the ingroup has always been a majority or at
least a non-minority. Unfortunately, Mullen (1991) does not deal with the
more telling case of the 'paradox of the minority outgroup'. Minority outgroups are precisely those groups which should be seen as most entitative
according to Mullen's model, but they are also the ones which should attract
attention by virtue of their stimulus distinctiveness. The idea that people
would have the least differentiated representation of the group to which they
pay the most attention seems implausible.

Hamilton and Sherman (1996) cite recent evidence that ingroups can have
prototype representations and suggest reasonably that it seems unlikely that
groups to which we belong would be seen to be less real and solid than groups
to which we do not belong. Essentially, these researchers argue for the role of
local contextual comparisons of the form that B. Simon and colleagues alert
us to. The presence of the personal self in the comparative context provides
a basis for differentiating between groups.

Nevertheless there is a consistent body of literature which suggests minorities are more entitative than majorities. An example is the meta-analysis by
Mullen and Hu (1989) which shows that smaller groups are more likely to be
seen as homogeneous than large groups.

Using a category verification paradigm (where participants respond as
fast as possible to a stimulus by saying whether it is a member of a particu-

lar category or not) Mullen et al. (1994) found strong evidence that describing a group as a minority led to faster responses to stimuli. Such a pattern is consistent with more entitative representations of minority groups. Brewer et al. (1995) used the who-said-what paradigm (where participants have to try to recall the source of a communication from a variety of choices) and found more intracategory errors for minority than majority sources.

It is important to note that in both cases the differences in relative group size were manipulated by telling the participants that the groups differed in size rather than demonstrating that they differ in size. Extending terminology used by Berndsen et al. (1998) this can be seen as an expectation-based (see Hamilton and Rose, 1980) rather than a data-based process. This is quite different to the illusory correlation paradigm where participants are told that the groups differ in size but they are also given more examples of the majority group than the other. In many respects the latter approach is probably closer to everyday life, in that we can have different expectations about small and large groups as well as having less experience of the smaller groups, but the Mullen et al. (1994) and Brewer et al. (1995) studies eliminate differing degrees of experience or the amount of information encountered as bases for explanations of the differences.

Bosveld et al. (1996) found that categories could be construed in different ways by ingroup and outgroup members. Thus the category *Christian* was construed more narrowly by Christians than non-Christians, even though knowledge of and expectations about Christians were fairly consensual across the two groups. The effect of this differing construal was to see the ingroup as less common. This stands in opposition to the common finding of false consensus and opens up the more general issue of *social projection*, the idea of seeing others as sharing one's own characteristics. Bosveld et al.'s results and the more general phenomenon of social projection suggest that 'subjectively' group size is not a stable factor but is changed by context. For example, Spears and Manstead (1990) argue that variations in social projection between ingroup and outgroup can reflect differentiation between social groups: projecting positive characteristics to the ingroup but not to the population in general or to the outgroup can enhance social identity.

Brewer's (1991) optimal distinctiveness model would suggest that the self would be seen more positively when associated with a smaller group, but increased social identification through a narrow construal of the ingroup can also emerge. One possibility is that a narrow construal of the ingroup enables members to assign marginal members with undesirable (i.e., non-normative) positions to the outgroup (i.e., the population in general). This process should increase intergroup differentiation for both Christians and non-Christians through the differing construals. We might also expect that undesirable ingroup characteristics would be seen as relatively common in the population (which would also be consistent with evidence of increased heterogeneity: see Doosje et al., 1995).

These arguments suggest that group size is important for group behaviour in two senses. First, group size can be a contributor to social context by creating expectancies about small and large groups (e.g., extremity or cohesion) which can heighten or reduce intergroup differentiation. Secondly, perceived group size can emerge as an outcome of intergroup differentiation thus contributing to social identity. These relations are shown in Figure 8.4.

However, this account needs some further linking concepts which enable us to tie in the evidence from the illusory correlation paradigm and related research about the differing levels of diagnosticity of social groups. Research by Krueger and Clement (1996) does much to articulate the links.

Krueger and Clement (1996) studied the process of generalizing characteristics from samples to populations in both the non-social and social domains. They explored the thesis that generalization will cross category boundaries unless those boundaries are made salient.

In experiment 1 participants were asked to estimate the proportion of blue chips in an urn that had earlier yielded a sample with a large proportion (9 out of 10) of blue chips. When the previous sample came from the same urn participants were able to distinguish that urn from another independent

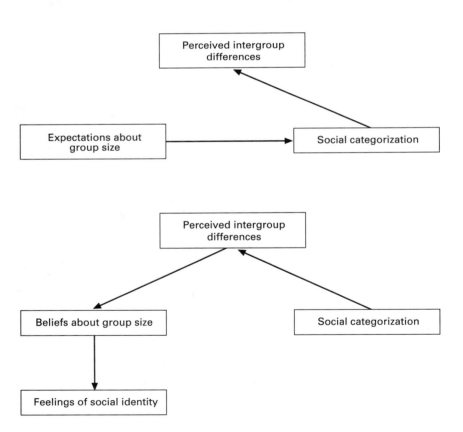

FIGURE 8.4   *Constraint relations involved in Bosveld et al.'s results*

and previously unsampled urn. Their estimates closely matched the optimum posterior percentages for the sampled and unknown urns.

When the two urns were combined into a larger urn participants' estimates also integrated their knowledge of the sampled urn and the range of possibilities in the unknown urn. These estimates also matched optimal estimates.

However, when the originally sampled urn was divided into two smaller urns participants' estimates were lower than the optima. Krueger and Clement (1996) do not explain this finding.

Most interestingly though, when the population was randomly divided into two *before* participants sampled from one of the sub-populations they did not generalize from one population to the other. Their estimates for the sampled population matched the optimum best estimates, but their estimates for the 'unknown' population did not differ from the prior probability of .5 (knowing as they did that the chips could be either red or blue). Krueger and Clement interpret this result as showing that salient categorizations reduce generalization across category boundaries.

Krueger and Clement studied social projection more directly in experiment 2. They manipulated social category salience in a minimal group study by means of the order of estimation. In order 1 (low salience) participants made population estimates before being assigned to a group. In order 2 (intermediate salience) participants made population estimates after being categorized but before group estimates. In order 3 (high salience) participants made population estimates last.

The task was for participants to present their own attitudes and then to estimate the percentage of group members and members of the population who shared the same attitude. For half the participants the target group was an outgroup, for the other half the target group was an ingroup. The authors found that participants projected their own attitudes to a target outgroup at the same low level as the population but that participants projected their own attitudes to a target ingroup at a higher level than the population, especially when salience was high. This was strong support for the authors' hypothesis that salience of category boundaries decreases generalization across categories.

Thus Krueger and Clement's (1996) work suggests that generalization could serve as the linking concept that integrates perceptions of group size with social context. Forming impressions of groups or individuals involves a process of generalization and impressions can be moderated by the amount of information available to generalize from as well as the nature of that information.

The idea of generalization therefore suggests a way to reconcile a coherent set of findings in terms of a single overview. A solution would be to suggest that minority status has a general effect of increasing salience but to replace the mechanism of determining salience in Mullen's formulation. This is essentially the view taken by Mullen of self-categorization theory:

> Self-categorization theory posits that the individual becomes 'depersonalized' whenever minority status makes their ingroup membership salient, whereas the individual becomes 'personalized' whenever majority status makes their ingroup membership salient. (1991: 316)

If we replace the words 'whenever' with 'if' then Mullen's reading of self-categorization theory appears correct. This qualification is necessary because no statement of self-categorization theory suggests that minority–majority status uniformly increases salience. The comparative fit principle in SCT is based on relative similarities and differences and not absolute numbers. To derive the prediction that minority status increases salience either some new principle needs to be added to the theory or the principles of normative fit or perceiver readiness need to be invoked. Certainly, it is possible that minority status could make perceivers more ready to use certain categorizations. It is also likely that certain categorizations will be more normatively consistent with certain types of beliefs. For example, holding extreme views or suffering discrimination may be more consistent with people's experience of what it means to be a minority member.

Although there can be beliefs about minorities which become part of the norms within a particular culture (this is the view adopted by Hamilton and Sherman, 1996), it is also true that large and small groups invite different responses by virtue of their differing sizes. McGarty et al. (1995) examined a number of variables that could be expected to differ between groups.

Our approach was informed by Campbell's (1958) analysis of entitativity in terms of the Gestalt principles of perception. Campbell expected groups to be seen to be entitative to the extent that people perceived the group members were perceptually alike (similarity), were close together (proximity), changed in the same ways (shared a common fate) and had a well-formed organization (pregnance). Importantly, Campbell also suggested that common fate would be a better source for drawing boundaries around a small group than a large group. The constructs of proximity and similarity can be linked to Medin's (1989) concept of psychological essentialism and Medin et al.'s (1993) analysis of similarity. Category formation proceeds on the basis of both intuitive theories about why things should be the same (including the theory that things share an underlying essence) and perceptions of similarity (closer to *proximity* in Campbell's treatment).

The key elements that are added from research on social categorization (Turner et al., 1987) are those of accentuation and intercategory contrasts. Similarity and proximity are not stable elements which are unaffected by categorization; rather perceptions of similarity and proximity are heightened by shared category membership. Secondly, the perception of commonality rests not just on perceived similarity but on perceived differences from other elements which do not share a category membership. These ideas are instantiated in the principle of meta-contrast discussed in Chapter 5.

There are several ways in which small and large groups can vary in terms of features which determine entitativity. Even when we hold pregnance and common fate constant we can still expect variations in qualities that relate to proximity and similarity.

One of the most important of these may be *diversity*: the richness or variety within a group. Although a large group and a small group can contain equal amounts of variability as measured by a variance measure, it will tend to be the case that the larger group will contain a greater number of different opinions. To take the simplest example: a group with one member can only occupy one position at any one time but a group with two members *can* occupy two positions. Thus larger groups contain more potential for diversity and, for a reasonably finely grained scale, can be expected to have more diversity. The implication is that if we perceive the same amount of diversity in a large and a small group we should expect the large group to be more entitative. This is because low diversity in a large group or high diversity in a small group should be diagnostic of the presence of some other factor that explains why the distribution of group members varies from that expected.

Diversity has some similarities to Linville et al.'s (1989) concept of probability of differentiation but that construct is independent of group size (except in the special sense that it is biased). Diversity, however, is a useful concept for framing discussions about the effects of group size on expectations about entitativity (and the following discussion is an elaboration of ideas developed by McGarty et al., 1995).

For example, knowing that group size is a predictor of diversity is a good reason to expect a better basketball team from a large school than from a small school. Even though the variability in height, aptitude and sporting interest could be identical in the two groups the pool of talented basketballers at school A with 1000 students will be larger than that at school B with 100 students (see also Schaller, 1992; 1994).

Assume that both schools select their teams from a squad made up of the 20 best basketballers on a normally distributed standardized measure of basketball ability (or by unbiased and reliable selectors). The mean standardized ability score of the top 20 students from a school of 100 students will be lower than the mean standardized ability score of the top 20 students from the school of 1000 students. By randomly sampling five individuals from this extreme group the large school will pick a more talented team than the small school (of course, if the schools were required to select from the other extreme tail the large school would pick a less talented team).

We would therefore be surprised if we found that there was no difference in ability between these two schools under such sampling conditions. However, we would be more surprised if we found that school A was particularly poor than if school B was particularly good. This is because if both schools are considered as samples drawn from the same population then it is less likely in statistical terms that a large sample will have a mean which deviates from the population mean than will a small sample. The paradox is therefore that large groups are more likely to have extreme tails but less likely to have extreme means. This reduces to the proposition that large groups can be expected to be less extreme on average but to contain more diversity.

If these expectations do hold then the implications of encountering varying levels of extremity and diversity on entitativity are quite extensive. If we
encounter a large group that contains very little diversity then this implies
that this group may be very entitative indeed because the lack of diversity is
very unlikely to have occurred by chance. This implies that some organizing
principle has constrained diversity. Similarly, a large extreme group also vio-
lates expectancies (as it is unlikely to have been produced by chance) and
therefore may also be seen to be entitative.

An intriguing feature of this analysis is that it suggests that small groups
need not be more entitative than large groups because the ability to form a
clear impression of a group may be a precondition for entitativity. Thus it
may be easier to make clear inferences about the nature (and the presence of
organizing principles) in large groups by virtue of the law of large numbers
(see Schaller, 1992). In terms used by Osherson et al. (1990) and by Gutheil
and Gelman (1997) samples of large size (monotonicity) and diversity 'cover'
the category more effectively and provide a stronger basis for inference.
Gutheil and Gelman note, however, that young children have difficulty using
sample size and diversity in this way.

Thus, although small groups should not be extreme on average they are
more likely to be extreme than are large groups, and although large groups
may be no more variable in terms of measures such as standard deviation
they will tend to be more diverse. However, extremity and low diversity are
both characteristics which could be expected to lead to high perceived entitativity. The fact that small groups can have these characteristics should
create the conditions whereby they are expected to be entitative; when we perceive cases where large groups have these characteristics then this should be
highly diagnostic of the group's true nature and contribute to perceptions of
very high entitativity.

Of course, these points are derived from statistical principles, and there is
no *a priori* reason to believe that exactly these principles should govern
people's perceptions. However, McGarty et al. (1995) demonstrated the
applicability of these ideas in two very simple experiments. Participants were
asked to judge the consistency or coherence of stimulus patterns which represented distributions of attitudes or persons' positions in a room. A
consistent finding over two studies was an interaction of size × diversity. The
effect of diversity on entitativity was greater for large groups than small
groups. Study 1 also demonstrated that diversity had an effect on group entitativity that was independent of group size, but it showed no interaction
between size and variability.

We therefore suggested that perceptions of entitativity are governed by the
following relationship:

$$E \propto N/D$$

That is, for a group of a particular size N the entitativity E will increase as the
diversity D or number of positions occupied by the group decreases, but for
a constant level of diversity the entitativity increases with group size. The

additional complications are that diversity and group size are themselves not probabilistically independent, and that this relationship does not appear to hold for variability.

One way of summarizing these ideas is to suggest that there are (at least) two relevant constructs here: entitativity and diagnosticity. We can define entitativity positively as Campbell did in terms of the features that increase it, or we can define it negatively and contrastively by defining what it is not. An entitative group is not a random collection of individuals who just happen to be together for no particular reason. Thus an entitative group is bound by some organizing principle; we can identify groups as entitative even without knowing what that principle is, however, if we observe that the distribution of members is not random. It follows that perceivers' entitativity judgements would be aided if they were able to distinguish between a random aggregation and a real group. It becomes critical therefore to establish the diagnosticity of some pattern in distinguishing between these possibilities.

The extent to which some aggregation of people can be seen to be entitative or not depends on how easy it is to detect any structure or organization within the aggregation when compared with a random pattern. It becomes easier to make this judgement with large groups than small groups, and therefore large groups will be diagnostic. That is, large groups make it easier to be confident that the pattern is entitative or random, and unless the pattern is sufficiently diagnostic there is no logical alternative other than to conclude that the pattern is random. If we encounter just a couple of violent members of a minority group, do we conclude that there is a tendency for violence in their group in general? Clearly people do make these stereotypical associations on some occasions and not on others. My suggestion is that the extent to which people make these associations depends in the first instance on the diagnosticity of the behaviour and that that will depend upon the amount of information encountered.

However, group size is also associated with expectations of high diversity and a low likelihood of extremity. Where these expectations are contradicted for sufficiently diagnostic stimulus patterns, large groups should be seen to be more entitative than small groups.

The remaining ideas, however, need to be qualified because they depend upon the particular hypotheses entertained by perceivers. When they are presented with two random patterns the smaller one will be seen as more entitative than the larger one. When they are presented with two organized patterns the larger one will be seen as more entitative than the smaller one.

These ideas can be applied directly to the illusory correlation paradigm. Participants are presented with two meaningful patterns of variation within groups. The large group is more diagnostic and it is easier to be confident about this pattern: group A contains more positive than negative behaviours. However, the small group is less diagnostic and therefore it is more difficult to reach a confident assessment. These hypotheses lead to the same predictions as the aggregation principle with the additional proviso that the differences between the groups are accentuated through processes of evaluative contrast and intergroup differentiation.

D. Other approaches to entitativity

Hamilton and Sherman (1996) have developed an account of variability in the perceived consistency of individual persons and groups. They start with the assumption that people expect coherence and consistency within individual persons. They suggest that people do not always expect such high consistency within groups.

The effect on processing of these differences is that individuals are more likely to be represented by on-line impressions and groups are more likely to be represented by memory-based impressions. The implication is that people's memory-based impressions are more likely to be biased because the information will have been processed less extensively.

They argue that distinctiveness-based illusory correlations are good examples of such memory-based impressions. If people went to the additional effort of processing the stimulus information more extensively, as they would if processing information about individual people, they would develop on-line impressions which would be less biased.

The representative research that Hamilton and Sherman cite for this idea is at best patchy. For example, research by Weisz and Jones (1993) which ostensibly compared target-based expectancies with category-based expectancies manipulated this variable by presenting participants with two pieces of information about one person or two pieces of information about two members of the same group. Hamilton and Sherman interpreted the results as showing that individuals were perceived to be more consistent than groups. However, the research only formally demonstrates that two people identified as members of one group may be perceived to be less consistent than is one person.

However, Hamilton and Sherman argue that groups vary in the extent to which their members are perceived to be consistent. These expectations of consistency define the entitativity or unity of the group. There is a continuum on which groups can be placed so that some groups are empirically harder and tighter than others. It follows therefore that some groups can even be perceived to be more consistent than individuals.

Better evidence for Hamilton and Sherman's approach comes from research by McConnell, Sherman and Hamilton (1997). These authors tested the hypothesis that coherent (entitative) groups would be processed on-line in a manner analogous to the processing of individual stimuli. Their research showed that when people *expected* coherence within the groups there was less stereotyping of the groups.

I find this idea to be highly counter-intuitive. The manipulation of expectations for coherence was to tell participants that 'the members of group A are quite similar to each other and do not differ in many ways from each other'. They were given similar information about group B. Under this formulation, expecting people to be the same as each other should produce detailed processing which reveals the differences between them. Since the work of Allport (1954) at least, stereotyping has been understood as perceiving members of groups to be similar to each other. I would anticipate that expecting people to be the same would lead to greater stereotyping and not to less stereotyping.

Put another way, Hamilton and Sherman's formulation runs into a problem analogous to that in Mullen's (1991) formulation. When perceivers are made aware of the similarities within a group they are less likely to perceive the stimuli to be similar. McConnell et al.'s (1997) results, however, are fully consistent with Hamilton and Sherman's analysis. Expectation-based coherence reduced the illusory correlation effect.

Berndsen et al. (1998), however, using a weaker manipulation of expectation-based coherence, found exactly the opposite result. They explain this state of affairs by positing that the interaction between data-based coherence and expectation-based coherence may produce a curvilinear relationship between coherence and illusory correlation. Such a curvilinear relationship between data-based coherence was in fact found by Berndsen et al. (1998, study 2).

A variant of this explanation may be even simpler. The extreme coherence that McConnell et al.'s participants are led to expect is a misrepresentation of the situation. The stimulus information provides the information necessary for the perceiver to test the idea that the differences within groups are very small and the experimentally induced expectancies can therefore be easily disconfirmed.

The crucial part of this argument is that the lack of illusory correlation arises not from the effect of the expectations *per se* but from the falsification of those expectancies and the reinterpretation of that information. Again as Berndsen et al. (1998) show, scope for reinterpretation of the information is a crucial precondition for illusory correlation. If the illusory correlation paradigm is thought of as an attempt by experimenters to get participants to distort reality then such attempts generally fail where the expectations induced are inconsistent with the data.

None of these points suggest an argument against the analysis of specific process suggested by Hamilton and Sherman (1996). McConnell et al.'s (1997) participants may well have been engaged in on-line processing. The reason for the on-line processing may be that they are scanning the information very closely because their prior expectations were disconfirmed or that they were perceiving and accentuating intragroup differences. To resolve these questions, measures of expectations for consistency and the fate of those expectations need to be taken.

It is important to note that Hamilton and Sherman see the entitativity of groups to be an enduring, stable feature of those groups. This continuity over time is a very important aspect to consider wherever expectancies are involved. There is very little point in having an understanding of something like a group unless it allows one to generate stable expectancies. There is, however, a tradeoff between having enduring expectancies and situationally appropriate expectancies. It is nevertheless the case that although expectancies should vary across situations there should also be relatively consistent expectancies every time people are in the same situation. The question that then develops is whether these expectancies are generated afresh for each situation or whether expectancies are stored with knowledge of that situation (this is analogous to the debate considered in Chapter 7 between approaches that stress knowledge activation and knowledge construction).

The question that Hamilton and Sherman do not address is the possibility of situational variations in the entitativity of groups from time to time. This defines the key difference between social category salience and Hamilton and Sherman's construct of entitativity. Any group can be seen to be more or less group-like and such transformations involve changes in perceptions of groups. For example, the enemy during a war will be seen as more entitative than they were beforehand.

Such changes can reflect changes in the perceived group (i.e., the enemy becomes more organized at times of war through processes of conformity and intergroup differentiation) but they can occur through changes in perception (see Oakes et al., 1994) which are independent of changes in the perceived group. Moreover, and consistent with the ideas of Jussim (1991), perceptions of groups can determine behaviour towards outgroups which can in turn solidify the boundaries between groups. This was essentially the point that Lewin (1948) made when he referred to common fate as the basis of group formation in the case of the Jews in Nazi Germany. The antecedent of the perceptions by Jews, and others, that Jews were an increasingly entitative group was their treatment by the Nazis (who identified Jewishness on the basis of ancestry rather than religious practices or behaviour).

Without such situational variation Hamilton and Sherman's continuum of entitativity would appear to relate more closely to the mooted SCT construct of relatively stable background knowledge. In the same way that strength of identification was argued to be a determinant of accessibility/readiness (Turner et al., 1987) so expectations of consistency within a group can be considered to be a relatively stable factor determining the salience of social categorizations. Castano and Yzerbyt (1998) assemble impressive evidence on this point. They manipulated factors related to four determinants of entitativity that were identified by Campbell (1958). They found that identification with the European Union was increased by increasing entitativity in each case but only for those with moderate initial attitudes to the European Union (see Chapter 9 though, where I interpret momentary identification as an outcome of a salient social categorization).

The work of Rothbart and Taylor (1992) which extends Medin's idea of psychological essentialism to social categories has generated considerable recent interest. Haslam et al. (1997) investigated variations in beliefs about social categories. They found that there are two orthogonal dimensions into which dimensions of essentialism can be divided. These were the extent that categories were understood to be natural kinds and the extent to which the categories were perceived to be coherent and unified entities. This is a surprising result in some ways and suggests the need for greater precision in theorizing on this point. Essentialism has been associated explicitly with entitativity by McGarty et al. (1995) and Yzerbyt et al. (1997) but it appears that the dimensions of *naturalness, immutability, discreteness* and *historical stability* cohere, as do the elements of *informativeness, uniformity, inherence* (having an underlying reality) and *exclusivity* (not allowing members to belong to other categories). The ambiguous element here is inherence. The extent to which category members share an underlying reality appears to have a great deal in common with the dimensions on the naturalness factor but had a zero loading. It is possible that this reflects a measurement issue because the dimension was labelled 'underlying reality or sameness'. The reference to sameness may have elicited a pattern of responses similar to that for the uniformity and exclusivity dimensions.

Evidence that the naturalness of social categories underlies variance in social categories also provides a limit on the claims of Rothbart and Taylor (1992). If it were the case that naturalness was a defining feature of social categories then we would expect very little variation in that feature. To take an example from natural object categories, the capacity to suckle young is a defining feature of mammal species but there is almost zero variation in suckling across mammals. Naturalness may thus be an important feature but it is not a defining feature for social categories.

Finally, as noted earlier, Yzerbyt et al. (1997) combine considerations of essentialistic categorization with the rationalizing/explanatory functions of stereotyping. They suggest abandoning the dominant view of stereotypes as simple lists of attributes. Instead, stereotypes ought to be considered as well-organized theoretical structures that comprise information not only as to what characteristics are related, but also as to *why* and *how* these characteristics are related. It follows that two persons cannot be considered to be members of the same category simply because they are similar in some absolute sense. Strictly speaking, any two objects with variable qualities can always be seen to differ from one another providing you select the right features. In line with recent theoretical developments on concept learning and categorization in cognitive psychology (e.g., Medin, 1989; Medin et al., 1993), these authors propose that similarity is a product rather than a cause of conceptual coherence. In other words, the real constraints on people's social categories are existing intuitive theories about the world. Surface similarities between stimuli do play a role in categorization but only in so far as they lead people into building up theories about the interconnectedness of these features. In this perspective, categorization and, for that matter, social categorization derive from the existence of *a priori* theories as to why particular stimuli should differ from or be similar to one another. Without such devices, it would simply be impossible to categorize in the first place. Stereotypes can best be seen as one particular example of such theories.

Essentialist beliefs provide excellent rationalizations for the treatment of and relative status of social groups. If unemployment is attributed to the laziness of the unemployed and this is seen as an enduring fixed characteristic of unemployed people then it makes little sense to change society to create opportunities for these people. If laziness were also seen as a genetically predisposed personality trait (perhaps because it has been stereotypically associated with one race) then it also makes little sense to try to change these characteristics. Such views, which echo the still more extreme views of colonial masters and slave owners throughout history, justify oppressive systems which benefit the powerful. On the other hand, an ideology which stresses economic and structural causes for unemployment provides a justification for social change (for discussions of the consequences of related ideologies see Augoustinos and Walker, 1996; Brown, 1999; Jost and Banaji, 1994; Moscovici, 1984).

As research by Schadron et al. and Yzerbyt et al. (both cited by Yzerbyt et al., 1997) demonstrates, different judgements are observed when participants are informed that a target group had been constituted on a purely random basis or on the basis of a series of personality, social and biographical questionnaires. Participants saw the group randomly assigned to an outstanding education programme or to unfavourable educational conditions. Results indicate that the fate of the group significantly affects the impression of the group members only when subjects believe the group comprises a homogeneous set of people. In other words, subsequent information about the group members is translated into enduring group-based characteristics only when subjects think that people's membership in a group is based on meaningful attributes and the group can therefore be perceived as an entity. These results are linked to people's beliefs in the existence of essential differences between members of meaningfully contrasting groups.

More recently, Yzerbyt et al. (1998b) have used a variation on Ross et al.'s (1977) quiz-game paradigm where participants saw persons who were asking questions based on their own general knowledge to be more knowledgeable than the people who were answering those questions (even though people had been randomly allocated to those roles). Yzerbyt et al. (1998b) found that perceptions of the questioners and answerers were moderated by whether the group of people asking the questions were presented as an aggregate (from three different colleges) or as an entitative group (from either their own college or another college). In general, the overattribution did not occur when the questioners or answerers comprised an aggregate. That is, when the entitativity of the groups provided a meaningful basis for differentiating between the groups there was a differentiation between the questioners and answerers. Intriguingly, although judges tend to give higher knowledge ratings to people from their own college there was nevertheless clear differentiation between entitative ingroup questioners and answerers.

The authors argue that their results show that the explanatory power of group memberships can lead to attributional errors. This may be too harsh a judgement, as I would make the point that the results suggest a similar interpretation to that made by McMullen et al. (1997). The provision of group memberships suggests to the participants that the task is 'about' the difference in knowledge between the members of different groups (see Higgins, 1997) and they therefore use that information to explain the apparent differences between questioners and answerers. Interestingly, entitativity in Yzerbyt et al.'s research plays the role that I attribute to diagnosticity earlier in this chapter. Entitativity is here a precondition for differentiation between questioners and answerers.

E. Reconciliation: variability, relative group size and entitativity

Some aspects of the very diverse research on perception of groups and their members afford a reconciliation. I think that the integrating elements that appear to be most important revolve around expectations of consistency and difference and the quasi-statistical models that perceivers use to make sense of the information they receive. A distinction must be made between the drawing of a data-based (to use Berndsen et al.'s, 1998, term) coherent impression of some group as a meaningful social entity which is distinct from other groups (entitativity) and the ease with which such impressions can be drawn from the available information (diagnosticity). The key reason why diagnosticity must be distinguished from entitativity is that diagnosticity is a precondition for perceiving entitativity: it is easier to draw an impression that a group is entitative or not when there is a sound basis for drawing an impression. Groups can then also be differentiated in terms of entitativity. When we say we or they are similar to each other we unavoidably say they are different from us.

There is also a rich variety of expectations about groups which affect entitativity. Some of these expectations relate to the naturalness of social groups, others relate to expectation-based coherence. Still other forms of expectation might relate to expectations about diagnosticity (i.e., is it likely that we will know whether some pattern is an organized social group?) but there is little concrete evidence about this last form of expectancy.

The reconciliation takes the form of five points. These reinforce the argument made here and elsewhere that judgements of social aggregations involve motivated attempts to make sense of similarities and differences between members in terms of social categories.

1   People expect groups that are labelled or identified in different ways to be different. Although the idea can be presented in a number of related ways (see e.g., Berndsen and Spears, 1997; McGarty et al., 1993a; Yzerbyt et al., 1997) I think the clearest articulation of this point is Brown's (1999) suggestion that different category labels provide a theory which generates expectations of intergroup differences and explains observed intergroup differences and similarities.

2   The distinction between minorities and majorities status takes on specific meanings in particular settings for a number of reasons. As Hamilton

et al. (1998) note, group size may be correlated with entitativity, but it is also correlated with other variables which independently determine entitativity:

(a) It is easier to draw conclusions with confidence about larger groups than smaller groups owing to the greater amount of information about a large group (see Schaller, 1992, for a discussion of the effect of the law of large numbers on judgements). This means that perceivers will tend to make more confident evaluations about large groups than small groups.

(b) For statistical reasons it is more likely that small and not large groups will occupy extreme positions within a frame of reference. People will therefore expect small groups to be more extreme and thus more entitative than large groups.

(c) As a rule, diversity can be expected to increase with group size. People will therefore expect diversity in large groups which will be associated with lower entitativity. This high diversity may be conflated with variability in the minds of perceivers. However, very low diversity relative to group size should suggest high entitativity.

3   Where a confident conclusion can be made about one group but not about some other comparison group we can expect that perceivers will accentuate the differences between the groups on the dimension that provides that clear impression.

4   Expectations of consistencies within groups and of differences between groups will only enhance entitativity where they are not contradicted by diagnostic stimulus information.

5   Perceived entitativity will increase with the ratio of the number of exemplars of a category to the diversity of the category.

These principles are shown in the constraint relations in Figure 8.5. For presentational purposes, new and/or updated knowledge is presented as a fourth box in the figure. Of course, such adjustments could serve to modify the future operation of subsequent categorization processes.

These relations all stress the importance of categorization for explanation and the limits on generalizing across categories. The ideas demand further consideration of the processes of causal explanation and covariation. I do this in Chapter 10, but before we consider these issues I wish to examine social constraints on the categorization process more closely.

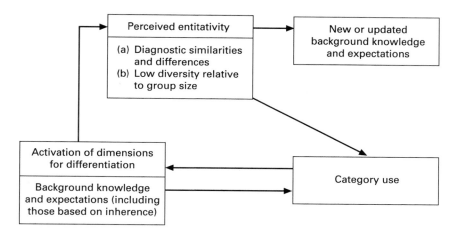

FIGURE 8.5   *Key constraint relations involved in perceptions of group entitativity and variability*

9 The Constraints of the Social Context on Categorization

Craig McGarty and Diana M. Grace

A. Distinguishing social categorization from social identification and social self-esteem

A continuing theme in social identity research is the problem of distinguishing the concepts of social categorization, social identification and social self-esteem. Conceptually, seeing oneself as being the *same as some class of persons* and different from others is distinguishable from feeling *one belongs to a group* and feeling *good about oneself as a group member*. This is the case even though social categorization is a necessary precondition for social identification and social self-esteem. We cannot feel we belong to a group without acknowledging the existence of that group in some sense.

Although correlation does not imply causation, causation implies correlation (providing that effects are not masked by other variables). It would be alarming therefore if the constructs of categorization, identification and self-esteem were unrelated.

However, Ellemers and van Knippenberg (1997) describe unpublished research by Ellemers, Korterkaas and Ouwerkerk in which these three constructs have been shown to be orthogonal principal components. What is more, they found that different variables affect each of the three components. Self-categorization changed as a function of the relative sizes of the groups (minority members showed stronger self-categorization than majority members), social self-esteem was influenced by group status (high status implying high esteem), but commitment to the group (identification) was higher for high-status groups and groups which were self-selected by the participants rather than assigned by the experimenter.

These results militate against the picture of salience that follows from self-categorization theory. Turner et al. (1987) discuss two related constructs: psychological group formation and the salience of social categories. The first relates to the extent to which people perceive themselves to share and define themselves in terms of some shared ingroup–outgroup categorization. Turner et al. make it clear that such categorizations can apply both to immediate and spontaneous group formation, as occurs when people form new groups, and to the internalization of preformed classifications that already exist within a cultural setting. The principle of group formation is the meta-contrast principle. People are more likely to perceive themselves as members of a group when they perceive differences between them to be less than differences between themselves and other people (psychologically) present in the setting (1987: 51, hypothesis 5). These comparisons are made on relevant dimensions selected from the self-category that includes all those being compared. Thus the idea of perceiver readiness is also encompassed in the hypothesis.

The salience of such ingroup–outgroup categorizations is the extent to which those categorizations are psychologically prepotent. As I discussed in Chapter 5, salience depends upon the interaction of perceiver readiness and fit, but a major component of the perceiver's readiness to use an ingroup–outgroup categorization is 'the degree of internalization of or identification with an ingroup–outgroup membership, the centrality and evaluative importance of a group membership in self-definition' (1987: 55).

Thus, SCT suggests a complex resolution. Group formation proceeds on the basis of the interaction of perceiver readiness and fit but once groups are formed the strength of identification and degree of internalization of that group become determinants of future readiness to perceive oneself in terms of that categorization.

The full model can be expressed as a path model which I have divided for convenience into three parts. The first is shown in Figure 9.1. Here long-term identification emerges from salient group memberships. The caveat is that I have depicted salience as the result of main effects of perceiver readiness and fit whereas formally it is defined as the interaction of the two.

Long-term identification is, in turn, one of many determinants of perceiver's readiness to use a social category, as shown in Figure 9.2.

The final path model in Figure 9.3 shows the outcomes of a salient social categorization. The salient social categorization leads to depersonalized self-perceptions which allow the self to be evaluated in terms of the norms provided by the group membership. To the extent that those comparisons show the group to be superior to relevant outgroups the perceiver will feel good about their group, and to the extent that group members perceive themselves as prototypical of the ingroup norms they will feel good about their

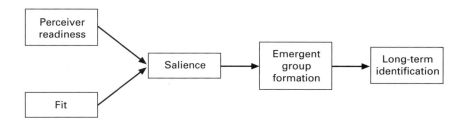

FIGURE 9.1   *Emergent group formation*

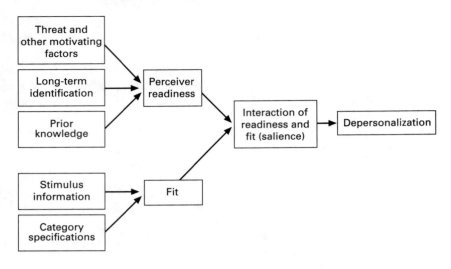

FIGURE 9.2   *The determinants of depersonalization*

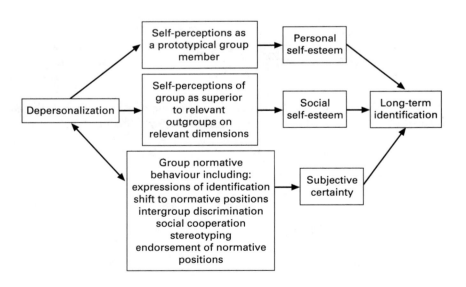

FIGURE 9.3   *Consequences of depersonalization*

own standing. Despite certain claims by Hogg and Abrams (1990) neither social identity theory nor self-categorization theory anticipate that self-esteem is a cause of social categorization (see Long and Spears, 1997).

Behaviour which is consistent with group norms also arises from salient social categorization. One common example of such group normative behaviour is the public statement or private recognition of one's identity as a group member. That is, under conditions of salient social categorization people are more likely to express identification with the group. In other words, if we measure identification under conditions of high social category salience we will find that identification is high.

This creates an important measurement problem. Long-term identification (a determinant of salience) is conceptually distinct from momentary identification which is an outcome of salience. The only solution to this measurement problem is to take a profile of identification across a wide range of periods and, in particular, to take measures of long-term identification well *prior* to the existence of the conditions that make the social categorization salient. High levels of long-term identification may also put a cap on any increases or changes in momentary identification (as the results of Castano and Yzerbyt, 1998, seem to suggest).

Subjective certainty is also presented as an outcome of group normative behaviour. Uncertainty reduction is anticipated by self-categorization theory to result from ingroup consensus. This is achieved by shift to ingroup norms or perceived validation of the current position by ingroup agreement (see McGarty et al., 1993b; Turner et al., 1987; Turner, 1991) or by taking action that is believed to be consistent with the norms of the group.

Contrary to Hogg and Abrams's (1993) model, uncertainty reduction is not a precursor to social categorization as such because both interpersonal and intergroup differentiation involve the single process of categorization. The attempt to reduce uncertainty and make sense of similarity and differences is not distinctively associated with social categorization and should not be expected to vary between intergroup and intragroup categorization. An analogy would be the role of oxygen in combustion. Oxygen is a crucial precondition for both forest and house fires and therefore we should not necessarily expect its presence to vary from one type of fire to the other (see the second section in Chapter 10). Similarly, regardless of whether the categories formed reflect a contrast between an individual and other individuals within that group, or between one's group and some other (or all other) groups, the process of categorization will reflect an attempt to make sense of the situation in terms of valid categories which should reduce uncertainty. Uncertainty should not of itself predispose perceivers to be more likely to use the social level of categorization.

Returning to the model in Figure 9.3, there are some substantial qualifications that should be made to this model which is derived relatively straightforwardly from SCT. First, it neglects what Reicher et al. (1995) refer to as the *strategic* dimension to behaviour, focusing instead on what they term the *cognitive* aspects (but could more properly be termed the *self-categorical* aspects) of social behaviour. That is, it does not include self-presentational behaviours which communicate to others that the perceiver's beliefs are other than what they really are.

Secondly, the overview does not make the subsidiary effects of group normative behaviour on self-esteem completely obvious. While depersonalization does not directly increase self-esteem and the primary path by which self-esteem is anticipated to be increased is through favourable social comparisons, the performance of group normative behaviours is itself a basis for evaluation of self and others. To the extent that actions by the individual are prototypical they contribute to increased respect, and to the extent that actions by the self and other ingroup members allow favourable intergroup comparisons they contribute to increased pride. This is shown in the model by the bidirectional causal arrow between depersonalization and group normative behaviour.

Another feature which is not encompassed within the model are the specific emotional reactions which can follow depersonalization under particular conditions. For example, Doosje et al. (in press) have shown that under conditions where unfavourable aspects of a group's history are made prominent, guilt can be evoked.

The final qualification I would make here is that Jetten et al. (1998) have shown that there is a curvilinear relationship between intergroup distinctiveness and positive group differentiation. In particular, the greatest differentiation between groups occurs when there is a low prior distinctiveness between groups but the groups are highly homogeneous so that they do not overlap. Jetten et al. explain these results in terms of a combination of the principle of comparative relevance drawn from social identity theory and comparative fit drawn from self-categorization theory. Most differentiation should occur when the groups can be clearly discriminated but where the outgroup is close in status to the ingroup and therefore relevant to comparison. I discuss this finding again in relation to Yaniv and Foster's (1995) arguments about the tradeoff between informativeness and accuracy in Chapter 10.

Overall, identification with (previously formed) groups is merely one of many determinants of perceiver readiness and this itself is but one determinant of salience. The indirect connection between long-term identification and salience means that a sizeable correlation cannot be expected, for the same reason that large correlations between general measures of attitude and specific behaviours cannot be expected (Fishbein and Ajzen, 1974).

Mummendey and Wenzel (1997) note that under different conditions intergroup similarity produces greater intergroup differentiation and that under other circumstances intergroup differences produce intergroup differentiation (see Jetten, 1997). Jetten (1997) suggests that this represents a theoretical contradiction, and Mummendey and Wenzel's solution to this contradiction is to point to the role of the hierarchical nature of the categorical system in shaping differentiation (the usefulness of hierarchies is considered in more detail in the first section in Chapter 10).

Consistent with both SIT and SCT, Mummendey and Wenzel (1997) argue that social discrimination is not an automatic consequence of social categorization but rests on the recognition of relevant differences between the groups. They argue that, under conditions where the outgroup's difference from the ingroup is evaluated to threaten the validity, positivity or superiority of the ingroup, hostility to the outgroup will be expressed. Thus they seek to explain why Serbs and Croats may express more hostility towards each other than say Serbs express to Mongolians or Navajo, despite the fact that Serbs and Croats might appear to a third party to be similar to each other.

The next step in their argument is to suggest that whether discrimination results from perceived intergroup differences depends on the conceptualization of the hierarchy involving these groups. Under conditions where (a) the ingroup and outgroup are seen to be equivalent at some superordinate level and (b) the attributes of the ingroup are seen as prototypical of that shared category, then the conditions for social discrimination exist. However, where the ingroup and outgroup are categorically distinct in the sense that they do not share a superordinate category membership, the conditions for intergroup tolerance exist. Thus Serbs and Croats may feel hostility towards each other in terms of their commitment to their common Slavic heritage and Christianity. Serbs or Croats, however, might look at the characteristics of Mongolians as interesting ethnographic curiosities and tolerate them. Thus the Orthodox Christianity of most Serbs might be seen as a heretical affront to the Catholicism of most Croats, but the Buddhism of most Mongolians might be looked upon benignly as a misunderstanding by people who could be expected to know no better.

I think that Mummendey and Wenzel have correctly identified some of the conditions for tolerance but they may have placed the wrong restrictions on discrimination. A shared superordinate category is only one way in which an outgroup becomes relevant. On one enduring and important dimension Serbs and Croats are far more different from each other than Serbs and Mongolians or Croats and Navajo. The recent treatment of Serbs by Croats and of Croats by Serbs has been characterized by hostility in much the same way that relations between Arabs and Jews in the twentieth century have been characterized by hostility. Thus in terms of the level of deliberately counter-normative behaviour completely contrary to the norms and values of the ingroup, a competing outgroup *is more different* than an unrelated outgroup. Thus the history of negative treatment by the outgroup and the negative views that the outgroup holds of the ingroup justify negative treatment of that outgroup and negative views about it. Each group should define acts which are consistent with its own norms positively and acts which are inconsistent with its own norms negatively. Outgroup members who discriminate against ingroup members are acting in a way that is maximally inconsistent with the norms of the ingroup but consistent with expectations of the outgroup. Thus Serbs who compete with Croats are acting in a way that is utterly inimical to the norms of Croats and must be confronted, but Mongolians who act in a way that is unrelated to Croat norms can be tolerated.

Thus, Mummendey and Wenzel are probably correct in suggesting that intergroup hostility will be maximized where the ingroup's characteristics are seen as prototypical, but it is probably not necessary for the ingroup and outgroup to comprise a superordinate group. Indeed all they need to have in common is a history of conflict.

An intriguing feature of Mummendey and Wenzel's analysis though is that the conditions for discrimination are also those which should favour superordinate group formation. To take a still more powerful example, Mummendey and Wenzel's account suggests that Arabs who perceive themselves to be Israeli citizens will either accept or discriminate against Israeli Jews, but those who see themselves as having nothing in common with Israel should tolerate them.

Although this seems paradoxical Mummendey and Wenzel's point may capture much of the tension in enduring historical conflicts. Action contrary to ingroup norms may be seen as more strongly counter-normative when the action is taken by those who have been seen to share an identity at some higher level. This would be consistent with the black sheep effect (Marques et al., 1988) that poor ingroup members are viewed more negatively than outgroup members. A former ingroup member, for example, who betrays the ingroup to a hostile outgroup is not only defying norms but defying expectations in a counter-normative manner. This could reinforce negative perceptions.

B. Social influences on the categorization process

Although there is a reasonably wide-ranging consensus that the same processes apply in the categorization of social and non-social objects, the balance of opinion seems to be that this is because the processes that apply to perceiving objects generalize to perceiving people. This is, of course, only one of the two possible causal directions. The alternative, that all categorization behaviour is socially mediated, is a basis for a deeper treatment of the social foundations of cognition.

This is because the way we go about categorizing things in the world may itself be determined by the social context. In social psychological and sociological traditions a continuing exposition of the social basis of thought categories has occurred in work on symbolic interactionism (Mead, 1934). Symbolic interactionists argue that the existence of mind and selfhood emerges through social interaction with relevant others, and this has continued to be addressed in the tradition of sociological social psychology (Stryker, 1997; Stryker and Statham, 1985). From a rhetorical/discursive standpoint, Edwards (1991) makes the point that categorization serves a rhetorical purpose: that is, categories are for talking.

Within psychological social psychology there has also been a recent surge of interest in the social foundations of cognition, and social influences on cognition. This includes, for example, the work of Hardin and Higgins (1996), Jussim (1991), Levine et al. (1993), Resnick et al., (1991), Ostrom (1984), Markus and Kitayama (1991; Markus et al., 1996), and the edited volumes by Nye and Brower (1996) and Semin and Fiedler (1992). Most of this work does not address the concept of categorization directly, but one quite detailed recent approach of interest here is the *shared reality perspective* of Hardin and Higgins (1996). They suggest that subjective experience becomes objective when it is shared with other people. Hardin and Higgins argue that one of the implications of their account is that it implies more fluid representations than many other approaches. Fluid representation seems plausible because the social context is diverse and complex. The persons we perceive ourselves to share a reality with will vary from context to context, so this implies that our understandings and interpretations of reality should vary from situation to situation. This argument has immediate implications for representation in general, and categorization in particular. As we saw in Chapter 1, if we accept that how we categorize objects is a function of how we interpret the current situation, then it follows that we should categorize in the same way as do people with whom we share a reality. Hardin and Higgins's account therefore has much in common with many of the arguments of SCT despite some claims made by these authors which are based on relatively common misunderstandings of social identity theory (see Turner and Bourhis, 1996).

This conclusion about categorization was made explicit by self-categorization theorists such as McGarty and Turner (1992), Oakes and Turner (1990) and Oakes et al. (1994). Self-categorization theorists (Turner et al., 1987) describe categorization as an adaptive, flexible, context-dependent, sense-making process which rests on fluid representations of available information. They also suggest that we should categorize the world in the same way as do relevant other people. The relevance of other people is itself social categorical, and depends on the context. The process of self-categorization means that to a greater or lesser degree we see ourselves as readily interchangeable with other people. It follows that consensus about the interpretation of context should exist with people whom we categorize as being (relatively) identical with self (ingroup members), even though the salient level of self-categorization can vary instantly from context to context.

Thus the self-categorization and shared reality perspectives both endorse the ideas that consensus should play a key role in thinking about both social and non-social objects, and they both suggest that this implies a fluid and dynamic representational system. The question which then arises is how it is possible to integrate these ideas in the social mediation of the categorization process.

One proposal along these lines was McGarty and Turner's suggestion that categories are social norms:

> This perspective takes for granted that the categories that people actually use originate and are acquired in social interaction and that the social context is a major constraint on the way in which we categorize things. It supposes that categorizing

is a social normative activity anchored in our reference group memberships, as well as a cognitive process. (1992: 256)

There are two problems with this proposal: (a) the formal evidence of such a social normative activity in categorizing is extremely sparse, and (b) the concept of a norm is itself ill-defined (Turner, 1991). The first issue can only be resolved by collecting more data. The second matter, however, is amenable to theoretical elucidation.

In everyday language a norm is a socially desirable behaviour or belief. A more minimal definition is that a norm is something which is customary or common. Sherif defined norms as 'customs, traditions, standards, rules, values, fashions, and all other criteria of conduct which are standardized as a consequence of the contact of individuals' (1936: 3). This is the definition he adopted in his famous study using the autokinetic effect where he demonstrated that groups developed norms collaboratively in order to resolve ambiguous situations.

Hovland et al. define norms as 'standards, shared among the members of a group and representing the behaviour and attitudes they expect of one another' (1953: 136). Also picking up on the expectation idea, Biddle and Thomas (1966) argue that a norm is a generalized expectation about behaviour that is learned in the course of interactions with other members of society.

Turner (1991) notes that, despite their crucial role in understanding social influence, there is as yet no definitive scientific theory of what social norms are. He does, however, observe a number of points that relate to the usage of the term in social psychology. Norms suggest similarities within groups and differences between groups, but these are more than just accidental regularities and this is because social groups act to achieve consensus. Furthermore, norms seem to involve prescriptive rules or social values. They are generally forms of thinking, feeling or behaving that are endorsed and *expected* by some social group because these are perceived to be the 'right thing' to do or believe. Thus norms are more than just likings or preferences; they are *prescriptions*. Turner argues that norms are descriptive and prescriptive, but we would add to this that they can also be predictive (relating to expectations) and most generally that they are *explanatory* (see also Tajfel, 1981). By invoking the concept of explanation/justification we mean that norms serve to add meaning, or to enlighten. Formally, explanations can be viewed as answers to 'how' and 'why' questions. We make no strong distinction here between explanation, justification and rationalization from the point of view of the explainer (but see Chapter 10). One person's sound explanation may be another's weak rationalization.

In one sense this is similar to Turner's observation that acting in terms of social norms leads to subjective validity (Festinger, 1950), the belief that one's opinions or percepts are correct. We elaborate this point, however, by arguing that feelings of correctness follow from the development of consensual understandings/explanations.

Self-categorization theory (e.g., Turner, 1987) also argues that normative positions reflect ingroup consensuses, and we endorse this position here. However, we believe that such a definition illustrates how norms come into existence rather than the role that norms play in regulating thought and behaviour. Our proposal is that, cognitively speaking, norms are representations of the mind's operation as an interpretive/explanatory system. In particular, norms are explanations of behaviours or beliefs, whether they be planned, past or current.

Thus norms provide explanations or justifications for action. To the extent that the action is appropriate it will be seen in a positive light (i.e., it will be understood to reflect some current ingroup consensus) and will provide a basis for that action. Where some group consensus is not seen to explain or justify action then this is not a true norm. Instead it reflects the operation of a power process, where the individual is opposed to the will of an outgroup.

Note that it is not critical that the *details* of the explanation be cognitively available to the social actor for it to be a norm. It is only necessary that the actor believe that some ingroup expert has the explanation available (cf. Turner, 1987). In the sense proposed by Moscovici (1976), the facts of individual cognition are social norms.

What sort of explanations are categorizations? We argue here that categories are explanations of similarities and differences between things. This builds on McGarty and Turner's (1992; see also Haslam et al., 1996a; McGarty et al., 1993a) idea of *differentiated meaning*, which refers to the knowledge that members of different categories are coherently and clearly different. The role of these explanations as norms can be illustrated by the case of attitudes to abortion.

Almost everybody in Western cultures believes infanticide is wrong. This is accepted with utter conviction even though we might have to take stock for a few moments to marshal the arguments that would support it, if we were confronted by an opposing view (e.g., that infanticide reduces population pressure, or that sex-linked infanticide is appropriate in cultures where one sex is more highly valued). However, we are all aware of the dilemmas and conflicting intergroup beliefs which arise when the concept of infanticide is applied to the issue of abortion. Under these circumstances the same belief, which is supposedly consensual for everybody, becomes highly partisan. Abortion is routinely condemned as infanticide by pro-life groups, but it could also be *defended* by pro-choice groups as reducing the risk of child death and suffering. The conflict rests on two completely orthogonal interpretations of reality. In the one case the fundamental truth is that a foetus is a child, that is, this conceptualization of reality rests on a *categorization* of the foetus as a child. The alternative conceptualization says that regardless of whether you see a foetus as a child or not, the fundamental issue is the right of a woman to decide whether to have a child. It would be impossible for this social conflict to be sustained unless there were competing views of the classification of the foetus and the implications of this classification. In the terms I introduce in Chapter 11, pro-life and pro-choice have competing normative frameworks, that is, they have opposed standards for deciding what is true or false in relation to this issue.

The purpose of this example is to illustrate that categorical norms can reflect complex and consensual interpretations, explanations and justifications of action. These may be framed in terms of appeals to overarching societal values because it would be highly dysfunctional for people to have beliefs that were palpably inconsistent. While there are many people who oppose abortion and who see it as infanticide, there is almost certainly nobody who is both pro-choice and simultaneously believes abortion is infanticide (they may, however, be unsure as to whether it is infanticide or not, or may maintain that the issue is 'not about infanticide', just as the pro-life advocates would assert that the right to life overrules other rights). In constraint relations terms (see Chapter 1) category use is constrained by the category assignments that are known to be consensual within some ingroup.

Moreover the normative belief that abortion is wrong becomes intertwined with the justification of protest against abortion, the vilification of those who practise abortion, and in some cases the condoning of violent action against them. None of these beliefs stand in isolation from the relevant social categorization of pro-life versus pro-choice. It is difficult to imagine, for example, a pro-life group accepting the membership of someone who was perceived to have pro-choice beliefs.

Doise expresses the idea that categorizations come to be shared with others who categorize themselves to be the same in this way:

> Differentiations produced by different social memberships, common to a number of individuals, associate individual differentiations with social differentiations. Category differentiation is therefore a social psychological process relating individual activities to social activities through intergroup evaluations and representations. (1978: 152)

One can also consider stereotypes to be explanations of relations between groups. Both categories and stereotypes are normally linked to other explanatory constructs: thus one's stereotype of the unemployed is almost certainly linked to one's explanation of the causes of unemployment (Brown, 1999; Oakes et al., 1994). Those who believe unemployment is caused by apathy on the part of prospective workers will be more likely to perceive the unemployed as lazy, and those who believe that unemployment is caused by macro-economic conditions should be more likely to see the unemployed as unfortunate. Each stereotype not only explains why unemployed people are the way they are, but also explains and justifies collective and individual behaviour towards the unemployed. Very similar ideas have been developed independently by Yzerbyt and colleagues (see Yzerbyt et al., 1997; Leyens et al., 1994; see also Fiske, 1993; Kunda, 1990; Kunda and Thagard, 1996; Wittenbrink et al., 1998) who argue that stereotypes are enlightening Gestalts or explanatory frameworks (see Chapter 6). These authors review a range of previous approaches that suggest that stereotypes serve explanatory functions.

The role of consensus in the development of such explanations is critical, and the reasons for this follow straightforwardly from self-categorization theory. If we assume that the purpose of categorizations is to develop psychologically valid representations which explain similarities and differences then these should correspond to the categorizations developed by (relevant) similar others and be different from those of outgroup members. To the extent that categories are normative understandings of the world they should be shared with similar others.

One of the problems with showing social influences on the categorization process is that any previously existing categorization will involve prior experience and validation. There is a potentially infinite number of possible self-categorizations that could be invoked as the perceiver engages in cognitive activity to interpret any disagreement created by an experimental manipulation. Perhaps the most obvious of these is the interpretation of the situation as an experimental deception: that is, where the participants decide that the sources of the information they receive are not real people.

McGarty and Grace (1996) investigated the consensual development of categorizations, and the implications of these categorizations for the judgement of self and others. In particular we wanted to find out whether consensual categorizations have the qualities that are conventionally associated with social norms. Do people endorse the categorizations of their own group over those of other groups? Do they judge themselves and others in terms of acceptance of those categorizations?

Our preliminary research on this issue involved giving participants attitude statements and asking each group to develop their own categorizations of the statements. The participants then rated their own group's categorization as well as the categorizations of other groups of participants in the same session. The results showed that ingroup categorizations were rated far more positively than outgroup categorizations and that these results were consistent with some of the highest levels of ingroup bias ever obtained in experimental settings (they would be the first and fourth largest effect sizes if they had been included in Mullen et al.'s, 1992, meta-analysis of ingroup bias).

Our initial concern was to provide some evidence of the development of consensual categorizations, a process of considerable importance that has received almost no attention in the published literature of experimental social psychology. To this end the results of these studies provide a starting point for the investigation of this topic. They show that consensually developed categorizations function in much the same way as do other norms, and that they provide a basis for normative judgements.

We believe that the strength of the effects that we obtained derived in part from the fact that our experimental procedure *required* the participants to develop a consensual understanding. Very nearly all other experimental paradigms attempt to assign these understandings, or assume that the participants have access to such shared understandings. In general, a manipulation of the salience of a social categorization involves the assumption that identification with a group implies access and commitment to the norms of the group. This will often be the case, and it may even tend to be the case on average, but any instances where group members do not have access to the norms, or do not feel committed to them, will increase the level of non-group stereotypic behaviour, and will therefore inflate random error.

All of this suggests the need to examine the concept of ingroup bias more closely. If the results are to be interpreted as evidence of ingroup bias then it is the case that both studies reveal extremely large ingroup bias effects. Those who take the view that the results are nothing more than a demonstration of ingroup bias are left with the question of why effects that were larger than those reported in the reviewed literature occur under conditions where the factors that have previously been identified as the major contributors to the ingroup bias effect were not present. In McGarty and Grace's experiments the groups were experimentally constructed; there was no competition for scarce resources; there was no difference in power or prestige of the groups; the targets of the judgement were personally identifiable (and were in some cases friends, and in all cases classmates, of the participants) and were thus able to be individuated. If the results are to be interpreted as ingroup bias then the massive effect sizes demand a close re-examination of the variables which cause ingroup bias, and the studies suggest a useful paradigm for investigating it further.

Why should the ingroup bias effect be particularly strong when evaluating group products of this form? We think that the reason for the strength of the effects has to do with features of judging beliefs. In discussing these features, we address the question of whether it is useful to describe our results as ingroup bias. If they are not mere ingroup bias, then they can constitute either something more specific than ingroup bias, or something more general.

The arguments can be illustrated with some simple thought experiments about which we do not believe there will be substantially differing interpretations. We have chosen the examples in the rest of this section to directly engage the reader. This is a deliberate strategy because part of our argument is that processes of differentiation between persons and groups become more puzzling if we try to put ourselves outside the context of the behaviour we are trying to observe.

Imagine that we have two groups, one of black separatists and one of white separatists. The black separatists believe that 'black is beautiful' and the white separatists believe that 'white is beautiful'. It is possible for us to avoid endorsing either view, by instead endorsing the composite view that 'both black and white are beautiful'. Indeed if we gave a group of white, Western social psychologists a questionnaire with the two statements 'black is beautiful' and 'white is beautiful' and asked them to express their agreement with each on a Likert scale, we would expect them to show very little bias towards whites, and this would be because they endorsed the non-discriminatory norms that are reflected in the statement 'both black and white are beautiful'. For the sake of argument, let us assume that this is the consensual group norm for white, Western social psychologists (a group that we have chosen for the purpose of the example, because we all know from personal experience, empirical research etc. that the norms of this group are inconsistent with racial discrimination). Thus the white, Western social psychologists do not show bias towards whites, and we should not expect that they would in this case anyway because 'white people' is not the relevant ingroup in this setting. The norms they appeal to are those shared by other reasonable, tolerant people for whom their fellow social psychologists provide but one representative sub-group on this issue. If you do not believe this, try suggesting to a group of social psychologists that you think that racism is a good thing and see what sort of reaction you get.

However, if the social psychologists were now confronted with separatist groups who claim that '*only* black is beautiful' or '*only* white is beautiful' they would be unable to reconcile the competing norms. The social psychologists cannot draw the conclusion that both 'we' and 'they' are right, because when truth claims are framed in an oppositional manner, truth becomes a single indivisible prize that cannot be shared by two winners. Endorsement of the opposing view necessarily implies that our own view is wrong.

If we were to conduct a second thought experiment and give our sample of white Western social psychologists a questionnaire with two items and ask them for their level of agreement with the two items 'black is beautiful and white is beautiful' (representing their own norm) and 'only white is beautiful' (representing the separatist norm), we would expect a difference between the means that would surpass even the effect sizes that were obtained by McGarty and Grace, because of the oppositional nature of the truth claims.

If these thought experiments were carried out we would have obtained evidence that white, Western social psychologists showed no ingroup bias towards whites, but that they showed the highest level of ingroup bias that had ever been obtained in endorsing their own values and rejecting the values of an outgroup (i.e., white separatists). Should we conclude that social psychologists are particularly biased? Certainly the participants in the study would be rather displeased that their own obviously anti-racist opinions were being enlisted as evidence of bias. Our point is that the term 'ingroup bias' will inevitably be misleading when applied to judgements of beliefs because any statement of opinion is simultaneously a statement *both about the world and about the correctness of other people's opinions*. It is impossible to say that something is true without also implying that everybody who shares this opinion is right and everybody who disagrees is wrong (or at best less correct). The alternative, to say that those who disagree with us are right, immediately implies that our own views are wrong. As McGarty et al. (1993b) show, agreement can be attributed to mutual correctness, but disagreement about the same thing implies that somebody must be wrong.

In this sense judging the validity of opinions is a zero-sum process for both intergroup and interpersonal evaluation. It is easier to reconcile other features and aspects of groups and individuals in ways that would be said to be unbiased. We can, for example, choose to rate both groups as equally intelligent, fair or wealthy. In most allocation tasks it is possible to give equal allocations to other groups (see Mummendey and Schreiber, 1983).

Is it never possible for two different views to be right? To return to the particular example we have chosen, is not beauty in the eye of the beholder? One answer to this emerges if we change the group attribute from beauty to intelligence. We would expect many social psychologists and others who endorsed non-discriminatory norms to show a similar level of 'ingroup bias' when asked to choose between endorsing the views that 'people of different races have equal capacities for intelligence' and that 'white people are generally predisposed to be more intelligent than black people': the so-called 'ingroup bias' in this case would involve endorsing the anti-discriminatory norm in clear opposition to a view that many social scientists would see as racially motivated and even contemptible. Regardless of their positions we suspect few psychologists would accept that *both* views were right. They might accept that there is evidence for one or other of the alternatives, but many of us would say that this specific evidence has been misused to support a general principle (e.g., we might argue that IQ tests showing whites to be more intelligent than blacks are not culturally fair). The implication that we wish to draw is that it may be no more useful to call the empirical results obtained by McGarty and Grace 'ingroup bias' than it would be to apply the label to the behaviour of social psychologists in our thought experiments.

The question arises therefore whether judgements of truth and validity only result in stronger effects because of their zero-sum nature, which requires that we support one position or neither, but not both. That is, we can say that both the ingroup and the outgroup are intelligent, but it is far more difficult to say that both the ingroup and the outgroup are equally correct when they disagree. Judgements of validity are forced choices which are far more stark than the choices conventionally offered in, for example, the matrices used in the minimal group paradigm (Tajfel et al., 1971). In such matrices participants are often given a choice between being fair and discriminating in favour of one group or the other. For judgements of validity there is no equivalent choice of fairness, other than to say that *both* groups are wrong. We can, of course, say we agree to disagree, but this means no more than to say that we wish to change the topic.

Such reinterpretation is not limited to ratings by groups of people. Any dispute over fact or belief can have the same all-or-none character, and this includes disputes in opinion between individuals. We can read a journal article, disagree with the arguments it contains and give it a lower evaluation than we would give a paper we have written ourselves. This reflects a dispute over opinion. It is no more or less helpful to call the differing evaluations the 'interpersonal bias effect' than it would be to call it 'ingroup bias' when the negative evaluations are made by a group of people. Disputes between groups over matters of fact and belief will in part be more obvious because of the regularity that consensual beliefs impose on situations. This is because all of the members of one group disagreeing with another group will be much easier to detect in statistical analyses than when many individuals disagree with each other on many different dimensions in different ways. This is for much the same reasons that a clump of trees can be seen from a plane more easily than the same number of individual trees strung randomly across the countryside (this is a diagnosticity-based argument: see Chapter 8). Although our view is that groups play a particularly powerful role in the establishment of validity (cf. Moscovici, 1976; Turner, 1991) it is not necessary to accept the truth of this position for the analysis of ingroup bias to hold.

Given that these facts apply to any dispute about validity, several important points need to be made. We all know that everybody believes things that are not true: that is, for practical purposes nobody believes that they or anyone else is infallible on every issue. However, the equivalence between ourselves and other people ends at this point. As we have suggested throughout this chapter, people do not believe things that they know to be false (even if they are not sure that their beliefs are true) but we cannot make an equivalent assertion about other people. We can believe, charitably, that they also believe nothing *they know* to be false, but that they will nevertheless believe things that we know to be untrue unless they only believe the same things as us, or only believe things that are unknown to us.

Inevitably then, whatever merits we may see in other people's beliefs, and however large the deficiencies in our own beliefs, they must be superior to those of other people in at least this sense. We might not know much but at least we do not believe known falsehoods. Our own beliefs may be shown to be wrong at some future time but that remains a prospect. In contrast, other people's errors are revealed to us as soon as they disagree (providing we believe that they are reliably informing us of their beliefs, that is, they may

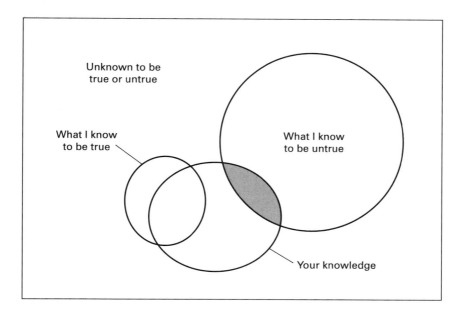

FIGURE 9.4 *Overview of what you and I, as individuals, know from my point of view*

even be mistaken about what they believe). The possibilities are shown in Figure 9.4. The relationships are shown for a dichotomous view of truth but the same arguments can be made about beliefs about which we are uncertain: I believe nothing that is probably untrue. I would add that the figure does not include all forms of ignorance and there are other intersections of the concepts that have been explored by Smithson (e.g., 1996) to deal with ignorance.

The problem with your knowledge from my point of view is that the shaded region is potentially non-zero (as it is also from your point of view when considering my knowledge). This is despite the fact that I assume here that the totality of your knowledge is greater than mine and that the two overlap considerably. The problem is not that you will continue to believe falsehoods after you discover them to be false, but that you can continue to believe falsehoods after *I* discover them to be false (especially if I do not inform you).

For the shaded region to be zero you have to believe nothing that I know that I do not also know to be untrue. Even if this condition did hold you would scarcely be able to convince me of it without revealing to me the entire contents of your knowledge (something which is scarcely practicable unless we constrain relevant knowledge in some way – see below). Thus we should all consider ourselves to be more faithful informants than anyone else, at least in the sense that we cannot make this sort of error.

The problem is compounded if we move from beliefs to assertions. If I say that 'Everything I say is a lie' or you say 'Everything I say is a lie' we create a logical paradox (the famous Cretan Liar's Paradox of Epimenides), but if you or I say 'Everything *you* say is a lie' we have made a harsh but perfectly intelligible judgement about the target's morality or psychopathology. I would make an additional claim here that disputes about validity create these logical paradoxes; in other words it is meaningless to make self-referential statements of falsehood because such statements do not relate to the logical possibilities that confront people in their everyday lives.

So-called ingroup or self-serving bias can therefore be seen as a rational response to the logical conditions confronting every individual. Does this mean that we should always see ourselves as more reliable informants than everybody else? Is this an argument for solipsism or scepticism?

Of course not. For a start, the shaded region may be rarely engaged when we deal with people who have different domains of knowledge. An astronomer who faithfully recounts his or her knowledge of certain stars to me may tell me very little that I know to be untrue because his or her knowledge may not contradict mine, or it may only contradict those beliefs about which I am already uncertain. The other person can know more than me, they can be right more often than I am, but nevertheless they are capable of making a specific error that I cannot.

Secondly, the representation of knowledge in Figure 9.4 represents a snapshot at a particular point of time. What we know to be true can vary from situation to situation with learning and context. Let us suppose you learn that I am angry at some time (something we both know). I later calm down without you becoming aware of it. Your knowledge of my emotional state, although correct at some earlier time, is now incorrect. I would suggest that a very large part of the shaded region relates to self-knowledge, that is, knowledge that pertains to the status of our own abilities, attitudes, emotions and behaviours.

Thirdly and very importantly, knowing or believing that something is true or untrue does not guarantee that it is true or untrue (see Chapter 11). In the example above, I may *think* that I am no longer angry but in fact still be angry. However, we are guided by our understanding of events in the world, that is, the facts as we know them and not the facts as they exist in the world (if we knew the facts to be otherwise we would change our beliefs). My argument is that a degree of scepticism is a rational response to the facts as they are known to the perceiver at that time, and that it is a logically respectable response to those facts and not to the world in general.

Finally, social categorization provides the means to align the domains of knowledge so that the shaded area is small or non-existent for our relations with members of a relevant ingroup. This is because the differences become irrelevant to the current situation. Disagreement draws our attentions to the false beliefs of others. The shaded region is a strong basis for differentiation between ourselves and other persons but it is also a strong basis for differentiating between ingroups and outgroups. Outgroups believe things that we *know* to be untrue, and what is more, they commonly persist in these beliefs despite exposure to the truth, and in fact frequently polarize or shift their own positions further from the truth when they are exposed to it (see discussions of the effects of group membership on group polarization and persuasion, e.g., Hogg et al., 1990; Mackie and Cooper, 1984; Mackie et al., 1990; McGarty et al., 1994; Turner et al., 1989; A. van Knippenberg and Wilke, 1988; D. van Knippenberg and Wilke, 1992; Wilder, 1990). On the other hand, ingroup members seek to minimize the degree of disagreement between ourselves and them through mutual influence. Thus, social categorization makes the 'shaded region' small or irrelevant for ingroup members and large or relevant for outgroup members.

If disputes about truth provide such a fundamental basis for differentiation, then it is not surprising that when we shift the focus of the disagreement from the evaluation of beliefs to behavioural and evaluative dimensions, the rational justification for interpersonal and intergroup differentiation becomes stronger. Outgroups are not just people who persist in wrong-headed beliefs but are frequently people who discriminate against us (though admittedly only where that is consistent with the norms of their groups). It is unreasonable to expect that people could lead their lives without developing expectations about the differences between the groups they belong to and those they do not in terms of their rationality and fairness.

Imagine the situation in these terms. You encounter two groups of people, and on the basis of your previous experience with groups you know that one of them is less likely to hold views which you know to be wrong, and that that group is also less likely to become *more entrenched* in false views when the truth is exposed to it, and that it is less likely to discriminate against you when it gets the opportunity. (The relative strengths of these factors could be of variable importance. The behavioural interaction model of Rabbie and colleagues assumes that the last of them has a determining role: see Rabbie et al., 1989, and Turner and Bourhis, 1996.) Which group would you prefer to support under those circumstances? Obviously the answer is the reasonable and fair one, and not coincidentally this will tend to be the one you belong to. The available research data suggest that in allocation tasks people tend to favour the ingroup (tempering this by fairness), but with minimal groups at least, they do not necessarily tend to punish the outgroup when given the opportunity (see Mummendey, 1995). People do not always discriminate against real or minimal outgroups in terms of allocations or punishment (even though their self-perception may be highly depersonalized) because there are alternative ways of expressing or obtaining a positive social identity which are consistent with the norms of certain groups (e.g., by being charitable or trying to understand the reasons for the disagreement: see Turner and Bourhis, 1996).

Discrimination against outgroups may thus be seen as a watered-down version of processes of differentiation between people in terms of the validity of their opinions. We say 'watered down' in the sense that discrimination or hostility towards some group is a possible response to the situation, but the experience that those who hold beliefs that you know to be wrong are themselves wrong and different is inevitable. Where their errors occur on particularly important dimensions, and in particular their errors lead to actions that challenge the norms of the ingroup though, hostility is inevitable.

Serendipitously then, McGarty and Grace's results may have been helpful in revealing the most powerful form of what is called ingroup bias because we focused on judgements of validity. These judgements make the connection between being different and being wrong most obvious. Other group judgement situations should make this oppositional nature less stark and produce weaker effects, but potentially any difference between any two people, or any two groups, on any attitudinal or normative dimension implies that one or both parties is wrong and this disagreement requires a resolution (Hogg and Abrams, 1993, have argued that uncertainty reduction is the basis of group motivation, but see the first section of this chapter). Thus the general phenomenon that subsumes ingroup bias appears to be the evaluation of disagreement, as disagreement inevitably implies that *somebody's* beliefs must be wrong. If we take the further step and assume that truth and validity are themselves derived from social normative processes within groups then we have the foundations of an analysis of the social influences of cognition, which returns us to the concerns with which we began this section. Regardless of whether these steps are taken, the strong implication of our analysis is that it is time for social psychologists to move beyond the term and the connotations of the 'ingroup bias' effect (see also Turner and Bourhis, 1996; Turner and Oakes, 1997).

Conclusion

This chapter dealt with two global issues in the study of social categorization. The first is that it is important and useful to distinguish social categorization from feelings of belongingness and from feeling good about belonging to a group. The approach adopted in the first section of this chapter involves a direct application of SCT principles with minor embellishments and suggests the prospect of a coherent overview.

The same degree of closure cannot be provided for the material in the second section of this chapter. The development of shared categorizations is a neglected area in the field and this is not surprising when we consider the complexities that exist. Having said that, the idea that categories are social norms and that social norms are explanations holds considerable promise.

Most importantly, in line with Doise's (1978) arguments, this discussion shows how categorical differentiation is a social psychological process because we categorize and evaluate in the same way as other people. The argument we have made here is that categorizations involving validity are inevitably shared or contested with others. Claims about truth which are shared with other people inevitably imply that either both we and they are right or both we and they are wrong. Disagreement demands that one or both of us are wrong, and given that we only hold beliefs which are correct it follows that we necessarily believe that others who disagree are wrong to that extent. There is a tendency in social psychology to refer to the inevitably more positive evaluations of our own views than those of others as 'ingroup bias' when those evaluations are shared with relevant others. This is a mistake in general and is highly ironic in particular if we take the view that the standards of truth and accuracy are themselves social norms which are shared with other people. We have made the strong claim though that conceptions of truth have powerful consequences for social interaction and the implications of categorizations. A large part of Chapter 11 is devoted to discussing the standards by which truth is assessed. Before we get there, though, the idea of covariation as a linking concept between categorization and explanation is discussed in Chapter 10.

10 Categorization, Covariation and Causal Explanation

Bruner (1957) and others have argued that categorization is a sense-making process, but it seems difficult to understand what this means unless we equate 'making sense of' with 'explaining'. The process of explanation has been widely held to depend on covariation too. The argument explored in this chapter therefore lies in answering the following double-barrelled question: do categorization and explanation both rest on the perception of covariation because categorization and explanation are really the same thing?

This answer to this question rests upon developments in cognitive and social psychology in relation to the process of covariation. I address these developments here. The first step in this chapter is to ask: if we take the idea that categorizations are explanations seriously, then how is the background knowledge that constrains categorizations organized? In the first section I therefore consider and reject the conventional assumption that background knowledge is hierarchically organized in terms of tree structures.

A. Hierarchies and overlap

One of the many difficult issues in the study of social categorization is the question of how to understand the structure of categorical systems and their constraining effect on category use. In some ways, these matters are simplified by SCT because it assumes (a) that the horizontal and vertical structure of categories is defined by fit principles, and (b) that categories are constructed spontaneously for particular needs rather than being recalled from memory.

Nevertheless a categorization scheme involves assumptions about structure even if those categories are not themselves long-lasting. SCT assumes, for example, that levels in a hierarchy can be defined in terms of inclusiveness, and that higher-order categories can include but never be included by lower-level categorizations. SCT also makes it clear that inclusiveness is the necessary feature to define the levels of a hierarchy and that position in a hierarchy cannot be determined by the attributes associated with a particular category.

Sloman (1998) presents several problems with class inclusion hierarchies clear. Logically speaking, every subordinate member of a superordinate category should have all of the properties that are shared by members of that superordinate category. Thus hierarchies should provide an unambiguous basis for inference. If we know that all birds have wings and that an exron is a bird then we can infer that an exron has wings. Nevertheless, the evidence of such inferences is tenuous. This is because reasoners, and in particular young children, have difficulty in making inferences of this form even when they have correctly identified the relevant categorical relations. One example of the problems involved is that class-inclusion hierarchies were often misunderstood to be part–whole relations. That is, superordinate categories were often assumed to be collections of things rather than classes of things. Children would, when asked to report an instance of a superordinate category like 'tree', give several instances. Similarly adult reasoners would accept that 'A car headlight is a kind of lamp' and that 'A lamp is a kind of furniture' but not that 'A car headlight is a kind of furniture.'

Sloman's own research has established evidence for *inclusion similarity* and *premise specificity*. Reasoners prefer inferences which involve subordinate categories which are typical of or similar to the superordinate, and reasoners prefer inferences where the premises are of a similar specificity to the target category. An example of the former would be that reasoners prefer inference from a feature of all birds to a feature of sparrows (typical bird) than to a feature of ducks (atypical). An example of the latter is that reasoners prefer to make inferences from a feature of all birds to sparrows than from all animals to sparrows even though in logical terms these arguments are equally strong.

In fact, Sloman points out the neglect of category inclusion makes little difference to reasoning because very few categories have a hierarchical organization that provides such a sound basis of inference. The world is full of exceptions and categories which are only partially distinct and only a small proportion of the classes we encounter have a hierarchy which is as clear as that of the biological taxonomy.

This, of course, returns us to Wittgenstein's observation that was at the core of the criticism of the classical view of categories. Useful superordinate categories such as 'game' do not have all-or-none defining features so it would be impossible in any case to make inferences about *all* of the members of these categories. Thus, if we were to reason about what features something like a game had we would probably assume that it involved competition and fun, without demanding that it must have either of those features. In the same way, we would expect something we knew to be a mammal to have fur and not to lay eggs. However, if we were to make inferences on the basis of class inclusion we would also make frequent errors and this applies even with biological categories. We expect dogs to have four legs but not *all* dogs have four legs. It makes sense therefore that human reasoning should be attuned to the fuzziness of classes in the world that perceivers encounter and the categories that they generate.

Oakes et al. (1994) use the example of the categorization of English speakers into sub-groups such as Australians, Britons and Americans with individual exemplars (i.e., people who make up these groups). I have reproduced a similar example in Figure 10.1.

I think that the tree diagram metaphor for category structure fails to

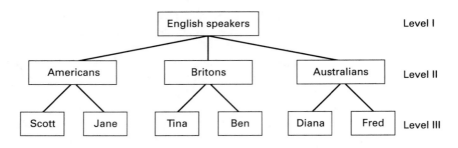

FIGURE 10.1   *An example of hierarchical categorical relations envisaged under SCT (after Oakes et al., 1994)*

capture much of the richness that is contained within any categorical system, and the self-categorization theory treatment of categorical systems partly reflects the limitations of this metaphor. Of course these criticisms apply to other formulations which assume that knowledge is hierarchically organized.

Self-categorization theory (assumption A.5 of Turner et al., 1987) holds that self-categorizations exist as part of a hierarchical system of classification so that each lower-level category is entirely included within one category at the higher level but is not exhaustive of it. The other important assumption in this context (A7.2) is that comparison between stimuli involves seeing them as the same or similar at some more abstract level that includes both of them. Comparison then occurs on dimensions that define their higher-level identity. Thus Scott and Jane would be compared as Americans whereas Scott and Ben would be compared as English speakers. I will term these three restrictions placed by SCT on categorical hierarchies as (a) the unique inclusion condition, (b) the exhaustion condition, and (c) the least abstraction condition. These conditions reflect some of the problems that can stem from the tree diagram metaphor (see also Sloman, 1998).

The unique inclusion condition is tenuous. Categories (of the mind and of the world) overlap at the same level of abstraction. Scott, for example, could be both Australian and American. Of course, non-overlapping categorizations can be derived through a process of meta-contrast, but this of itself implies that unique inclusion should be a function of salience and not a pre-determined and fixed property of the hierarchy. Where the American–Australian social categorization is salient, the perceived overlap of the categories should be reduced and Scott should be seen to be less proto-typical of Australians to the degree that he is also seen to be American. Put simply, the problem with unique inclusion echoes the old problem that categories do not have defining features (Wittgenstein, 1974) and that categories do not have fixed boundaries (Rosch, 1978).

Similar problems were addressed in 1970s research in categorization through the concept of *cue validity* (Rosch et al., 1976a). The cue validity of a feature *i* is the conditional probability that an entity belongs to category *j* given that feature *i* is present.

To illustrate the problems for any construct in SCT which were to be used as a substitute for cue validity, consider the natural object hierarchy in Figure 10.2, where there are animals belonging to five different species and there are six categories/attributes. I presume here that the categorical system relates to some perceiver's knowledge of the world at some instant.

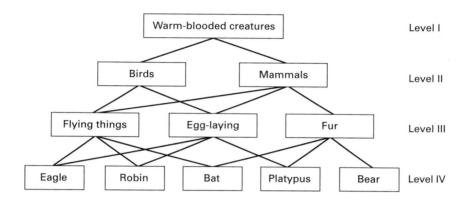

FIGURE 10.2   *Overlapping, hierarchical categorical relations*

This hierarchy fails the unique inclusion condition because lower-level categories belong to more than one higher-level category. It is important to note that as soon as such overlap between categories exists the inclusion relations become ambiguous for level I and level II. That is, we could redraw the system with the category 'bird' as an element of the categories 'flying things' and 'egg-laying' and so on.

Is it possible to consider hierarchies that could meet the SCT conditions for this natural object category system? The answer is that it is, but only if we introduce an additional level as in Figure 10.3.

This structure satisfies the unique inclusion condition but now fails the exhaustion condition because certain lower-level categories are exhaustive of higher-level categories. The first conclusion I would draw is that SCT's exhaustion condition should be relaxed. It serves no apparent purpose for the theory and potentially introduces some errors. For this categorical system the conjunction of egg-laying and flying is an all-or-none defining feature for birds, and fur is an all-or-none defining feature for mammals. Although such defining features may be extremely rare, categorical systems should have the facility to incorporate them where they do exist. Sloman's (1998) experiment 4 showed that people do take full account of inclusion relations when the inclusion relations are made accessible.

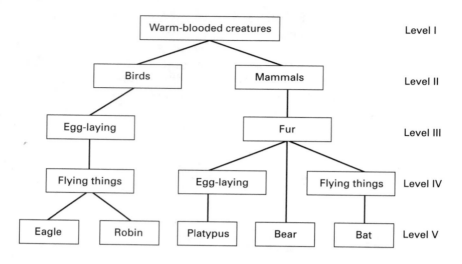

FIGURE 10.3   *An overlapping hierarchy reordered into a tree structure*

However, the least abstraction prediction is counter-intuitive for this system. If flying is treated as a separate feature of all birds and some mammals then this implies that eagles and bats can be compared as warm-blooded creatures and not as flying creatures. Of course, it might be argued that making a comparison between bats and eagles will invoke a different hierarchy, but this begs the question of what the hierarchy is for. If certain comparisons lead to the categorical system being supplanted by another hierarchical system that is more suitable for comparison, then we are entitled to ask: what do we need hierarchies for? The answer seems to be, surprisingly little.

A series of critical questions about hierarchies needs to be put. Is it plausible, given the prevalence of overlapping categories, that perceivers would develop categorical hierarchical systems which dealt with overlap so poorly?

Still other questions relate to differences between particular levels of self-categorizations. Higher-order categories can be seen as attributes of lower-order categories – thus English speaking can be seen as an attribute of Americans – but it is also the case that lower-order categories with high cue validity can be seen as attributes of higher-order categories. Thus, fur can be seen as an attribute of mammals, and mammalian can be an attribute of furry creatures. The same is not true where the reciprocal cue validity relations do not hold. Thus egg-laying is an attribute of birds, but bird-like is not an attribute of egg-laying creatures. This is because being a bird implies a creature lays eggs, but laying eggs does not imply a creature is a bird.

Whether cue validity relations are reciprocal or not is highly informative about possible causal relations. Egg-laying is an all-or-none defining feature for birds in this hierarchy, but birds are not the only egg-laying creatures. This implies that something about being a bird could lead to egg-laying. However, it is not true that some feature of egg-layers makes them birds. Note that relations like the first one satisfy the unique inclusion condition. This implies that although SCT may have been overly restrictive in imposing this condition on hierarchies, unique inclusion does allow strong inferences about possible causal relations.

There are also limits to the possible level of covariation between categories at the bottom of the hierarchy. Elements at the bottom of a hierarchy can only be seen to be the same to the extent to which they share some higher-order category. Higher-order categories, however, can be the same (overlap) to the extent that they share *subordinate members*. Thus eagles and robins are the same in the overlapping version of the hierarchy depicted in Figure 10.3 to the extent that they are both flying birds. Flying creatures and egg-laying can be seen to be similar to the extent that they are both attributes of birds, but the categories are also the same to the extent that they share some of the same exemplars (eagles and robins).

When we replace the tree diagram metaphor with a metaphor that does deal with overlap then many of the logical problems disappear. The alternative is, of course, Venn diagrams as used in classical and fuzzy set theory (Zadeh, 1965; and in fact tree diagrams are special cases of Venn diagrams). When we use Venn diagrams to show overlap we do not have to make any assumption about the hierarchical ordering of categories other than that the things belong to categories. The only knowledge that perceivers need to have therefore is of overlap between categories and membership of exemplars within those categories. From this, knowledge of association, hierarchies can be deduced but hierarchies are not necessary for logical inference.

Thus for the natural object categories the set of Venn relations in Figure 10.4 serves to capture knowledge.

Up to this point I have skirted around the temporal status of the categorical system. SCT holds that the actual categorizations used are created for particular purposes rather than being retrieved from memory. It also holds that these categories are derived in part from background knowledge which is relatively enduring. I suggested in Chapters 5 and 7 that even if categories are constructed afresh on every occasion the background knowledge must itself take account of categories (and it would seem strange if we could not store categorical knowledge). To take an example from Chapter 9, long-term identification cannot contribute to perceivers' readiness to see themselves as belonging to some group unless perceivers know what that group is and associate themselves with that category.

It is also important to note though that classical set theory is not immune to problems in relation to overlap. As Osherson and Smith (1981) argued, and others have demonstrated, the intersection of two sets does not necessarily behave in a manner that would be well understood by classical set theory.

To summarize the section so far, hierarchical categorical systems with tree structures provide deficient models for representing relatively enduring background knowledge. This suggests to me that background knowledge instead takes the form of knowledge of the features of exemplars and knowledge of

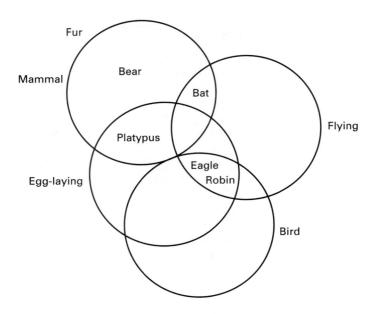

FIGURE 10.4   *A Venn diagrammatic representation of the hierarchy*

covariation/association between features. I use the term 'feature' here to refer to a characteristic in background knowledge; I will retain the term 'category' for the recognition that some set of exemplars shares a feature.

This approach is a compromise between SCT and Smith and Zárate's (1992) exemplar model of social judgement in that a role for abstraction-level phenomena (covariation between features) is retained. However, the idea of a hierarchy is dispensed with except in two senses: (a) categories can include exemplars but exemplars cannot include categories, and (b) hierarchies can be abstracted from the categorical system in particular circumstances, and can guide understanding once developed, but they have no central causal role. Thus a hierarchy may reflect our current understanding of some set of objects (as the biological taxonomy does), and a hierarchy may be used to make inferences where it has been developed (as biologists would do), but the hierarchy does not reflect how we come to understand those objects.

The usefulness of the Venn diagram approach for self-categories can be seen if we return to the example from Chapter 5 of the quote from Einstein:

> If my theory of relativity is proven successful, Germany will claim me as a German and France will declare that I am a citizen of the world. Should my theory prove untrue France will say I am a German and Germany will declare that I am a Jew.

According to Einstein the category he is assigned to will depend upon social comparative relations between himself and particular perceivers. Although the structure that is implied in this system appears to be elegantly described by a hierarchical system there are in fact some problems which allow us to elaborate the issues raised above.

First, there appears to be a well-described hierarchical relationship so that citizens of the world, Germans and Jews are categories of decreasing inclusiveness (and that this categorical system could even be consensually shared by all people). The response of a person who seeks to differentiate themselves from Einstein-the-failure should be to accentuate perceived differences between self and Einstein by assigning Einstein to a category that does not include the self. For German non-Jews that category is *Jew*, for the French that category is *German*. The response of the person who seeks to associate self with Einstein should be to assign him to the least abstract category which includes the self. For Germans this is Germans and for the French it is citizens of the world.

The problem with this structure is the overlap between the categories 'German' and 'Jew' and the ambiguity about the differing inclusiveness of these categories. Would Germans (non-Jews) perceive Einstein as a German Jew or as a Jew? The point is that the overlap between the categories makes the level of inclusiveness of these categories ambiguous (Feldman, 1988, and the earlier example make clear that such overlap may be equally common with natural object categories). The problem arises because Jew is simultaneously a sub-group of Germans, non-Germans and citizens the world.

In Figure 10.5 the letter E represents Einstein in the intersection of the sets Germans and Jews. In Figure 10.6 the category to which Einstein is assigned by the perceiver under conditions of success and failure is shown by cross-

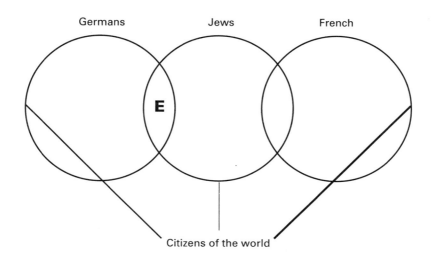

FIGURE 10.5   *Possible characterizations of Einstein (E)*

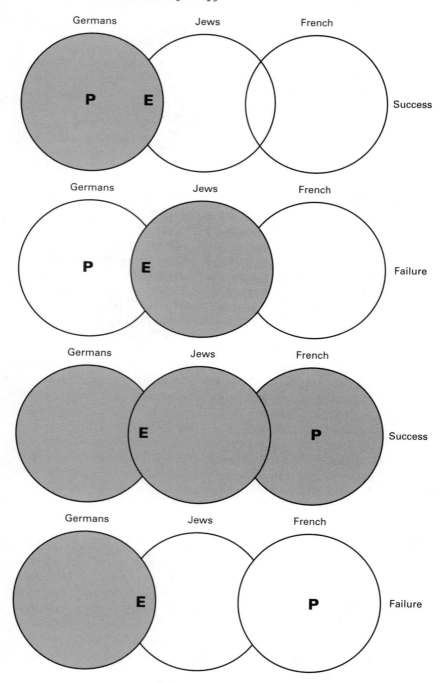

FIGURE 10.6   *Characterizations of Einstein (E) by the Germans and the French (perceivers P) under conditions of success and failure*

hatching and the position of the perceiver is represented by the letter P. For ease of representation 'citizens of the world' are limited to the French, Germans and Jews of those and other nations.

This representation requires us to differentiate between background knowledge about membership of social groups and the specific categorization that is salient. As I have pointed out previously, this knowledge must itself take a categorical form and must be informative about category memberships, category overlap and covariation. Developments on the theory-coherence approach discussed in Chapter 3 have stressed the importance of correlated attributes and, given the importance of covariation and overlap, the link between the two must be explored. This is something I do in the next section. For the moment though, I suggest that knowledge of covariation helps us to make attributions. If we know that there is a weak association between being Jewish and being German we will not expect to meet many Jews in Germany and we can make informed guesses about whether some person we meet in Germany is likely to be Jewish. Similarly, on the basis of knowledge of relations between minorities and majorities elsewhere we might be able to generate expectations about the role and place of Jews in German society (these features are, of course, part of what makes the quote from Einstein memorable and significant).

If we dispense with hierarchies as organizing principles (with the caveats noted) then this suggests that the third condition imposed by SCT also needs to be relaxed. SCT's least abstraction prediction holds that in order for objects to be compared they must be seen as identical at some superordinate level. The current covariation approach places no restrictions on comparison other than knowledge of whether or not the two things share some feature.

For this purpose I need to distinguish features from attributes. Under this view attributes are attributions. That is, attributes are perceived covariations between categories which serve *to explain* the similarities and differences between groups. Returning to the example above, the difference between self and other that must be explained when Einstein fails is his failure. This failure is attributed to a relevant difference between self and other, the attribute that becomes relevant to explain this failure (being wrong) is 'Jewish' for Germans and 'German' for French. When Einstein succeeds (being right) the attribute that explains the success is the shared identity as a citizen of the world (for the French) or as a German. These ideas were clearly anticipated by Oakes et al. (1991) who argued that the fit between a social categorization and an individual's behaviour contributes most to salience when it implies a meaningful explanation of the person's behaviour. Of course, this argument can be readily extended to features other than behaviour.

In summary, hierarchies appear to be a defective system for understanding the ways in which background knowledge constrains categorization. Venn diagrams which allow us to describe covariation appear to be more helpful, and it is to the broad issue of covariation that we now turn.

To close this section though, the idea that hierarchies are a possible outcome of the categorization process rather than an antecedent or organizing principle for categorization does have some positive implications for creating the conditions for cooperation between groups. Presentations of SCT and developments on it such as the work of Mummendey and Wenzel (1997) suggest that a hierarchy is a precondition for comparison. My argument is that hierarchies are outcomes of comparison and differentiation that are highly useful in particular circumstances. I agree entirely with the SCT perspective that the creation of effective long-term cooperation rests on forming a superordinate categorization. The positive aspect of my suggestions is that those superordinate categorizations will commonly represent completely new understandings of relations between people rather than engaging dormant ones (see Eggins, forthcoming). I would argue, for example, that the success or failure of the environmental movement in creating a global conscience hinges on developing in people a new understanding of themselves as citizens of the world rather than engaging a previously dormant superordinate level.

B. Categorization and covariation

Cheng (1997) addresses the way in which reasoners abstract causal links from covariation. She sees previous attempts as being derived from two approaches: statistical contingency theories (following Hume) and causal power theories (following Kant).

The former advocate the idea that the mind can abstract cause from statistical regularities. This idea is at the core of Kelley's (1967) ANOVA model of causal attribution in social psychology. The models hold that if reasoners note that some event i precedes some other event e then this allows them to conclude that i is the cause for e, especially where it is also true that e does not occur in the absence of i. The chief problem with these models is that such covariation, even where completely reliable, does not demand that i causes e. This can be illustrated by the oft-quoted example of roosters and sunrise. Although roosters always crow before the sunrise this does not mean that crowing causes the sun to rise.

Kelley's (1967) attribution theory is an example of a covariational approach. This theory assumes that everyday explanations of people's responses to stimuli at particular times can be distinguished in terms of dimensions related to the person, the stimulus and the occasion. If we consider a piece of behaviour such as 'Mary laughed at the comedian' then the attribution of this behaviour to something about Mary, something about the comedian, or something about the occasion, or some conjunction of these factors, can be considered as resulting from a process of analysis of variance (ANOVA). If the reasoner had enough data they should be able to identify the cause with confidence. Thus, if the reasoner saw that Mary commonly laughed at the clown they could conclude that it was nothing to do with this particular occasion, and if the reasoner saw that everybody laughed at the clown on this occasion that it was nothing to do with Mary.

One problem with this account is that it does not deal with commonly reported tendencies for reasoners to give greater prominence to causes to do with persons than to causes involving the occasion or stimulus that were of ostensibly equal importance. Cheng and Novick's (1990) probabilistic contrast model deals with this problem. This model holds that, providing some candidate cause occurs prior to the effect, a cause's contingency can be evaluated over a (contextually determined) set of events that the reasoner uses as inputs to the covariation process. This set of inputs is called the *focal set* and it is contextually determined in the sense that it is a selected subset of the universal set of events. For simple events the degree of covariation perceived depends on the contrast (or difference) between the probability of the event given the candidate cause minus the probability of the event in the absence of the candidate cause.

The probabilistic contrast model explains the tendency for perceivers to favour explanations involving persons rather than situations. This reflects not so much a bias but the different focal sets used by experimenters and participants in social psychological experiments. In short, participants include events in their focal sets that are drawn from relevant personal experiences. That is, their focal sets are broader than the experimenters intended them to be. Although the actual content of these personal experiences varies from person to person, and might be expected to be a source of random error rather than bias, the effect of personal experiences in most cases is to broaden the range of the focal set. Broadening of any kind is likely to affect causal judgements in the same way. Cheng and Novick (1990) demonstrated the effect of these factors by showing that causal judgements were affected by manipulating information that experimenters customarily treat as irrelevant.

The probabilistic contrast model also allows a distinction between causes and enabling conditions (Cheng and Novick, 1991; 1992; cited by Cheng, 1997). A causal candidate *i* is an enabling condition for a cause *j* if it is constantly present in some focal set, but covaries with the effect *e* in some other focal set. The example Cheng uses is that oxygen would be seen to be an enabling condition for forest fires and not a cause of them. However, in a broader focal set that included environments which were oxygen-free, the contrast provided by oxygen would be noted and it could be seen as a cause.

The other class of theories relies less on statistical regularities and more on reasoners' background knowledge and their search for mechanisms which make it possible for event *i* to be the cause for event *e*. This knowledge includes the general principle that all events have causes. Thus, as no mechanism exists by which rooster crowing could be a plausible cause for sunrise, it is not seen to be a cause.

Cheng's first criticism of the causal power approach is that it is non-computational. She articulates this by saying that the way in which the general knowledge that 'all events have causes' constrains inferences made in specific settings has not been made clear.

The other criticism is that the definition of causal power is circular. How do we know that crowing is not an adequate mechanism to produce the sunrise, if we have not previously made some causal inference about what crowing can and cannot do? That is, the causal power theories assume that causal inferences are based on prior causal inferences. This pushes back the issue of how causal inferences are made one step in time. Suppose that the inference that crowing does not produce the sunrise is based on the knowledge that crowing (or making noises of any kind) does not have the power to affect massive objects at a distance such as the sun. This then raises the question of how the reasoner came to make this inference about the limits on the power of crowing, and suggests the possibility of infinite regression. Cheng suggests that the only alternative to this regression is for knowledge of causal powers to be innate.

Such problems of infinite regression can be overstated and I think Cheng does this here. It could be the case that all causal inferences made by an adult reasoner rest upon prior causal inferences. The problem of regression can be pushed back to some point where the reasoner has used some other process to make causal inferences such as a contingency-based process. Thus, another solution to the circularity problems with causal power theory could be a developmental shift from causal inference based on covariation to causal inference based on causal power. The proviso being that as the method of causal inference changes, the prior inferences would be retained as a basis for future inferences despite the fact that the method they were derived from may subsequently be considered questionable. The original source of even a solar astronomer's knowledge that the sun is far away may be the authority of a parent or an illustrated story book. Ahn et al. (1995, experiment 2) shows that reasoners in an information-seeking task who sought covariational information tended to do so in the early stages of the reasoning process. This suggests that covariation may provide a source of heuristics for generating mechanism-based information.

Cheng probably unfairly includes Ahn et al. (1995) as examples of researchers who adopt the causal power approach. In fact, these authors argued for a mechanism-based approach that was complementary to the covariation approach, and which includes ideas which are very similar in parts to some of the ideas developed by Cheng (1997) discussed below. Ahn et al. (1995) also suggest that as covariation- and mechanism-based processes play different roles it is meaningless to argue that one is more important than the other.

Ahn et al. (1995) argue that one of the best but as yet neglected empirical approaches to causal inference is to look at reasoners' preferences for information in reasoning settings. If it is the case that reasoners engage in a form of statistical reasoning then this should be reflected in the type of information that reasoners seek out from the environment.

They distinguished between two broad classes of information: ANOVA-type information and mechanism information. ANOVA-type information relates to information about the variation of factors that are potentially implicated in causing some effect (as per Kelley's, 1967, attribution theory). Mechanisms relate to explanatory processes that could bring about the effect e when candidate cause i occurs.

To justify this idea Ahn et al. (1995) cite Gopnik and Nellman's distinction between empirical generalizations and theoretical entities. Empirical generalizations involve orderings of evidence using the same basic vocabulary that is used to describe the evidence. Theoretical entities are causal, explanatory entities that use a different vocabulary to the evidence. Although it is possible to push the vocabulary-based distinction too far, this would seem consistent with linguistic variations that are predicted by the linguistic category model (Semin and Fiedler, 1988). Researchers using the linguistic category model have found that concrete terms such as descriptive action verbs (like 'John *hit* Ben') are used to describe behaviours which are inconsistent with stereotypic expectations, and that abstract language is used to describe behaviours which are consistent with stereotypic expectations (e.g., 'John *punished* Ben'; see Maass and Arcuri, 1992). In terms of Ahn et al.'s arguments the abstract language involves a theoretical entity that serves to explain the action.

For Ahn et al. (1995) causal explanation involves looking for covariations and mechanisms which would produce them. People believe covariations without such mechanisms are spurious and therefore look for the underlying mechanisms. They contrast this idea with the information-seeking strategy predicted by the covariation approach. When explaining a single event, the covariation-based reasoner should start out with candidate causes and seek information about the covariation between candidate factors and effects. The mechanism-based reasoner instead searches for information about that particular event that suggests a mechanism.

We can contrast these two approaches as being molar on the one hand and molecular on the other. The covariational approach involves attempting to establish the existence of explanatory principles by stepping back to look at the big picture. The mechanism-based approach involves tightening the focus of observation on the specific event.

In their empirical research Ahn et al. (1995) find that information-seeking reasoners have a clear and strong preference for mechanism-based information over covariation information. Thus, when given an event to explain such as 'Harry punched Jack', participants were more likely to request information of the form 'Does Harry dislike Jack?' than information of the form 'Has Harry punched Jack on other occasions?', 'Has Harry punched other people?' or 'Have other people punched Jack?'

Moreover when reasoners were given contradictory evidence (experiment 4) about the causal influence of some factor (person, stimulus or occasion), mechanism-based information had approximately twice as much impact on causal inferences as did covariational information. Thus, when participants were given an event of the form 'Harry punched Jack', mechanism-based information such as 'Harry is a violent person' (i.e., some underlying feature of Harry which could cause physical aggression) rather than covariational information such as 'Jack is much more likely than other people to get punched' had more impact on whether Harry or Jack was seen as the cause of the event.

Why should mechanism-based information be both preferred by reasoners and more influential when it is received? First, covariational information may often not be available in everyday situations. Where some novel or unusual event occurs it may be very difficult to reproduce the conditions and/or vary the factors involved. After all, this is true even for experimental social psychologists who use the ANOVA model for causal inference under conditions where factors are unconfounded. If they obtain some unusual or unexpected effect most experimenters' first and pragmatic reaction would be to seek to find some mechanism within the data that they already have rather than immediately attempt to replicate the study with the same factors. Indeed where we could not identify this mechanism (e.g., through mediator analyses) any replication that we did conduct would be likely to include a further manipulation of some factor or additional measures which we had a hunch were implicated in our effect. If mechanism-based information is to be preferred in controlled experiments where confounds are eliminated there is all the more reason to expect an even stronger preference in everyday causal reasoning where confounds are almost invariably present, rendering all covariational information potentially spurious.

Secondly, Ahn et al. (1995) make the point that the mechanism-based information is easier to express in words than covariational information. They suggest that this is evidence that mechanism-based information occurs more readily in natural language. Certainly, mechanism-based information should match conversational pragmatics. If we ask 'Why did Harry punch Jack?' then an answer at the level afforded by covariational analysis would only be acceptable if the mechanism was revealed to be unknown, irrelevant or obviously implied by the covariational information (Hilton, 1991). If we are told 'Harry punches everybody' then the implied mechanism that Harry is violent does not need to be spelled out for us to know we should avoid Harry. If we were told that 'Harry has only ever punched Jack' then we would be more likely to accept this as evidence that our informant is unable or unwilling to provide us with a mechanism, but that s/he might be entertaining a hypothesis, perhaps along the lines that there is ill-feeling towards Jack from Harry. Although covariational information may serve to tell us that the cause is associated with Jack or Harry or the situation, no amount of covariational information can uniquely point to a mechanism. In one sense then, Ahn et al.'s results should not be surprising: given that a covariational account could never be seen as a satisfactory explanation unless it implies a mechanism, reasoners should prefer mechanism-based information, because in the absence of such information they would need to develop their own mechanism-based account anyway.

The most important insight developed by Ahn et al. (1995) is that the relationship between mechanism- and covariation-based causal analysis is of the same kind as the relationship between similarity and theory (e.g., Murphy and Medin, 1985) that has been a recurring theme in this book. Ahn et al. (1995) argue that similarity-based concept formation is similar to covariation-based causal inference in that both involve abstracting common features and ignoring different features. Theory-based concept formation and mechanism-based causal reasoning both involve applying general principles to a target case.

In terms of the constraint relations formulation that I have adopted throughout this book, theories and mechanisms involve the constraint of knowledge on category use whereas covariations and similarities involve the constraint of perceived equivalence on category use. To this I would add the caveat that knowledge and perceived equivalence can also constrain each other, both indirectly through category use and through the direct link.

I would use Ahn et al.'s evidence and arguments to make a stronger claim. Causal reasoning has the same form as categorization because (a) similarity-based categorization is founded on covariation, (b) causal reasoning is a special case of categorization which involves identifying categories of events and, most importantly, (c) categorizations are explanations of relevant similarities and differences (Oakes et al., 1991). When we identify some mechanism to be the cause of some event then we automatically identify the event as belonging to a particular class that allows us to predict that the same event will occur in the future should the same causes occur. In large part the seemingly banal idea that causation implies correlation means that we can be confident in such predictions about the future.

Cheng's (1997) model shares some ideas with the approach of Ahn et al. (1995). She argues that the relationship between causal power and covariation is the same as the relationship between a researcher's theory and a model that is explained by that theory. This metaphor sits very comfortably with the discussion so far. A satisfactory explanation is often seen to be one which is not redescriptive, that is, one which accounts for events in terms other than those observed. Thus, people have a model of how events in the world are related as well as a theory of why they should be related.

Cheng argues that Cheng and Novick's model of probabilistic contrast (PC) serves as the best available description of the way that people see events in the world to be related and that her causal power theory explains how they come to see some of these relations as causal. She assumes that people believe that events have causes and that there can be both generative and preventive causal powers.

The mathematical relations envisaged by Cheng are reasonably complex and can be simplified considerably by applying Venn diagrams which I use to draw some further implications for categorization from Cheng's work. If we consider a candidate cause i and the sum of all possible alternatives to i, termed a, but where i and a can both be present in the same event, then the relationships for generative causal powers can be shown as in Figure 10.7.

An event (corresponding to the regions v, w and x) can occur in the presence of either or both i or a but not in the absence of both of these. However, events may fail to occur when either or both is present. Covariation is perceived to exist where the odds of an event given i (v and w) are greater than the odds of an event in the absence of i (x). A causal relation is inferred where some causal power is seen to explain this covariation.

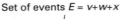

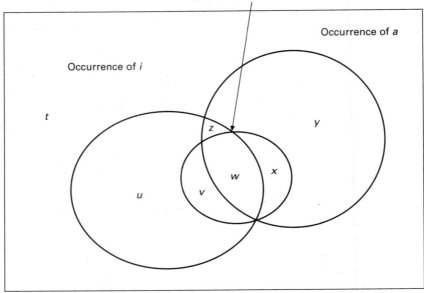

FIGURE 10.7   *The possible outcomes that enable the perception of cause from covariation in Cheng's formulation*

Here the probability of an event *e* is estimated by the frequency of events over the frequency of events and non-events:

$$P(e) = p_i P(i) + p_a P(a) + p_i P(i) p_a P(a)$$

Here $P(i)$ is the probability of a causal candidate *i* and $P(a)$ is the probability of all possible (known and unknown) alternative causal candidates *a*. The two factors in lower case are the causal powers of the candidate cause and all alternatives. These causal powers are entities hypothesized by reasoners to explain the occurrence of an event. A causal power is the probability with which a candidate cause produces an event given that the cause is present. Causal powers behave like probabilities. The causal power will differ from the conditional probability of the event given the cause if the event ever occurs in the presence of both the candidate cause and its alternatives.

The probabilistic contrast ΔP_i is the difference between the probability of the event given cause *i* minus the probability of the event in the absence of cause *i* (not –*i* or *ī*) It can be shown that this difference is given by the formula (in this case for generative power):

$$\Delta P_i = p_i + p_a P(a \mid i) + p_i p_a P(a \mid i) - p_a P(a \mid \bar{i})$$

The implication of this relation is that probabilistic contrast which has been shown to be related to the detection of covariation is explained in terms of causal powers which are hypothesized by the reasoner. Cheng notes further that where a occurs independently of i conditions the probabilistic contrast can provide an estimate for the causal power of i. This is important because the probabilistic contrast can be empirically determined providing that the reasoner knows when e occurs and i is present or absent. The chief attraction of the formulation is therefore that it provides a justification for inferring cause from covariation.

Without seeking to belittle what is a significant achievement, there are some problems with this formulation. The assumption that the causes are independent seems to be an unreasonable restriction on reasoning as reasoners seem to be able to infer cause without independence. Also the power PC theory seems to imply that reasoners should have difficulty inferring p_i when a is constantly present. Having said that, the formulation has a number of strong implications for categorization.

Inferring cause, that is explaining events, is based on a contrast between support for an entity and its alternatives. In other words, explanation involves a process of differentiation. If we apply the formulation to the illusory correlation paradigm, and if we think of group membership as a cause of desirable or undesirable behaviour, then for this special case where the cause (group A) and the alternative (group B) are independent and mutually exclusive the ΔP_i reduces to $p_i - p_a$ (because $P(a \mid i) = 0$ and $P(a \mid \bar{\imath}) = 1$). If reasoners start with the assumption that $p_i <> p_a$ then this provides a justification for perceiving covariation. As we saw in Chapter 8, there are several reasons why that contrast may be resolved in favour of p_i (i.e., group A).

The argument we have developed is that reinterpretation of the stimulus information leads perceivers to perceive a correlation between group membership and behaviour because the nature of the instructions and the task leads participants to expect that there should be such a relation (e.g., partly owing to the conversational logic of the experimental situation – see Bless et al., 1993 – which implies to participants that their task involves looking for something rather than looking for nothing).

The illusory correlation research, however, also points to another factor that is missing from the ΔP relation but is dealt with in Cheng and Holyoak's (1995; cited by Cheng, 1997) version of the causal power formulation of the probabilistic contrast model. This is what they term *confidence of assessment of contrast* and what I referred to as diagnosticity in Chapter 8. It should be easier to perceive covariation and to infer causality with large amounts of information than with small amounts of information. Cheng (1997) assumes that confidence of contrast increases monotonically with the number of cases observed. The caveats I would add to this though are that (a) the increase in confidence/diagnosticity will have an asymptotic relationship with the number of cases, and (b) where a causal mechanism is identified which allows generalization/projection to other similar situations there can be very high confidence despite what appears to be a small amount of information. In

Cheng's terms the latter caveat involves a change in focal set: reasoners can recruit instances from past experience as evidence of a causal connection and in doing this they may be going beyond the information given by experimenters.

However, the formulation also assumes that the contrasts that reasoners resolve involve multidimensional contingency tables. I think this is questionable because such contingency relations are often decomposed into smaller contrasts (Fiedler, 1991). The reason that this is most important is because the idea of covariation is insufficient to account for a crucial feature of relations between groups that needs explanation, and that is category overlap.

We saw why overlap was important in the previous section when I discussed hierarchies and inclusion. As we have just seen in this section, overlap of causal candidates creates difficulties for inferring cause.

Let us return to social categorization and the use of group memberships and their attributes by reasoners to explain states of affairs in the world. Reasoning problems can proliferate when there is a disparity in size between groups under comparison. As we saw in Chapter 8, this can be seen to be a consequence of the law of large numbers. Disparities in size between groups, however, also make possible containment or inclusion relations and, for a given context, disparities in group size can be created by overlap.

These two conditions are actually quite simple. Complete or near complete overlap between groups means that minorities can be contained within a majority, and incomplete overlap between two frequently occurring groups can create minority status. Neither containment nor overlap is well described by covariation between group memberships. Consider the contingency table below, where members of group B are a minority within a society dominated by group A. The question of whether unemployment is explained by group membership is answered poorly by the contingency table.

	Employed	Unemployed
Group A	1000	100
Group B	5000	0

This contingency table yields a very low probabilistic contrast ($\Delta P_i = 0.09$) and correlation coefficient ($\phi = -.27$) for the relation between group membership and unemployment even though group membership could explain unemployment very well. On the other hand, group membership is a poor explanation of employment. There are several important points to make here. Covariations can conceal information that is contained within low-frequency rows or columns of contingency tables, and therefore we should expect reasoners to ignore contingencies which deal with less relevant features of their environment. This occurs in everyday reasoning and scientific reasoning. Very high-frequency non-events are ignored in the process of explaining many events. In seeking to explain road accident deaths we spend little time in pondering the <u>rate</u> of successfully completed journeys because this figure barely changes from year to year (we might consider the <u>total</u>

though when we wonder if there are more deaths because there are more cars on the road).

In line with this, covariation and probabilistic contrast are insensitive to very large changes in the group B employed cell. If this increases from 5000 to 50,000 the change in ϕ or ΔP_i is very small because the proportion of events (unemployed persons) is already zero.

As well as producing possible containment/inclusion relations, overlap between groups also creates the conditions for minority status within a group. In a way that is relatively independent of covariation, minority group memberships represent plausible explanations of some phenomena but not of others. In particular, minority groups can serve to explain minority trends but not majority trends. In the table above it is in principle possible for minority group membership to be a unique explanation of a low-frequency phenomenon such as unemployment, but it can never be a unique explanation of a high-frequency phenomenon such as employment. In other words, the match between the overall frequency of the cause and the event puts limits on the scope of the explanation. Such scope considerations are not revealed by covariation statistics.

Cheng relies on formal probability theory for her derivations. This is problematic because she has attempted to account for causal inferences by humans and other species. We know, however, that people's probability estimates do not correspond to the additive specifications of probability theory. For example, Tversky and Koehler's (1994; Rottenstreich and Tversky, 1997) support theory was developed explicitly for the purpose of dealing with the observation that many probability estimates do not sum to the values that probability theory suggests.

To take an example, the conjunction of two events is often seen as more likely than either event on its own. Thus, a major flood which could kill 1000 people in the US is seen as a very unlikely event by American reasoners, but it is seen as far more likely when the possibility of a major earthquake which could cause such a flood is raised. Tversky and Koehler's solution is to suggest that subjective probability estimates are attached not to events but to hypotheses which are descriptions of events. Hypotheses can be implicit or explicit, and unpacking a hypothesis by pointing to some of its components tends to increase the support for that hypothesis by increasing its availability. For example, the earthquake becomes more available when it is given a plausible cause. The effect of this is that where there are fine partitions of a hypothesis, the sum of the judged probabilities of a hypothesis and its alternatives will be greater than one.

A particular form of unpacking that Tversky and Koehler consider, which is very important for my purposes, is *categorical unpacking*. This involves partitioning some superordinate into a set of sub-categories. Bar-Hillel and Neter (1993) found that such superordinates could be seen to be less likely than their sub-categories.

For an approach such as Cheng's the non-additive probability formulations and the results they set out to explain pose some problems. Conditional properties are used extensively in the power PC theory. Although support theory does not rule out the existence of quantities that we can call 'probabilities' which must be distinguished from subjective probability estimates, there is a need to explain what the relation between the two is. This is especially the case given that willingness to bet on outcomes seems to be closely related to the subjective probability estimates: that is, the processes which produce subjective probability estimates also relate to the apparent confidence with which reasoners hold those beliefs and have real consequences for behavioural choices. A mathematical formalism that could deal with both areas (causal reasoning and subjective probability estimates) therefore seems preferable.

The general implication that I wish to draw about unpacking, however, is that probability estimates (which are in effect expressions of the degree of perceived truth of some hypothesis) are powerfully constrained by the psychological context that is made salient to the perceiver. This is quite consistent with Krueger and Clement's (1996) finding that generalization was moderated by relevant category boundaries. Tversky and Koehler (1994) make the point that unpacking reflects a cognitive process which has much more general implications than setting probability estimates.

We can see this by returning to the issue of covariation and overlap. Although covariation is implicated in causal explanation the idea of correlation is insufficient to account for causal explanation. This is because relations between variables involve both main effects and interactions and to understand these we need to unpack relations.

The idea of categorical unpacking also helps to explicate aspects of relative homogeneity effects. Given that subjective probability estimates need not sum to one, the same argument can be made about frequency estimates (but see Gigerenzer, 1991). Given that unpacking an alternative makes it appear more likely or more frequent the increased heterogeneity of either outgroups or ingroups can be understood as the unpacking of one or the other category. When we focus on the ingroup we unpack the ingroup, when we focus on the outgroup we unpack both the outgroup and the ingroup. This works well as an elaboration of the SCT account of outgroup homogeneity (Haslam et al., 1995b; 1996c).

Leaving aside for the moment the role of covariation in causal explanation we should bear in mind that covariation is also integral to prediction (and we are presumably most likely to make predictions about things we understand). Yaniv and Foster (1995) have provided some insights into a judgement process that is relevant to categorization and prediction by using an imprecise probability model.

Their work focuses on the tradeoff between accuracy and informativeness in making decisions. In particular, whether a judge makes fine-grained (precise) or coarse-grained (vague) decisions will depend upon two competing objectives. If we ask when some task will be finished and receive the answer 'in the future' that may be accurate but it is presumably too imprecise to be useful. However, a very precise answer has a high probability of being wrong.

Analysis of preference for judgements shows that the tradeoff appears to be additive.

Importantly, the form of the tradeoff varies from conditions of certainty and uncertainty. Where there is no uncertainty the estimates should reflect pragmatic considerations. Conversational norms would imply that communicators would provide an estimate that was informative for the receiver of the information. When asked the distance to the moon an astronomer might respond 'a long way away' to a small child but with a precise distance at a particular time to an astronaut or ballistic scientist. Similarly, when one is asked what something is, then under conditions of certainty the category label chosen should be of a form that reflects the conversational context.

Yaniv and Foster (1995) suggest that under conditions of uncertainty, category use should reflect the tradeoff between informativeness and accuracy. This implies that a more abstract categorization will be adopted under the same conditions that a coarse-grained decision would be made.

These concepts suggest some further elaborations of ideas that I have dealt with earlier in this book. First, the idea of diagnosticity that I discussed extensively in Chapter 8 is also explicable in these terms. I argued that a precondition for the perception of entitativity is diagnosticity and that groups were more likely to be seen as entitative where it was possible to diagnose the nature of the group (in Yaniv and Foster's, 1995, terms this is judgement under certainty). That is, specific categorical inferences are most probable where the conditions suit such clear judgements.

Similarly, some of the conditions discussed by Jetten et al. (1998; see Chapter 9) appear to relate to such circumstances. Overlapping groups that are indistinct allow two possible resolutions: they can be perceived to be the same group (and assimilated to each other) or they can be contrasted from each other. The only way to resolve relatively indistinct groups that do not overlap, however, is to contrast them from each other.

From this discussion it is clear that covariation defection provides a platform for many aspects of the categorization process. It appears to provide the necessary groundwork for considering issues of hierarchical relations and the ambiguities provided by overlap. Theories of covariation also suggest that the perception of causal relations should be aided by the development of clear and separable categories.

Having said that, it is also the case that the principle of covariation, even when augmented by causal mechanisms, is insufficient to account for a variety of important group relationships. The idea of covariation needs to be augmented by a consideration of mechanism-based knowledge, unpacking, containment/inclusion relations, and tradeoffs between accuracy and informativeness. Nevertheless, covariation clearly merits close consideration and in the next section we look at social psychological research which has sought to model covariation in a way that can be applied to categorization.

C. Modelling covariation and causal explanation

Causal explanation is probably the area of social psychology which has experienced the most direct impact of connectionist social psychology (see Read et al., 1997; E. R. Smith, 1996). A major paper on this topic was published by Read and Marcus-Newhall (1993) in which the authors sought to demonstrate that a parallel constraint satisfaction (PCS) model could provide an account of causal reasoning in human subjects (van Overwalle, 1998: 326, note A1, suggests that such models should be called interactive activation and competition models if one is to follow Rumelhart and McClelland's, 1986, nomenclature, but I will follow the social psychological convention in calling them constraint satisfaction models).

Parallel constraint satisfaction systems involve units which represent underlying concepts that are linked to other concepts by both excitatory and inhibitory links. Such models are parallel in that many different units can be activated simultaneously, and they are constraint satisfying in that the activation of units reciprocally affects the activation of linked units either positively or negatively. One popular source of such models is the work of Thagard (1989) on explanatory coherence and this has been used by Kunda and Thagard (1996) to account for impression formation. Note that contrary to many other connectionist implications the nodes are symbolic, that is, they involve the activation of concepts that can be experienced and potentially communicated.

Such models involve a series of nodes that are connected by positive or negative links to each other. On each cycle of activation the contribution of nodes to other nodes is calculated. The level of activation is intended to reflect the strength of belief of an explanation. An example of such a system is shown in Figure 10.8 which deals with the case of an unemployed person refusing a job offer.

Note that some nodes are linked to a special *observed* node. This is normally clamped (i.e., fixed) to a particular value such as 1.0. The nodes linked to the observed node can be termed evidence nodes. The evidence here is that an unemployed person refused a job offer. The other nodes can be termed explanatory nodes. In this case, two competing explanations are considered: the person was lazy, or the person was over-qualified for the position. The laziness explanation is activated by both evidence nodes but over-qualified is activated only by refusing the job offer. Note also that the explanations are competing in that they are negatively linked. To the extent that one explanatory node is activated it will suppress or inhibit the other.

Such systems tend to be associated with convergence on a stable compromise level of activation across the system after a number of iterations. The simple system in Figure 10.8, for example, rapidly converges on higher levels of activation for *lazy* rather than *over-qualified*. This is not true of the somewhat more complex system in Figure 10.9. In this case, *over-qualified* tends to be activated more strongly than it was in the previous system, and *lazy* is activated less strongly. This is because *lazy* is no longer linked to the unemployed

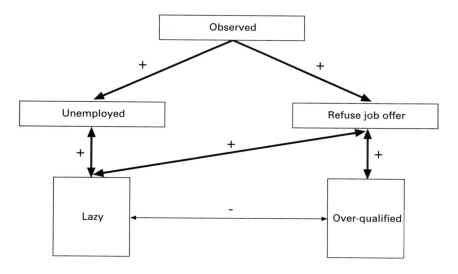

FIGURE 10.8   *An example of a (simple) parallel constraint satisfaction network model*

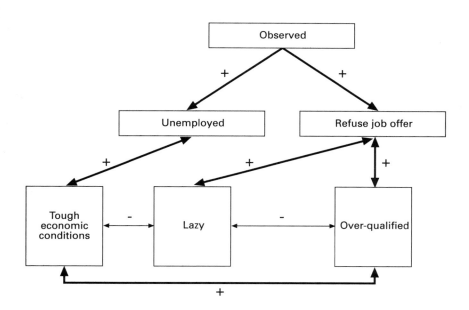

FIGURE 10.9   *A more complex example of a parallel constraint satisfaction model*

evidence node and because of the presence of the other explanation (*tough economic conditions*) that inhibits *lazy* and excites or augments *over-qualified*.

Read and Miller (1993) considered such systems in the light of Thagard's (1989) explanatory coherence account. According to Thagard (1989) coherent explanations are those which have the characteristics of breadth (explain much evidence), simplicity (involve few explanatory nodes), the ability to be explained themselves (by other explanatory nodes), the avoidance of unexplained data, and unification (jointly explain all the evidence rather than uniquely explain many), and are supported by analogies to other causal systems with the same structure. The merits of coherent explanations are relative; a good explanation is thus one which is relatively more coherent than its alternatives.

Read and Miller apply a model based on the parallel constraint satisfaction model to a range of phenomena in person perception including work drawn from Gilbert's (1989) model of cognitive busyness and Trope's (1986) model of dispositional inference. The model was applied by Read and Marcus-Newhall (1993) to causal inference in social psychology. These authors found that broader and simpler explanations were perceived to be more satisfactory by perceivers and that the parallel constraint satisfaction models were successful in simulating the data obtained by human participants.

However, van Overwalle (1998) has challenged the relevance of the parallel constraint satisfaction model for causal explanation by demonstrating through simulations and mathematical proofs that parallel constraint satisfaction models cannot detect covariation between cause and effect even for a simple case of one cause and one effect. The problem is that such networks do not learn well, especially when they are required to learn multiplicative relations such as those required to learn covariation (see previous section).

Van Overwalle (1998; van Overwalle and van Rooy, 1996) has proposed a feedforward model of causal explanation. This model is based on the flow of activation through a system of nodes from inputs to outputs. The feedforward model is thus similar to Gluck and Bower's (1988) categorization model which was presented in Chapter 3.

The system that was modelled in Figure 10.8 can be reconsidered as a feedforward system as in Figure 10.10. Note that the key differences are that all links are positive and that all links flow from input to output. Note here that the inputs to the system are causes and the outputs are events. The system works by taking the outputs it obtains and comparing them with observed events. If it is unable to achieve a match between its outputs and observed reality the contribution of the inputs is adjusted in the direction of achieving a closer match.

The system can therefore be seen as generating predictions based on known causes which are tested against the evidence. If the evidence is not consistent with the predictions the contribution of those causes is adjusted.

In fact, the presentation of the system as in Figure 10.10 ignores the learning algorithm involved. The system shown also fails to detect covariation

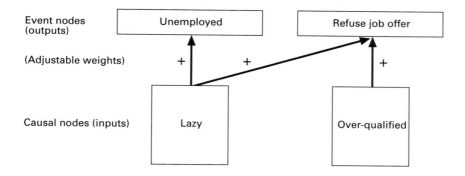

FIGURE 10.10   *Certain aspects of a feedforward model*

without important adjustments. The connection strengths do not have a fixed value as they do in the PCS model but these strengths are learned from experience by comparing the predicted activation of some output to observed events. Thus, the values of two types of parameters are being altered on successive iterations of the network. The activations of output nodes are being incremented, as are the values of the links between inputs and outputs. The latter process is not shown in Figure 10.10.

The increments are calculated by setting the activation of causes which are observed to be present to a default activation level of 1 and the connection strengths to 0. The activation of output nodes is incremented by the sum of the products of activation level and connection strength. This will initially be zero because the connection strengths are zero. The activation of the output nodes is then compared with an external teaching signal (also not shown in Figure 10.10) which is set to 1 when the event has occurred and 0 when the event has not occurred. Where there is a discrepancy between the prediction and observed events the connection strengths are either incremented or decremented to bring the obtained activation in line with the observed event.

Thus, despite the appearance of a similar architecture to the PCS model there is a lot more going on behind the scenes in the feedforward model. In the PCS model all of the nodes, whether evidence or explanatory, are symbolic and are potentially available for introspection. Moreover the flow of activation from evidence nodes to explanatory nodes means that the PCS system will tend to result in one or more explanations being activated by the evidence. The PCS suggests the prospect that some explanation in symbolic terms will emerge from the system such as 'The unemployed person refused the job offer because s/he was lazy.' This is a specific statement of the more general abstraction 'The observed event occurred because of the most strongly activated explanatory node linked to it.'

In the feedforward model the flow that is actually shown in the model is from explanation to evidence. This is counter-intuitive in the sense that although causes lead to effects, in causal reasoning the output of the system should be explanations (though we should expect explanations that are already activated to affect the interpretation of evidence). To deal with this van Overwalle (1998) takes the output of the system to be the activation of events. Note that this is an interpretational complexity rather than a limitation of feedforward models in general as models could be constructed which had evidence, and previously activated explanations, as inputs and current explanations as outputs.

The prospect exists, however, that the two types of model are dealing with different aspects of the explanation process. The symbolic PCS model may actually be providing a better model of the way reasoners understand their own explanations than of the way they actually form explanations. I will refer to this less automatic process as *justification* rather than reasoning. Justification involves *giving reasons*, it is necessarily a process that is symbolic to enable communication (see Kunda and Oleson, 1995, for a treatment of justification).

It is reasonable to expect that the explanations that reasoners proffer for some state of affairs would involve dynamic excitatory and inhibitory relations. To the extent that perceivers see generative or preventive connections between candidate causes and events these causes should be more or less prominent. Similarly, to the degree that one cause is seen to be more prominent it should inhibit other alternative explanations. Note that giving reasons and reasoning *per se* are distinguishable in terms of the detection of covariation. A reasoner can come to believe that the unemployed are lazy on the basis of some background knowledge or ideology. They may nevertheless say that the unemployed are lazy because they refuse job offers even where covariation does not hold in general because disconfirming instances are dealt with as special cases (e.g., see Rothbart and Lewis's, 1988, discussion of the statement: 'There are no good women rock climbers'). Similarly, an explanation could be based on covariation, but be justified on the basis of background knowledge. In neither case need we assume that the reasoner is being dishonest; it is just unsafe to assume that reasoners have full, uninterrupted access to the reasoning process. However, it would be equally unsafe to assume that the products of conscious mental life are *unrelated* to the processes which produce them.

The feedforward model may be doing a better job at explaining the process by which participants actually derive explanations. This would seem to follow from the demonstration that the feedforward model can detect covariation. Alterations are necessary to the PCS model that allow it to learn before it could be used for the same purpose.

This implies that a two-stage architecture may be required to model both explanation and justification. The assumption I make is that inputs to justifications can include the explanations that are developed by the reasoning process. Reasoning relates to the process by which people come to hold some belief X, whereas justification relates to the answers that people give to questions like 'Why do you believe X?' or 'Why does factor Y cause X?' or 'Why does evidence Y lead you to believe X?' Reasoning can be characterized as a process of detecting covariation and causal agents, whereas justification is a dynamic process which involves competition between competing explanations in terms of evidence. Explanations and evidence can have inhibitory or excitatory connections in such a system. Thus where there was a highly activated explanation this would tend to suppress competing evidence and explanations and activate supporting evidence and explanations. However, the justification process could also serve to inhibit some highly activated explanation. For example, the process of answering the question 'Why do you believe X despite evidence Y which disconfirms it?' could suppress X to the extent to which Y was well supported. Thus, strong reciprocal links between justification and explanation should be expected.

Thagard's (1989) ECHO model which is instantiated in terms of the PCS model may work quite well as a model of justification, and this should not be surprising given that a major focus of the model was scientific explanation. Scientific explanation certainly appears to have the characteristics of justification: it is symbolic and involves communication. However, the special status of evidence nodes might need to be dropped from models of justification. Logically, either evidence or explanations could have high initial activations.

Van Overwalle's (1998) feedforward model performs equally well in modelling data from human participants as does the PCS model used by Read and Marcus-Newhall (1993). It also matches the breadth and simplicity coherence principles that are anticipated by ECHO. Given that it can predict covariation it should be preferred to the PCS model for causal explanation (but not justification which requires symbolic elements).

Given that the models do equally well in modelling data from human participants but only one of them is capable of detecting covariation, this implies that detection of covariation is not essential for modelling causal explanation in humans. If we accept the thesis that human causal explanation really involves two correlated processes – explanation and justification – then this potential logical problem disappears. Rating the extent to which an explanation is satisfactory (the task performed by Read and Marcus-Newhall's, 1993, human participants) is much closer to the process of justification, but as I have argued above, justification is predicated upon the development of explanations that can be considered as inputs to the process. In a process of justification an explanation will be seen to be better than its alternatives to the extent that it matches the explanation that we have developed, and inferior to alternatives to the extent that it differs.

The logic of this argument is independent of the mechanisms of either of these models. If a person develops an explanation A and you ask the person to rate their satisfaction with explanation A and explanation B, you should expect the rating of explanation A to be higher than that for explanation B (see Chapter 9, section B). Thus a model that predicts which explanation a person develops should also be able to predict which explanation is preferred in a rating task in broad terms. This does not mean that explanation is the same as justification, however. The explanation model does not explain how the explanation (once developed) is justified to be superior relative to its alternatives (in terms of highly activated representations of supporting and disconfirming evidence). Of course, the feedforward model could be adjusted to include a further stage of competition in order to model justification, but it would start to look very much like the PCS model. In line with the results obtained by Ahn et al. (1995) I would anticipate that justifications would tend to stress mechanism-based information.

These arguments suggest that causal explanation and the process of attribution are best understood as the intersection of two processes: explanation and justification, where explanation is seen as an input to justification (i.e., the explanations that can be justified are those which reasoners have developed themselves or are presented with as alternatives). Whereas explanation can be seen to be omnipresent, justification is most likely to be present where explanations are registered in symbolic terms in conscious thought. This should apply most commonly where reasoners seek to communicate explanations to other people.

The autoassociator alternative

Although it satisfies the requirements for perceiving covariation, the feedforward model is only one possible model. Still another possibility for predicting covariation is E. R. Smith and de Coster's (1998) autoassociative model which employs the same learning rule as van Overwalle's model (the delta learning rule).

The autoassociative model involves a distributed system where many subsymbolic nodes are linked to all of the other nodes in the network with positive or negative connections. The nodes accept an external input and then excite or inhibit each other. Following this exchange, the levels of activation of these nodes are checked against the external input. Those which differ from the external input have their connections with positively contributing nodes increased and connections with negatively contributing nodes decreased. Thus, the key differences from the feedforward model are that (a) there are bidirectional links between all nodes, (b) these links can be positive or negative, and (c) the representation of the input by the system is distributed across the entire system. The last point is particularly important: unlike the other two models considered the autoassociator does not have specific nodes associated with a specific piece of evidence or construct. Rather, the representation of some piece of evidence or construct reflects the response of the entire system to the new input.

A simple four-unit system is shown below in Figure 10.11, with thicker lines representing stronger links.

Smith and de Coster (1998) suggest that such a model is most useful for modelling preconscious conceptual interpretation. They apply the autoassociator to the assignment of idiosyncratic characteristics of a well-known person to some new rather similar person; learning group stereotypes from exposure to exemplars; learning multiple knowledge structures and applying them in combination to infer new characteristics; and accessibility effects.

External inputs

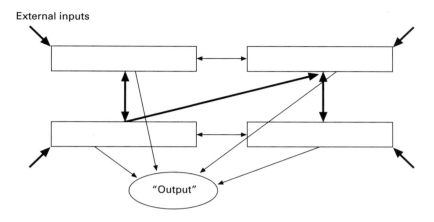

FIGURE 10.11   *A simple autoassociator*

These are all concepts that are within the purview of categorization research; the immediate question is whether such an autoassociator could detect covariation.

Logically, the feature of the feedforward model that allows it to detect covariation is the learning rule. The autoassociator incorporates the learning rule, therefore it should be able to detect covariation.

As it turns out though, the question of whether the autoassociator can detect covariation is not well formed. Smith and de Coster's autoassociator is designed to learn a set of inputs and then to produce outputs when prompted with new inputs. If one set of inputs were defined to be a piece of evidence then such a system would certainly produce similar outputs when prompted with similar evidence. If one makes the logical assignment that the outputs are causes then it follows that the autoassociator can detect covariation.

Thus at least one and possibly two different architectures can detect covariation amongst stimuli. These systems would also enable reasoners to derive causal explanations and also to generate outputs which could be used as symbolic inputs to systems of justification for the explanations developed.

Although the actual structures of the systems that might be used for causal explanation and justification are well beyond the scope of this book, the fact that it is possible that structures exist which serve these functions has tantalizing implications for our understanding of the categorization process. Some of these implications are considered in the next section.

Conclusion

In the concluding section of this chapter I wish to demonstrate that causal explanation and covariation underpin the categorization process. To do this,

I draw upon ideas presented in the two previous chapters and attempt to place them within the structure of a logical argument.

When I say that causal explanation and covariation underpin categorization I am really trying to turn some common assumptions made by social psychologists like myself into some currency that is more useful than slogans such as 'categorization is an adaptive sense-making process' or 'categorization is a flexible process' or 'stereotypes create expectancies'. To do this I argue that many other important ideas can be derived from just four propositions:

1   Categorizations are explanations.
2   Causation implies correlation (or at least containment/inclusion relations).
3   Causal explanations are derived from the detection of covariation and prior causal explanations.
4   Categorizations are derived from background knowledge.

If categorizations are explanations then categories should form through the process of causal explanation. From the discussion in this chapter there are good reasons for believing that this process can be modelled by an inductive (possibly distributed) process whereby explanations are obtained from inputs which include evidence and previously activated explanations.

If causation implies correlation and categorizations are explanations then categorizations should be useful for prediction and expectancy generation. That is, if some category which is believed to be a causal power (mechanism) can be identified then it should be useful for predicting future events. If laziness is accepted as an explanation of an unemployed person refusing a job offer then (a) that person will be categorized as lazy in those circumstances, and (b) laziness could be used to predict the conjunction of unemployment and refusing job offers (and possibly each of these things individually), but only under those conditions where that explanation is highly activated. However, if categories are to have a predictive function then they must have some long-term representation. As Smith and de Coster demonstrate, this of itself does not require that there be a localized unit to represent the category.

If causal explanations are derived from the detection of covariation (with the qualifications made in the second section of this chapter in relation to categorical unpacking, informativeness and containment/inclusion) and prior explanations, and categorizations are derived from background knowledge, then it follows that background knowledge must take the form of knowledge of covariation and other causal relations. When we add to this the idea that covariation knowledge is also useful for dealing with overlapping categories and for subsuming the concept of hierarchical categorical organization then a plan for articulating the links between categorization, explanation and prediction emerges. These can be seen in the by-now-familiar constraint relations formulation in Figure 10.12.

We need models of the six key constraint relations which are labelled (a) through to (f) in Figure 10.12.

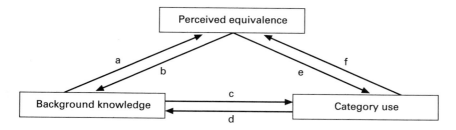

FIGURE 10.12   *Constraint relations in categorization and explanation to be modelled*

(a) We need a model which shows how perceived equivalence emerges from detected covariation and prior explanations without categories necessarily being invoked. Autoassociator and feedforward models show how exemplars known to share similar features can be seen to be equivalent.

(b) Autoassociator models in particular provide good models of how knowledge of perceived equivalence between exemplars can be stored in a distributed form. However, there is no great difficulty in modelling such a process in many other connectionist architectures. Note that the term *categorization* would rarely be invoked to describe links (a) or (b) on their own. These links do not involve the use of category memberships by the system in symbolic terms. Having said that, relations involving category use can be mediated through these links.

(c) We need a model of how previously stored knowledge of covariation and causal mechanism is activated to create categorizations for immediate use. Smith and de Coster's autoassociator model again captures the direct link well. Note though that link (c) is equivalent to link (a) followed by link (e). For this latter purpose an instantiation of the causal power theory of probabilistic contrast should work well as a model. Models incorporating the delta learning rule such as van Overwalle's (1998) feedforward model appear to be plausible candidates, but the application of van Overwalle's model would be easier to work with conceptually (for this purpose at least) if explanations were depicted as outputs and evidence as inputs.

(d) We need a model of how these categories once formed are stored for use in future explanations. Again autoassociator models such as that proposed by Smith and de Coster (1998) show that distributed sub-symbolic representations can reproduce category-level and exemplar-level information and thus demand further attention.

(e) As noted above, when link (e) is considered in conjunction with link (a) then this process is modelled well by a large number of different connectionist architectures that rely on flow from evidence to categories (for examples see developments on Gluck and Bower's, 1988, work, e.g., Shanks and Gluck, 1994).

(f) Finally there is the constraining effect of category use on perceived equivalence. Although none of the models I have considered in this chapter actually describe this process formally it is in fact very easy to model in terms of autoassociator, feedforward, parallel constraint satisfaction networks, or other systems such as Kashima et al.'s (1998) tensor product model. For example, although it is not formally a model of cognitive processes, and even though it is used to develop almost the opposite argument, the vector model proposed by Fiedler (1996) for his BIAS model neatly captures the constraining effect of category use on perceived equivalence.

However, the central argument of this chapter is that even if we were able to model all these links we would still have an insufficient account of categorization/explanation. This is because these models do not cover the process whereby categorizations/explanations which appear in consciousness in symbolic terms are justified, compared and communicated with other people. As Edwards (1991) argues from a discourse analytic perspective: categories are for talking. What I have called justification in this chapter is actually also the subject matter of social psychological research in the related areas of social attribution (e.g., Hewstone, 1989) and lay explanation (D.J. Hilton and Slugoski, 1986).

There are two dividends from examining the nexus between categorizations and explanations. As I have discussed above, the first of these is that this treatment shows how categorizations help us make sense of the world. The other dividend is that it helps us to understand the competitive and contrastive nature of explanations by reference to the contrastive and competitive nature of categorizations. We should expect that to the extent that one explanation is preferred, other alternative explanations will be contrasted away from it. This is the role that justification serves in this overview. The development of coherent and separable statements of categorizations/explanations depends upon recognizing the differences between explanations and their alternatives. This process of competitive justification appears to be modelled elegantly by parallel constraint satisfaction models such as those used by Read and Marcus-Newhall (1993) and Kunda and Thagard (1996) because they incorporate the prospect of negative links to prominent (highly activated) conflicting explanations and evidence and positive links to prominent supporting explanations and evidence.

In terms of the constraint relations formulation the operation of competitive justification should be seen as an articulation of processes operating within the broad domain of category use. That is, the constraint relations formulation is one level too general to show the details of these processes.

In summary the thesis developed in this chapter is as follows. There are two processes which are normally grouped under the broad heading of explanation. I term these explanation and justification, and the process of categorization is fully subsumed by these two processes. Explanation involves detecting and using perceived covariations. The operation of this process

FISH

and ask you what you see. You can respond by saying 'I see the word FISH' or 'I see the four letters F, I, S and H'. The first response uses words as categories and the second uses letters. Both are perfectly valid categorical representations; they simply rely on different levels of abstraction. Neither is more accurate until some normative framework is applied in some particular setting. For example, the second would be judged to be an incorrect response in a test of reading ability. However, if I then wrote:

TROVT

and you answered that you saw TROUT or T, R, O, U and T (presumably because I had just primed the category 'fish') then we have a more interesting error. Your response would be inaccurate in terms of a normative framework that we both accept, and your answer probably does not reflect a change in your acceptance of some normative framework. Rather you have been tricked into making an error. My argument is that equivalent errors can be produced by tricking participants into <u>not</u> using categorizations, and that, in a word recognition task, the use of such categories (words) normally leads to efficiencies and improvements in accuracy when compared against a base rate of, for example, reading individual letters.

When I show you a group of rioters or a football team and ask you what you see, then the response 'I see a set of individuals' or 'I see a group' can be right or wrong as a description of the facts of social organization and self-perceptions of the targets (from the point of view of a social scientific normative framework) in a way in which the letter or word representation is unlikely to be wrong. Perceiving people as individuals or as a group is a more or less accurate representation of real (psychological) states of affairs in the world in a way that a word or a letter is not.

Again the notions of expectation and inference are critical here. The interpretation of the rioters as a set of individuals may be a *psychologically valid* experience but that is largely irrelevant to the consideration of whether it is correct with respect to some normative framework. The interpretation is wrong in terms of a normative framework that holds that groups are real (a normative framework that is itself contested by reductionists) and it has a high probability of leading to errors (judged against normative frameworks that are shared by just about everybody) in predicting the future actions of the rioters. Yet other errors will be made by assuming that the rioters' unity of purpose does not change over time. The toughest standards for accuracy therefore do not necessarily relate to being able to interpret what something is in the present, but in being able to predict what it will do in the future. Incorrect attributions about other people's self-categorizations will lead to a high rate of incorrect predictions about their future behaviour.

Even if the overall rate of inferences is not improved much by categorization, certain very important inferences will be. To borrow Barsalou and

Medin's (1986) example, imagine that someone were to make the incorrect inference that all snakes are poisonous. We might make many mistakes about whether a particular snake is poisonous but we would not make the (fatal) mistake of assuming that no snakes are poisonous. In the terms used by Fiske and Leyens (1997) we can deploy a sufficiency rule and not a necessity rule here. It is *sufficient* for something to be known to be a snake for it to be seen as potentially dangerous. It is not *necessary* for it to be known to be a poisonous snake. As Krueger and Clement (1996) demonstrate, categories place limitations on generalization. We need not infer that all creatures are poisonous or dangerous because snakes are. The explanatory success of a categorical system rests on being able to place appropriate limits on generalization/inference.

In line with Chapter 10, categorizations can also be considered in terms of inferences based on premises. If categorization can be shown to lead to unsound inferences from premises then categorization would be shown to be leading to internal inconsistency. Suppose we consider a syllogism of the form:

> Whites score higher than blacks on IQ tests.
> IQ tests are not valid measures of intelligence.
> Whites are more intelligent than blacks.

Evidence that salient categorizations produce internally incoherent inferences of this form would be strong evidence of categorization leading to error. I do not believe that the literature reveals that categorization leads to this form of error.

Here the categorization of blacks and whites on the dimension of intelligence can be wrong from the point of view of the perceiver in the sense that either of the first two statements is inconsistent with what the perceiver knows to be true. I agree with Oakes et al. (1994) that most of the research that has sought to show inaccuracy and biases in social perception has actually relied on misleading participants (see also McMullen et al., 1997).

However, given that categories are used for making inferences, a particularly common form of error may involve memory for distinguishing information. Using categories leads to the perception of equivalences/nonequivalences on certain dimensions and the activation of certain forms of knowledge at a particular time (e.g. when the stimulus is first encountered). This knowledge might not be the knowledge that is important at some later time. If a perceiver is required to recall information that was not attended to, then errors (in terms of, say, a normative framework that is actually shared by an experimenter and a participant) will occur. Demonstrating such errors is a popular activity for many social psychologists. I would argue that the activity would be of much greater value if the researchers also sought to demonstrate when category use leads to superior recall of equivalences between persons and a stronger basis for inferences of relatedness of members and predictions about social interaction.

A final and very interesting criterion for accuracy is accuracy of prediction. This is used only rarely by social psychologists (but see e.g., Funder, 1987). Prediction relies on considering the time course of the perception. If it could be established that prediction is impaired by categorization then this would be strong evidence that categorization produces errors. I think that even though there is only a limited amount of evidence on this topic in the formal literature a clear picture will emerge. It is possible to mislead perceivers by getting them to categorize inappropriately so that categorization will lead to impaired predictions. However, when we categorize targets in a way which captures the target's current self-categorization we are likely to be able to predict their behaviour more accurately than we would if we did not accurately reflect the target self-categorization. Imagine how difficult it would be to predict which direction a player would pass the ball in a football game without knowing which team they were on. This example makes it easy to see the importance of the adaptive and rational functions of categorization that have been highlighted by cognitive and social psychologists alike (Anderson, 1991; Bruner, 1957; Tajfel, 1981; Turner et al., 1987). Indeed as Krueger and Clement (1994) note, categorization can improve prediction *despite* the loss of information.

These complex arguments demand some recapitulation. Three chief criticisms can be made of the idea that categorization leads to distortion: (a) demonstrations of errors produced by categorization have not been tested against appropriate standards; (b) categorizing at different levels is appropriate at different times because reality is complex and variable and is inevitably partial and relative and (c) there are no appropriate standards to demonstrate error that can be derived from psychological measurement. I argued that only the first and second of these are relevant to the issue of categorical distortion, and that the third can serve to marginalize the other points, without an attempt to define standards as is done here.

Importantly though, I also argued that reality is not only variable and complex but it is variably variable and complex (cf. Kraus et al., 1993: 23). Perceivers need to be able to differentiate between those features of the world which remain stable despite changes in interpretation, and those where there is no reason to assume such stability. If perceivers did not differentiate in this way they would not be able to generate accurate expectancies. The belief that black and white people belong to the same category (human beings) for the dimension of intelligence might lead someone to believe that blacks and whites achieve *more similar* scores on IQ tests than they actually do. Such constraints on perceived equivalence are relatively trivial; the much more powerful and interesting effect on their cognition is, after witnessing evidence of group differences in IQ scores, whether a perceiver who expects no differences will come to question whether IQ tests accurately measure intelligence. That is, will there be a change in the normative framework? The more interesting psychological process therefore is not the changes in memory or judgement of the numerical values of the scores, but the interpretation of what those scores *mean* and what intelligence *is*. This is very different to what seems to occur in the Tajfel and Wilkes (1963) paradigm. It seems implausible to me that their participants were challenging the normative framework when they judge lines labelled A to be shorter than lines labelled B. Rather, in the absence of precise information about the match of their perceptions to the normative framework, perceivers do the best they can.

Characteristics of the world which are believed to be stable such as IQ scores and height, however, have a different quality to aspects of the social world which are changeable. Most importantly, changes occur in reality owing to psychological group formation that perceivers can track by inferring group memberships. The only way to do this *accurately* is to identify the appropriate level for categorizing the target in terms of that target's self-perception. Perceivers do make mistakes in this task, but generally they do well enough. This is I feel the key point that the SCT analysis has to offer in building upon the work of the Gestalt theorists, but as I say, it has at times been understated owing to the emphasis paid to the metaphysical critique and the failure to distinguish consensus from normative frameworks.

In summary then, the question of whether categorization produces errors is most meaningful if we restrict our discussion to errors in terms of some normative framework which is uncontested by the categorizer, that is, where the process of categorizing does not shift or change the normative framework. These errors could include erroneous logical inferences and predictions about the future behaviour of the object of categorization. I suggest that such errors are rare and when they do arise they occur as frequently from *not* treating a stimulus as a member of some category as from treating it as such. That is, errors of inference and prediction may stem from categorizing inappropriately rather than from categorizing *per se*.

Final note

Although solutions to some of the field's problems are suggested by exploring the proposition that categorization is explanation, it is also true that categorization researchers have much to learn about the process of explanation. The weight of the field, however, is shifting in this direction. As we have seen in the previous chapters, researchers in the fields of impression formation, stereotype formation and group entitativity are emphasizing in a variety of ways the importance of meanings derived by perceivers. However, where social categorization researchers do deal with explanation they are usually concerned with causal attributions about particular targets' behaviour rather than explanation of the attributes of the categories (though work by authors such as Berndsen et al., 1998; Wittenbrink et al., 1998; and Yzerbyt et al., 1997, represents exceptions).

In my opinion progress in this direction rests in asking just how far it is possible to push the equation between categorization and explanation. This involves exploring the proposition that not only is categorization based on background knowledge and theory but categorization is the process by which background knowledge and theory are formed. More tantalizing still, the process by which background knowledge is constrained by the social context without it being directly exchanged remains a central scientific problem for the field.

References

Abrams, D. & Masser, B. (1998). Content and social self-regulation of stereotyping: perception, judgement and behaviour. In R.S. Wyer Jr (Ed.), *Advances in social cognition* (Vol. 11, pp. 53–67). Mahwah, NJ: Erlbaum.

Ahn, W-K., Kalish, C.W., Medin, D.L., & Gelman, S.A. (1995). The role of covariation versus mechanism information in causal attribution. *Cognition, 54*, 299–352.

Alloy, L.B. & Tabachnick, N. (1984). Assessment of covariation by human and animals: the joint influence of prior expectations and current situational information. *Psychological Review, 91*, 112–149.

Allport, G.W. (1954). *The nature of prejudice*. Reading, MA: Addison-Wesley.

Andersen, S.M. & Klatzky, R.L. (1987). Traits and social stereotypes: Levels of categorization in person perception. *Journal of Personality and Social Psychology, 53*, 235–246.

Anderson, J.R. (1991). The adaptive nature of human categorization. *Psychological Review, 98*, 409–429.

Anderson, J.R. & Fincham, J.M. (1996). Categorization and sensitivity to correlation. *Journal of Experimental Psychology: Learning, Memory, and Cognition, 22*, 259–277.

Arcuri, L. (1982). Three patterns of social categorization in attribution memory. *European Journal of Social Psychology, 12*, 271–282.

Asch, S.E. (1952). *Social Psychology*. Englewood Cliffs, NJ: Prentice-Hall.

Asch, S.E. & Zukier, H. (1984). Thinking about persons. *Journal of Personality and Social Psychology, 46*, 1230–1240.

Augoustinos, M. & Walker, I. (1996). *Social cognition: an integrated introduction*. London: Sage.

Bargh, J.A. (1994). The four horsemen of automaticity: awareness, intention, efficiency, and control in social cognition. In R.S. Wyer, Jr. & T.K. Srull (Eds.) *Handbook of social cognition* (2nd ed., pp. 1–40). Hillsdale, NJ: Erlbaum.

Bargh, J.A. (1996). Automaticity in social psychology. In E. T. Higgins & A. W. Kruglanski (Eds.), *Social psychology: handbook of basic principles* (pp. 169–183). New York: Guilford

Bar-Hillel, M. & Neter, E. (1993). How alike is it versus how likely is it: a distinction fallacy in probability judgements. *Journal of Personality and Social Psychology, 65*, 1119–1131.

Barsalou, L.W. (1987). The instability of graded structure. In U. Neisser (Ed.), *Concepts and conceptual development: ecological and intellectual factors in categorization* (pp. 101–140). Cambridge, New York: Cambridge University Press.

Barsalou, L.W. (1990). Access and inference in categorization. *Bulletin of the Psychonomic Society, 28*, 268–271.

Barsalou, L.W. (1991). Deriving categories to achieve goals. In G.H. Bower (Ed.), *The psychology of learning and motivation: advances in theory and research* (Vol. 27). New York: Academic Press.

Barsalou, L.W. (1993). Challenging assumptions about concepts. *Cognitive Development, 8*, 169–80.

Barsalou, L.W. & Medin, D.L. (1986). Concepts: static definitions or context-dependent representations. *Cahiers de Psychologie, 6*, 187–202.

Bassok, M. & Medin, D.L. (1997). Birds of a feather flock together: Similarity judgments with semantically rich stimuli. *Journal of Memory and Language, 36*, 311–336.

Berndsen, M. (1997). *Some illusions about illusory correlation.* PhD thesis, University of Amsterdam.

Berndsen, M. & Spears, R. (1997). Reinterpreting illusory correlation: from biased covariation to meaningful categorisation. *Swiss Journal of Psychology, 57*, 127–138.

Berndsen, M., van der Pligt, J., Spears, R., & McGarty, C. (1996). Expectation-based and data-based illusory correlation: the effects of confirming versus disconfirming evidence. *European Journal of Social Psychology, 26*, 899–913.

Berndsen, M., Spears, R., McGarty, C., & van der Pligt, J. (1998). The dynamics of differentiation: similarity as a precursor and product of stereotype formation. *Journal of Personality and Social Psychology, 74*, 1451–1463.

Biddle, B.J. & Thomas, E. J. (Eds.) (1966). *Role theory: concepts and research.* New York: Wiley.

Biernat, M., Vescio, T.K., & Manis, M. (1998). Judging and behaving toward members of stereotyped groups: a shifting standards perspective. In C.R. Sedikides, J. Schopler, & C.A. Insko (Eds.), *Intergroup cognition and intergroup behaviour* (pp. 151–175). Mahwah, NJ: Erlbaum.

Billig, M. (1997). Discursive, rhetorical and ideological messages. In C. McGarty & S. A. Haslam (Eds.), *The message of social psychology: perspectives on mind in society* (pp. 36–53). Oxford, UK and Cambridge, MT: Blackwell.

Birnbaum, M.H. (1982). Controversies in psychological measurement. In B. Wegener (Ed.), *Social attitudes and psychophysical measurement* (pp. 401–486). Hillsdale, NJ: Erlbaum.

Blair, I. & Banaji, M. R. (1996). Automatic and controlled processes in stereotype priming. *Journal of Personality and Social Psychology, 70*, 1142–1163.

Bless, H. & Schwarz, N. (1998). Context effects in political judgement: assimilation and contrast as a function of categorization processes. *European Journal of Social Psychology, 28*, 159–172.

Bless, H., Strack, F., & Schwarz, N. (1993). The informative functions of research procedures: bias and the logic of conversation. *European Journal of Social Psychology, 23*, 149–165.

Bodenhausen, G.V. & Macrae, C.N. (1998a). On social judgment and social justice: further reflections on stereotyping and its avoidance. In R.S. Wyer (Ed.), *Advances in social cognition* (Vol. 11, pp. 243–256). Mahwah, NJ: Erlbaum.

Bodenhausen, G.V. & Macrae, C.N. (1998b). Stereotype activation and inhibition. In R. S. Wyer (Ed.), *Advances in social cognition* (Vol. 11, pp. 1–52). Mahwah, NJ: Erlbaum.

Bodenhausen, G.V., Sheppard, L.A., & Kramer, G.P. (1994). Negative affect and social judgment: The differential impact of anger and sadness. *European Journal of Social Psychology, 24*, 45–62.

Bosveld, W., Koomen, W., & van der Pligt, J. (1996). Estimating group size: effects of category membership, differential construal and selective exposure. *European Journal of Social Psychology, 26*, 523–535.

Bourhis, R.Y., Turner, J.C. & Gagnon, A. (1997). Interdependence, social identity and discrimination. In R. Spears, P. J. Oakes, N. Ellemers & S. A. Haslam (Eds.), *The social psychology of stereotyping and group life* (pp. 273–295). Oxford: Blackwell.

Bower, G.H. (1967). A multicomponent theory of the mental trace. In K.W. Spence & J.T. Spence (Eds.), *The psychology of learning and motivation: advances in research and theory* (pp. 230–327). New York: Academic Press.

Brewer, M.B. (1988). A dual process model of impression formation. In T.K. Srull & R.S. Wyer, Jr. (Eds.), *Advances in social cognition: a dual process model of impression formation* (Vol. 1, pp. 1–36). Hillsdale, NJ: Erlbaum.

Brewer, M.B. (1991). The social self: on being the same and different at the same time. *Personality and Social Psychology Bulletin, 17*, 475–482.

Brewer, M.B. (1993a). Social identity, distinctiveness, and in–group homogeneity. *Social Cognition, 11*, 150–164.

Brewer, M.B. (1993b). The role of distinctiveness in social identity and group behaviour. In M.A. Hogg & D. Abrams (Eds.), *Group motivation: Social psychological perspectives* (pp. 1–16). London: Harvester Wheatsheaf.

Brewer, M.B. (1994). Associated systems theory: if you buy two representational systems, why not many? In R.S. Wyer (Ed.), *Advances in social cognition* (Vol. 7, pp. 141–147). Hillsdale, NJ: Erlbaum.

Brewer, M.B. & Harasty, A. S. (1996). Seeing groups as entities: the role of perceiver motivation. In R.M. Sorrentino & E.T. Higgins (Eds.), *The handbook of motivation and cognition: the interpersonal context* (Vol. 3, pp. 347–370). New York: Guilford.

Brewer, M.B. & Miller, N. (1984). Beyond the contact hypothesis: theoretical perspectives on desegregation. In N. Miller & M.B. Brewer (Eds.), *Groups in contact: the psychology of desegregation*. New York: Academic Press.

Brewer, M.B., Weber, J.G., & Carini, B. (1995). Person memory in intergroup contexts: categorization versus individuation. *Journal of Personality and Social Psychology, 69*, 29–40.

Brown, P.M. (1999). *Category fit and theories in the formation of stereotype content.* Unpublished PhD thesis, Australian National University.

Brown, P.M. & Turner, J.C. (1998). *Making different background theories accessible: the impact on judgements of prototypicality and stereotype content.* Paper presented at the New Zealand Meeting of the Society of Australasian Social Psychologists. Christchurch, New Zealand, April.

Bruner, J.S. (1957). On perceptual readiness. *Psychological Review, 64*, 123–152.

Bruner, J.S. (1983). *In search of mind: essays in autobiography of Jerome Bruner*. New York: Harper and Row.

Campbell, D.T. (1956). Enhancement of contrast as a composite habit. *Journal of Abnormal and Social Psychology, 53*, 350–355.

Campbell, D.T. (1958). Common fate, similarity, and other indices of the status of aggregates of persons as social entities. *Behavioral Science, 3*, 14–25.

Carey, S. (1982). Semantic development: the state of the art. In E. Wanner & L.R. Gleitman (Eds.), *Language acquisition: the state of the art* (pp. 347–389). Cambridge: Cambridge University Press.

Carlston, D.E. (1994). Associated systems theory: a systematic approach to cognitive representations of persons. In T. K. Srull & R. S. Wyer (Eds.), *Advances in social cognition* (Vol. 7, pp. 1–78). Hillsdale, NJ: Erlbaum.

Carlston, D.E. & Smith, E.R. (1996). Principles of mental representation. In E.T. Higgins & A.W. Kruglanski (Eds.), *Social psychology: handbook of basic principles* (pp. 184–210). New York: Guilford.

Carlston, D.E. & Sparks, C.W. (1994). AST revisited: on the many facets of impressions and theories. In R. S. Wyer (Ed.), *Advances in social cognition* (Vol. 7, pp. 169–225). Hillsdale, NJ: Erlbaum.

Castano, E. & Yzerbyt, V.Y. (1998). *We are one and I like it: the impact of ingroup entitativity on social identification.* Unpublished manuscript, Catholic University of Louvain at Louvain-la-Neuve.

Cheng, P.W. (1997). From covariation to causation: a causal power theory. *Psychological Review, 104*, 367–405.

Cheng, P.W. & Novick, L.R. (1990). A probabilistic contrast model of causal induction. *Journal of Personality and Social Psychology, 58*, 545–567.

Cho, J.-R. & Mathews, R. C. (1996). Interactions between mental models used in categorization and experiential knowledge of specific cases. *Quarterly Journal of Experimental Psychology, 49A,* 572–595.

Claire, T. & Fiske, S.T. (1998). A systemic view of behavioral confirmation:

Counterpoint to the individualist view. In C. Sedikides, J. Schopler & C.A. Insko (Eds.), *Intergroup cognition and intergroup behavior* (pp. 205–231). Mahwah, NJ: Erlbaum.

Collins, A. & Loftus, E.F. (1975). A spreading activation theory of semantic processing. *Psychological Review, 82*, 407–428.

de la Haye, A.–M. (1998). *False consensus and the out-group homogeneity effect: interference in measurement or intrinsically dependent processes?* Unpublished manuscript, Université de Poitiers.

Deschamps, J.-C. & Doise, W. (1978). Crossed category memberships in intergroup relations. In H. Tajfel (Ed.), *Differentiation between social groups* (pp. 141–158). Cambridge, UK: Cambridge University Press.

Devine, P.G. (1989). Stereotypes and prejudice: their automatic and controlled components. *Journal of Personality and Social Psychology, 56*, 5–18.

Doise, W. (1978). *Groups and individuals: explanations in social psychology.* Cambridge: Cambridge University Press.

Doosje, B.J., Spears, R., & Koomen, W. (1995). When bad isn't all bad: the strategic use of sample information in generalization and stereotyping. *Journal of Personality and Social Psychology, 69*, 642–655.

Doosje, B.J., Haslam, S. A., Spears, R., Oakes, P.J. & Koomen, W. (1998). The effect of comparative context on central tendency and variability judgments and the evaluation of group characteristics. *European Journal of Social Psychology, 28*, 159–172.

Doosje, B. J., Branscombe, N., Spears, R., & Manstead, A.S.R. (in press). Guilty by association: when one's group has a negative history. *Journal of Personality and Social Psychology.*

Edwards, D. (1991). Categories are for talking: on the cognitive and discursive bases of categorization. *Theory and Psychology, 1*, 515–542.

Eggins, R.A. (forthcoming). *Social identity processes in negotiation.* Unpublished PhD thesis, Australian National University.

Eiser, J.R. (1971). Enhancement of contrast in the absolute judgement of attitude statements. *Journal of Personality and Social Psychology, 17*, 1–10.

Eiser, J.R. (1980). *Cognitive social psychology: a guidebook to theory and research.* Maidenhead: McGraw Hill.

Eiser, J.R. (1986). *Social psychology: attitudes, cognition and social behaviour.* Cambridge: Cambridge University Press.

Eiser, J.R. (1990). *Social judgment.* Milton Keynes: Open University Press.

Eiser, J.R., & Stroebe, W. (1972). *Categorization and social judgement.* London: Academic Press.

Eiser, J.R., van der Pligt, J., & Gossop, M.R. (1979). Categorization, attitudes and memory for the source of attitude statements. *European Journal of Social Psychology, 9*, 243–251.

Eiser, J.R., Martien, C., & van Schie, E. (1991). Categorization and interclass assimilation in social judgement. *European Journal of Social Psychology, 21*, 493–505.

Ellemers, N. & van Knippenberg, A.F.M. (1997). Stereotyping in social context. In R. Spears, P. J. Oakes, N. Ellemers, & S. A. Haslam (Eds.), *The social psychology of stereotyping and group life* (pp. 208–235). Oxford: Blackwell.

Estes, W.K. (1950). Towards a statistical theory of learning. *Psychological Review, 57*, 94–107.

Estes, W.K. (1991). Cognitive architectures from the standpoint of an experimental psychologist. *Annual Review of Psychology, 42*, 1–28.

Feldman, J. (1988). Objects in categories and objects as categories. In T.K. Srull & R.S. Wyer, (Eds.), *Advances in social cognition: a dual process model of impression formation* (Vol. 1, pp. 53–63). Hillsdale, NJ: Erlbaum.

Festinger, L. (1950). Informal social communication. *Psychological Review, 57*, 271–282.

Festinger, L. (1954). A theory of social comparison processes. *Human Relations, 7,* 117–140.

Fiedler, K. (1991). The tricky nature of skewed frequency tables: an information loss account of distinctiveness-based illusory correlations. *Journal of Personality and Social Psychology, 60,* 26–36.

Fiedler, K. (1996). Explaining and simulating judgment biases as an aggregation phenomenon in probabilistic, multiple-cue environments. *Psychological Review, 103,* 193–214.

Fiedler, K., Russer, S., & Gramm, K. (1993). Illusory correlations and memory performance. *Journal of Experimental Social Psychology, 29,* 111–136.

Fillmore, C. (1982). Towards a descriptive framework for spatial deixis. In R.J. Jarvella & W. Klein (Eds.), *Speech, place and action: studies in deixis and related topics* (pp. 31–59). Chichester: Wiley.

Fishbein, M. & Ajzen, I. (1974). Factors influencing intentions and the intention–behavior relation. *Human Relations, 27,* 1–15.

Fiske, S.T. (1993). Social cognition and social perception. *Annual Review of Psychology, 44,* 155–194.

Fiske, S.T. & Leyens, J.-P. (1997). Let social psychology be faddish or, at least, heterogeneous. In C. McGarty & S. A. Haslam (Eds.), *The message of social psychology: perspectives on mind in society* (pp. 92–112). Oxford, UK and Cambridge, MA: Blackwell.

Fiske, S.T. & Morling, B. (1996). Stereotyping as a function of personal control motives and capacity constraints: the odd couple of power and anxiety. In R.M. Sorrentino & E.T. Higgins (Eds.), *Handbook of motivation and cognition: Vol. 3 The interpersonal context* (pp. 322–346). New York: Guilford.

Fiske, S.T. & Neuberg, S.L. (1990). A continuum of impression formation, from category-based to individuating processes: influences of information and motivation on attention and interpretation. *Advances in Experimental Social Psychology, 23,* 1–74.

Fiske, S.T. & Pavelchak, M.A. (1986). Category-based versus piecemeal-based affective responses: developments in schema-triggered affect. In R.M. Sorrentino and E.T. Higgins (Eds.), *Handbook of motivation and cognition: Foundations of social behavior* (pp. 167–203). New York: Guilford.

Fiske, S.T., Lin, M. & Neuberg, S. L. (in press). The continuum model: ten years later. In S. Chaiken & Y. Trope (Eds.), *Dual process theories in social psychology*. New York: Guilford.

Ford, T.E. & Stangor, C. R. (1992). The role of diagnosticity in stereotype formation: perceiving group means and variances. *Journal of Personality and Social Psychology, 63,* 356–367.

Ford, T.E., Stangor, C.R., & Duan, C. (1994). Influence of social category accessibility and category–associated trait accessibility on judgements of individuals. *Social Cognition, 12,* 149–168.

Forgas, J.P. (1994). The role of emotion in social judgments: an introductory review and an Affect Infusion Model (AIM). *European Journal of Social Psychology, 24,* 1–24.

Fried, L.S. & Holyoak, K.J. (1984). Induction of category learning: a framework for classification learning. *Journal of Experimental Psychology: Learning, Memory, and Cognition, 10,* 234–257.

Funder, D.C. (1987). Errors and mistakes: evaluating the accuracy of social judgment. *Psychological Bulletin, 101,* 75–90.

Fyock, J. & Stangor, C. (1994). The role of memory biases in stereotype maintenance. *British Journal of Social Psychology, 33,* 331–343.

Gaertner, S.L., Mann, J., Murrell, A., & Dovidio, J.F. (1989). Reducing intergroup bias: the benefits of recategorization. *Journal of Personality and Social Psychology, 59,* 692–704.

Gelman, S. & Medin, D.L. (1993). What's so essential about essentialism? A different perspective on the interaction of perception, language, and conceptual knowledge. *Cognitive Development, 8*, 157–167.

Gentner, D. (1983). Structure mapping: a theoretical framework for analogy. *Cognitive Science, 7*, 155–170.

Gentner, D. & Medina, J. (1998). Similarity and the development of rules. *Cognition, 65*, 263–297.

Gibson, J.J. (1966). *The senses considered as perceptual systems*. Boston: Houghton-Mifflin.

Gibson, J.J. (1979). *The ecological approach to perception*. Boston: Houghton–Mifflin.

Gigerenzer, G. (1991). How to make cognitive illusions disappear: beyond 'heuristics and biases'. *European Review of Social Psychology, 2*, 83–115.

Gilbert, D.T. (1989). Thinking lightly about others: automatic components of the social inference process. In J.S. Uleman & J.A. Bargh (Eds.), *Unintended thought* (pp. 189–211). New York: Guilford.

Gilbert, D.T. & Hixon, J. G. (1991). The trouble of thinking: activation and application of stereotypic beliefs. *Journal of Personality and Social Psychology, 60*, 509–517.

Gluck, M.A. & Bower, G.H. (1988). From conditioning to category learning: an adaptive network model. *Journal of Experimental Psychology: General, 117*, 227–247.

Goldstone, R.L. (1995). Effects of categorization on color perception. *Psychological Science, 6*, 298–304.

Goldstone, R.L. (1998). Perceptual learning. *Annual Review of Psychology, 49*, 585–612.

Goldstone, R.L. & Barsalou, L.W. (1998). Reuniting perception and conception. *Cognition, 65*, 231–262.

Greenwald, A.G. & Banaji, M.R. (1995). Implicit social cognition: attitudes, self-esteem, and stereotypes. *Psychological Review, 102*, 4–27.

Gutheil, G. & Gelman, S.A. (1997). Children's use of sample size and diversity information within basic-level categories. *Journal of Experimental Child Psychology, 64*, 159–174.

Hamilton, D.L. (Ed.) (1981). *Cognitive processes in stereotyping and intergroup behaviour*. Hillsdale, NJ: Erlbaum.

Hamilton, D.L. & Gifford, R.K. (1976). Illusory correlation in intergroup perception: a cognitive basis of stereotypic judgments. *Journal of Experimental Social Psychology, 12*, 392–407.

Hamilton, D.L. & Rose, T. L. (1980). Illusory correlation and the maintenance of stereotypic beliefs. *Journal of Personality and Social Psychology, 39*, 832–845.

Hamilton, D.L. & Sherman, S.J. (1989). Illusory correlations: implications for stereotype theory and research. In D. Bar–Tal, C.F. Graumann, A.W. Kruglanski, & W. Stroebe (Eds.), *Stereotyping and prejudice: changing conceptions*. New York and London: Springer.

Hamilton, D.L. & Sherman, S.J. (1996). Perceiving persons and groups. *Psychological Review, 103*, 336–355.

Hamilton, D.L., Sherman, S.J., & Lickel, B. (1998). Perceiving social groups: the importance of the entitativity continuum. In C. Sedikides, J. Schopler & C.A. Insko (Eds.), *Intergroup cognition and intergroup behaviour* (pp. 47–74). Mahwah, NJ: Erlbaum.

Hampson, S.E. (1988). The dynamics of categorization and impression formation. In T.K. Srull & R.S. Wyer (Eds.), *Advances in social cognition* (Vol. 1, pp. 77–82). Hillsdale, NJ: Erlbaum.

Hardin, C. & Higgins, E.T. (1996). Shared reality: how social verification makes the subjective objective. In R.M. Sorrentino & E.T. Higgins (Eds.), *The handbook of motivation and cognition: the interpersonal context* (Vol. 3, pp. 28–84). New York: Guilford.

Harnad, S. (1987). *Categorical perception: the groundwork of cognition.* Cambridge: Cambridge University Press.

Haslam, N. (1994). Mental representation of social relationships: dimensions, laws, or categories? *Journal of Personality and Social Psychology, 67,* 575–584.

Haslam, N., Rothschild, L., & Ernst, D. (1997). *Essentialist beliefs about social categories.* Unpublished manuscript, New School for Social Research.

Haslam, S.A. (1997). Stereotyping and social influence: foundations of stereotype consensus. In R. Spears, P.J. Oakes, N. Ellemers, & S.A. Haslam (Eds.) *The social psychology of stereotyping and group life* (pp.119–143). Oxford: Blackwell.

Haslam, S.A. & McGarty, C. (1998). *Doing psychological research: an introduction to methodology and statistics.* London: Sage.

Haslam, S.A. & Turner, J.C. (1992). Context-dependent variation in social stereotyping. 2: The relationship between frame of reference, self-categorization and accentuation. *European Journal of Social Psychology, 22,* 251–277.

Haslam, S.A. & Turner, J.C. (1995). Context-dependent variation in social stereotyping. 3: Extremism as a self-categorical basis for polarized judgement. *European Journal of Social Psychology, 25,* 341–371.

Haslam, S.A., Oakes, P.J., McGarty, C., Turner, J.C., & Onorato, R. (1995a). Contextual changes in the prototypicality of extreme and moderate outgroup members. *European Journal of Social Psychology, 25,* 509–530.

Haslam, S.A., Oakes, P.J., Turner, J.C., & McGarty, C. (1995b). Social categorization and group homogeneity: changes in the perceived applicability of stereotype content as a function of comparative context and trait favourableness. *British Journal of Social Psychology, 34,* 139–160.

Haslam, S.A., McGarty, C., & Brown, P.M. (1996a). The search for differentiated meaning is a precursor to illusory correlation. *Personality and Social Psychology Bulletin, 22,* 611–619.

Haslam, S.A., Oakes, P.J., McGarty, C., Turner, J.C., Reynolds, K., & Eggins, R. (1996b). Stereotyping and social influence: the mediation of stereotype applicability and sharedness by the views of ingroups and outgroup members. *British Journal of Social Psychology, 35,* 369–397.

Haslam, S.A., Oakes, P.J., Turner, J.C., & McGarty, C. (1996c). Social identity, self-categorization and the perceived homogeneity of ingroups and outgroups: the interaction between social motivation and cognition. In R. M. Sorrentino & E. T. Higgins (Eds.), *Handbook of Motivation and Cognition* (Vol. 3, pp. 182–222). New York: Guilford.

Haslam, S.A., Oakes, P.J., Turner, J.C., McGarty, C., & Reynolds, K.J. (1998). The group as a basis for emergent stereotype consensus. *The European Review of Social Psychology, 8,* 203–239.

Hastie, R. & Park, B. (1986). The relationship between memory and judgment depends on whether the judgment task is memory-based or on-line. *Psychological Review, 93,* 258–268.

Hayes, B.K. & Taplin, J.E. (1992). Developmental changes in categorization processes: knowledge and similarity-based modes of categorization. *Journal of Experimental Child Psychology, 54,* 188–212.

Hayes, B.K. & Taplin, J.E. (1995). Similarity-based and knowledge-based processes in category learning. *European Journal of Cognitive Psychology, 7,* 383–410.

Heider, E.E. & Olivier, D. (1974). The structure of the color space in naming and memory for two languages. *Cognitive Psychology, 3,* 337–354.

Helson, H. (1964). *Adaptation-level theory.* New York: Harper.

Hewstone, M. (1989). *Causal attribution: from cognitive processes to collective beliefs.* Oxford, UK and Cambridge, MA: Blackwell.

Hewstone, M. & Brown, R. (Eds.) (1986). *Contact and conflict in intergroup encounters.* Oxford: Basil Blackwell.

Hewstone, M. & Lord, C. (1998). Changing intergroup cognitions and intergroup behaviour: the role of typicality. In C. Sedikides, J. Schopler, & C.A. Insko (Eds.), *Intergroup cognition and intergroup behaviour* (pp. 367–392). Mahwah, NJ: Erlbaum.

Higgins, E.T. (1996). Knowledge activation: Accessibility, applicability, and salience. In E.T. Higgins & A.W. Kruglanski (Eds.), *Social psychology: handbook of basic principles* (pp. 133–168). New York: Guilford.

Higgins, E.T. (1997). Biases in social cognition: 'Aboutness' as a general principle. In C. McGarty & S.A. Haslam (Eds.), *The message of social psychology: perspectives on mind in society* (pp. 182–199). Oxford, UK & Cambridge, MA: Blackwell.

Higgins, E.T. & Brendl, C.M. (1995). Accessibility and applicability: some 'activation rules' influencing judgement. *Journal of Experimental Social Psychology, 31*, 218–243.

Higgins, E.T. & King, G. (1981). Accessibility of social constructs: information processing consequences of individual and contextual variability. In N. Cantor & J.F. Kihlstrom (Eds.), *Personality, cognition, and social interaction* (pp. 69–121). Hillsdale, NJ: Erlbaum.

Higgins, E.T., Bargh, J.A., & Lombardi, W.L. (1985). Nature of priming effects on categorization. *Journal of Experimental Psychology: Learning, Memory, and Cognition, 11*, 59–69.

Hilton, D.J. (1991). A conversational model of causal explanation. *European Review of Social Psychology, 2*, 51–81.

Hilton, D.J. & Slugoski, B. (1986). Knowledge-based causal attribution: the abnormal conditions focus model. *Psychological Review, 93*, 75–88.

Hintzman, D.L. (1986). 'Schema abstraction' in a multiple-trace memory model. *Psychological Review, 93*, 411–428.

Hogg, M.A. & Abrams, D. (1990). Social motivation, self-esteem and social identity. In D. Abrams & M.A. Hogg (Eds.), *Social identity theory: constructive and critical advances* (pp. 28–47). London: Harvester Wheatsheaf.

Hogg, M.A. & Abrams, D. (1993). Towards a single-process uncertainty-reduction model of social motivation in groups. In D. Abrams & M.A. Hogg (Eds.), *Group motivation: social psychological perspectives* (pp. 173–190). London: Harvester Wheatsheaf.

Hogg, M.A., Turner, J.C. and Davidson, B. (1990) Polarized norms and social frames of reference: a test of the self-categorization theory of group polarization. *Basic and Applied Social Psychology, 11*, 77–100.

Holyoak, K.J. & Spellman, B.A. (1993). Thinking. *Annual Review of Psychology, 44*, 265–315.

Hovland, C.I., Janis, I. L., & Kelley, H.H. (1953). *Communication and persuasion: psychological studies in opinion change*. New Haven, CT: Yale.

Howard, J.W. & Rothbart, M. (1980). Social categorization and memory for in-group and out-group behaviour. *Journal of Personality and Social Psychology, 38*, 301–310.

Huber, G.L. & Sorrentino, R.M. (1996). Uncertainty in interpersonal and intergroup relations: an individual-differences perspective. In R.M. Sorrentino & E.T. Higgins (Eds.), *The handbook of motivation and cognition* (Vol. 3, pp. 591–619). New York: Guilford.

Hunt, R.R. (1995). The subtlety of distinctiveness: what von Restorff really did. *Psychonomic Bulletin and Review, 2*, 105–112.

Huttenlocher, J., Hedges, L.V., & Duncan, S. (1991). Categories and particulars: prototype effects in estimating spatial location. *Psychological Review, 98*, 352–376.

Isen, A.M. (1987). Positive affect, cognitive processes, and social behavior. *Advances in Experimental Social Psychology, 20*, 203–253.

Isen, A.M. (1993). Positive affect and decision making. In M. Lewis & J.M. Haviland (Eds.), *Handbook of emotions* (pp. 261–277). New York: Guilford.

Isen, A.M., Niedenthal, P.M., & Cantor, N. (1992). An influence of positive affect on social categorization. *Motivation and Emotion, 16,* 65–78.

Jenkins, J.L. (1992). The organization and reorganization of categories: the case of speech perception. In H.L. Pick, P. van den Broek, & D.C. Knill (Eds.), *Cognition: conceptual and methodological issues* (pp. 11–31). Washington, DC: American Psychological Association.

Jetten, J. (1997). *Dimensions of distinctiveness: intergroup discrimination and social identity.* Amsterdam: Thesis.

Jetten, J., Spears, R. & Manstead, A.S.R. (1998). Defining dimensions of distinctiveness: group variability makes a difference to differentiation. *Journal of Personality and Social Psychology, 74,* 1481–1492.

John, O.P., Hampson, S.E., & Goldberg, L.R. (1991). The basic level in personality-trait hierarchies: studies of trait use and accessibility in different contexts. *Journal of Personality and Social Psychology, 60,* 348–361.

Jones, S.S. & Smith, L.B. (1993). The place of perception in children's concepts. *Cognitive Development, 8,* 113–139.

Jost, J.T. & Banaji, M.R. (1994). The role of stereotyping in system-justification and the production of false consciousness. *British Journal of Social Psychology, 33,* 1–27.

Judd, C.M. & Park, B. (1988). Outgroup homogeneity: judgments of variability at the individual and group levels. *Journal of Personality and Social Psychology, 54,* 778–788.

Judd, C.M. & Park, B. (1993). Definition and assessment of accuracy in social stereotypes. *Psychological Review, 100,* 109–128.

Jussim, L. (1991). Social perception and social reality: a reflection-construction model. *Psychological Review, 98,* 54–73.

Kahneman, D. (1973). *Attention and effort.* Englewood Cliffs, NJ: Prentice-Hall.

Kahneman, D. & Miller, D.T. (1986). Norm theory: comparing reality to its alternatives. *Psychological Review, 93,* 136–153.

Kashima, E.S. & Kashima, Y. (1993). Perceptions of general variability of social groups. *Social Cognition, 11,* 1–21.

Kashima, Y., Woolcock, J., & King, D. (1998). The dynamics of group impression formation: the Tensor Product Model of exemplar-based social category learning. In S.J. Read & L.C. Miller et al. (Eds.), *Connectionist models of social reasoning and social behaviour* (pp. 71–109). Mahwah, NJ: Erlbaum.

Kelley, H.H. (1967). Attribution theory in social psychology. In D. Levine (Ed.), *Nebraska symposium on motivation.* Lincoln, NE: University.

Kelly, C. (1989). Political identity and perceived intragroup homogeneity. *British Journal of Social Psychology, 28,* 239–250.

Kobrynowicz, D. & Biernat, M. (1998). Considering correctness, contrast, and categorization in stereotyping phenomena. In R. S. Wyer (Ed.), *Advances in social cognition* (Vol. 11, pp. 109–126). Mahwah, NJ: Erlbaum.

Kraus, S., Ryan, C.S., Judd, C.M., Hastie, R., & Park, B. (1993). Use of mental frequency distributions to represent variability among members of social categories. *Social Cognition, 11,* 22–43.

Krueger, J. (1991). Accentuation effects and illusory change in exemplar-based category learning. *European Journal of Social Psychology, 21,* 37–48.

Krueger, J. (1992). On the overestimation of between-group differences. *European Review of Social Psychology, 3,* 31–56.

Krueger, J. & Clement, R.W. (1994). Memory-based judgments about multiple categories: a revision and extension of Tajfel's accentuation theory. *Journal of Personality and Social Psychology, 67,* 35–47.

Krueger, J. & Clement, R.W. (1996). Inferring category characteristics from sample characteristics: inductive reasoning and social projection. *Journal of Experimental Psychology: General, 125,* 52–68.

Krueger, J., Rothbart, M., & Sriram, N. (1989). Category learning and change: differences in sensitivity to information that enhances or reduces intercategory distinctions. *Journal of Personality and Social Psychology, 56,* 866–875.

Kruglanski, A.W. (1996). Motivated social cognition: principles of the interface. In E.T. Higgins & A. W. Kruglanski (Eds.), *Social psychology: handbook of basic principles* (pp. 493–520). New York: Guilford.

Kruglanski, A.W. & Webster, D.M. (1991). Group members' reactions to opinion deviates and conformists at varying degrees of proximity to decision deadline and of environmental noise. *Journal of Personality and Social Psychology, 61,* 212–225.

Kunda, Z. (1990). The case for motivated reasoning. *Psychological Bulletin, 108,* 480–498.

Kunda, Z. & Oleson, K.C. (1995). Maintaining stereotypes in the face of disconfirmation: constructing grounds for subtyping deviants. *Journal of Personality and Social Psychology, 68,* 565–580.

Kunda, Z. & Sherman-Williams, B. (1993). Stereotypes and the construal of individuating information. *Personality and Social Psychology Bulletin, 19,* 90–99.

Kunda, Z. & Thagard, P. (1996). Forming impressions from stereotypes, traits and behaviors: a parallel-constraint-satisfaction theory. *Psychological Review, 103,* 284–308.

Kunda, Z., Sinclair, L., & Griffin, D. (1997). Equal ratings but separate meanings: stereotypes and the construal of traits. *Journal of Personality and Social Psychology, 72,* 720–734.

Lakoff, G. (1987). *Women, fire and dangerous things: what categories tell us about the nature of thought.* Chicago: University of Chicago Press.

Lakoff, G. & Johnson, M. (1980). *Metaphors we live by.* Chicago: University of Chicago Press.

Lassaline, M.E. & Murphy, G. L. (1998). Alignment and category learning. *Journal of Experimental Psychology: Learning, Memory, and Cognition, 24,* 144–160.

Lee, Y.T., Jussim, L., & McCauley, C.R. (1993). *Stereotype accuracy: towards appreciating group differences.* Washington, DC: American Psychological Association.

Lepore, L. & Brown, R. (1997). Category and stereotype activation: is prejudice inevitable? *Journal of Personality and Social Psychology, 72,* 275–287.

Levine, J.M., Resnick, L.D., & Higgins, E.T. (1993). Social foundations of cognition. *Annual Review of Psychology, 44,* 584–612.

Lewin, K. (1948). *Resolving social conflicts.* New York: Harper and Row.

Lewin, K. (1951). *Field theory in social science* (edited by D. Cartwright). New York: Harper and Row.

Leyens, J.-P., Yzerbyt, V.Y., & Schadron, G.H. (1992). Stereotypes and social judgeability. *European Review of Social Psychology, 3,* 91–120.

Leyens, J.-P., Yzerbyt, V.Y., & Schadron, G.H. (1994). *Stereotypes and social cognition.* London: Sage.

Lin, E.L. & Murphy, G.L. (1997). Effects of background knowledge on object categorization and part detection. *Journal of Experimental Psychology: Human, Perception and Performance, 23,* 1153–1169.

Lingle, J.H., Altom, M. W., & Medin, D.L. (1984). Of cabbages and kings: assessing the extendibility of natural object concept models to social things. In R.S. Wyer & T. Srull (Eds.), *Handbook of social cognition* (Vol. 1, pp. 71–117). Hillsdale, NJ: Erlbaum.

Linville, P.W. & Fischer, G.W. (1998). Group variability and covariation: effects on intergroup behavior and judgment. In C. Sedikides, J. Schopler, & C.A. Insko (Eds.), *Intergroup cognition and intergroup behavior* (pp. 123–150). Mahwah, NJ: Erlbaum.

Linville, P.W. & Jones, E.E. (1980). Polarized appraisals of outgroup members. *Journal of Personality and Social Psychology, 38,* 689–703.

Linville, P.W., Salovey, P., & Fischer, G.W. (1986). Stereotyping and perceived distributions of social characteristics: an application to ingroup–outgroup perception. In J.F. Dovidio & S.L. Gaertner (Eds.), *Prejudice, discrimination, racism: theory and research* (pp. 165–208). New York: Academic Press.

Linville, P.W., Fischer, G.W., & Salovey, P. (1989). Perceived distributions of the characteristics of in-group and out-group members: empirical evidence and a computer simulation. *Journal of Personality and Social Psychology, 57,* 165–188.

Linville, P.W., Fischer, G.W., & Yoon, C. (1996). Perceived covariation among the features of ingroup and outgroup members: the outgroup covariation effect. *Journal of Personality and Social Psychology, 70,* 421–436.

Livingston, K.R., Andrews, J.K., & Harnad, S. (1998). Categorical perception effects induced by category learning. *Journal of Experimental Psychology: Learning, Memory, Cognition, 24,* 732–753.

Long, K. & Spears, R. (1997). The self-esteem hypothesis revisited: differentiation and the disaffected. In R. Spears, P.J. Oakes, N. Ellemers & S.A. Haslam (Eds.) *The social psychology of stereotyping and group life* (pp. 296–317). Oxford: Blackwell.

Lord, C.G., Desforges, D. M., Ramsey, S.L., Trezza, G.R., & Lepper, M.R. (1991). Typicality effects in attitude–behavior consistency: effects of category discrimination and category knowledge. *Journal of Experimental Social Psychology, 27,* 550–575.

Lorenzi-Cioldi, F. (1993). They all look alike, but so do we . . . sometimes: perceptions of in-group and out-group homogeneity as a function of sex and context. *British Journal of Social Psychology, 32,* 111–124.

Lorenzi-Cioldi, F., Eagly, A.H., & Stewart, T.L. (1995). Homogeneity of gender groups in memory. *Journal of Experimental Social Psychology, 31,* 193–217.

Maass, A. & Arcuri, L. (1992). The role of language in the persistence of stereotypes. In G. R. Semin & K. Fiedler (Eds.), *Language, interaction, and social cognition* (pp. 129–143). Newbury Park, CA: Sage.

Mackie, D.M. & Cooper, J. (1984). Attitude polarization: the effects of group membership. *Journal of Personality and Social Psychology, 46,* 575–585.

Mackie, D., Worth, L.T., & Asuncion, A.G. (1990). Processing of persuasive in-group messages. *Journal of Personality and Social Psychology, 58,* 812–822.

Macrae, C.N., Hewstone, M., & Griffiths, R.J. (1993). Processing load and memory for stereotype-based information. *European Journal of Social Psychology, 23,* 77–87.

Macrae, C.N., Bodenhausen, G.V., Milne, A.B., & Jetten, J. (1994). Out of mind but back in sight: stereotypes on the rebound. *Journal of Personality and Social Psychology, 67,* 808–817.

Macrae, C.N., Bodenhausen, G.V., & Milne, A.B. (1995). The dissection of selection in person perception: inhibitory processes in social stereotyping. *Journal of Personality and Social Psychology, 69,* 397–407.

Macrae, C.N., Bodenhausen, G.V., Milne, A.B., & Ford, R.L. (1997). On the regulation of recollection: the intentional forgetting of stereotypical memories. *Journal of Personality and Social Psychology, 72,* 709–719.

Macrae, C.N., Bodenhausen, G.V., & Milne, A.B. (1998). Saying no to unwanted thoughts: self-focus and the regulation of mental life. *Journal of Personality and Social Psychology, 74,* 578–589.

Manis, M., Paskewitz, J., & Cotler, S. (1986). Stereotypes and social judgement. *Journal of Personality and Social Psychology, 50,* 461–473.

Markus, H. & Kitayama, S. (1991). Culture and self: implications for cognition, emotion and motivation. *Psychological Review, 98,* 224–253.

Markus, H.R. & Wurf, E. (1987). The dynamic self-concept: a social psychological perspective. *Annual Review of Psychology, 38,* 299–337.

Markus, H.R., Kitayama, S., & Heiman, R.J. (1996). Culture and 'basic' psychological principles. In E. T. Higgins & A. W. Kruglanski (Eds.), *Social psychology:*

handbook of basic principles (pp. 857–913). New York: Guilford.

Marques, J.M., Yzerbyt, V.Y., & Leyens, J.-P. (1988). The 'Black Sheep Effect': extremity of judgments towards ingroup members as a function of group identification. *European Journal of Social Psychology, 18*, 1–16.

Martin, L.L. (1985). *Categorization and differentiation: a set, re-set, comparison analysis of the effects of context on person perception.* New York: Springer-Verlag.

Martin, L.L. & Tesser, A. (Eds.) (1992). *The construction of social judgments* (pp. 217–245). Hillsdale, NJ: Erlbaum.

Martin, L.L., Seta, J.J., & Crelia, R.A. (1990). Assimilation and contrast as a function of people's willingness and ability to expend effort in forming an impression. *Journal of Personality and Social Psychology, 59,* 27–37.

Massaro, D.W. (1992). Broadening the domain of the fuzzy logical model of perception. In H.L. Pick, P. van den Broek, and D.C. Knill (Eds.), *Cognition: Conceptual and methodological issues* (pp. 51–84). Washington, DC: American Psychological Association.

McConnell, A.R., Sherman, S.J., & Hamilton, D.L. (1994). Illusory correlation in the perception of groups: an extension of the distinctiveness-based account. *Journal of Personality and Social Psychology, 67,* 414–429.

McConnell, A.R., Sherman, S.J., & Hamilton, D.L. (1997). Target entitativity: implications for information processing about individual and group targets. *Journal of Personality and Social Psychology, 72,* 750–762.

McGarty, C. (1990). *Categorization and the social psychology of judgement.* Unpublished PhD thesis, Macquarie University.

McGarty, C. & de la Haye, A.-M. (1995). *Stereotype formation: beyond illusory correlation.* Paper presented to the Joint Meeting of the European Association of Social Psychology and the Society of Experimental Social Psychology, September, Washington, DC.

McGarty, C. & de la Haye, A.-M. (1997). Stereotype formation: beyond illusory correlation. In R. Spears, P. J. Oakes, N. Ellemers & S. A. Haslam (Eds.), *The social psychology of stereotyping and group life* (pp. 144–70). Oxford: Blackwell.

McGarty, C. & Grace, D.M. (1996). *Categorization, explanation and group norms: reconsidering the nature of ingroup bias.* Unpublished manuscript, Australian National University.

McGarty, C. & Haslam, S.A. (1997). Introduction and short history of social psychology. In C. McGarty and S. A. Haslam (Eds.), *The message of social psychology: perspectives on mind in society* (pp. 1–19). Oxford: Blackwell.

McGarty, C. & Penny, R.E.C. (1988). Categorization, accentuation and social judgement. *British Journal of Social Psychology, 22,* 147–157.

McGarty, C. & Turner, J.C. (1992). The effects of categorization on social judgement. *British Journal of Social Psychology, 31,* 253–268.

McGarty, C., Turner, J.C., Hogg, M.A., Davidson, B., & Wetherell, M.S. (1992). Group polarization as conformity to the prototypical group member. *British Journal of Social Psychology, 31,* 1–20.

McGarty, C., Haslam, S.A., Turner, J.C., & Oakes, P.J. (1993a). Illusory correlation as accentuation of actual intercategory difference: evidence for the effect with minimal stimulus information. *European Journal of Social Psychology, 23,* 391–410.

McGarty, C., Turner, J.C., Oakes, P.J., & Haslam, S.A. (1993b). The creation of uncertainty in the influence process: the roles of stimulus information and disagreement with similar others. *European Journal of Social Psychology, 23,* 17–38.

McGarty, C., Haslam, S.A., Hutchinson, K.J., & Turner, J.C. (1994). The effects of salient group memberships on persuasion. *Small Group Research, 25,* 267–293.

McGarty, C., Haslam, S.A., Hutchinson, K.J., & Grace, D.M. (1995). Determinants of perceived consistency: the relationship between group entitativity and the meaningfulness of categories. *British Journal of Social Psychology, 34,* 237–256.

McMullen, M.N., Fazio, R.H., & Gavanski, I. (1997). Motivation, attention and judgment: a natural sample spaces account. *Social Cognition, 15*, 77–90.

Mead, G.H. (1934). *Mind, self and society*. Chicago: University of Chicago Press.

Medin, D.L. (1988). Social categorization: structures, processes and purposes. In T. K. Srull & R. S. Wyer (Eds.), *Advances in social cognition: a dual process model of impression formation* (Vol. 1, pp. 1–36). Hillsdale, NJ: Erlbaum.

Medin, D.L. (1989). Concepts and conceptual structure. *American Psychologist, 44*, 1464–1481.

Medin, D.L. & Barsalou, L.W. (1987). General knowledge categories and categorical perception. In S. Harnad (Ed.), *Categorical perception: the groundwork of cognition*. Cambridge: Cambridge University Press.

Medin, D.L. & Ortony, A. (1989). Psychological essentialism. In S. Vosniadou & A. Ortony (Eds.), *Similarity and analogical reasoning* (pp. 179–195). New York: Cambridge University Press.

Medin, D.L. & Schaffer, M.M. (1978). Context theory of classification learning. *Psychological Review, 85*, 207–238.

Medin, D.L. & Schwanenflugel, P.L. (1981). Linear separability in classification learning. *Journal of Experimental Psychology: Human Learning and Memory, 7*, 355–368.

Medin, D L. & Smith, E.E. (1984). Concepts and concept formation. *Annual Review of Psychology, 40*, 113–138.

Medin, D.L. & Thau, D.M. (1992). Theories, constraints, and cognition. In H.L. Pick, P. van den Broek, & D.C. Knill (Eds.), *Cognition: conceptual and methodological issues* (pp. 165–187). Washington, DC: American Psychological Association.

Medin, D.L. & Wattenmaker, W.D. (1987). Category cohesiveness, theories, and cognitive archeology. In U. Neisser (Ed.), *Concepts and conceptual development: ecological and intellectual factors in categorization* (pp. 25–62). Cambridge/ New York: Cambridge University Press.

Medin, D.L., Goldstone, R.L., & Gentner, D. (1990). Similarity involving attributes and relations: judgements of similarity and difference are not inverses. *Psychological Science, 1*, 64–69.

Medin, D.L., Goldstone, R.L., & Gentner, D. (1993). Respects for similarity. *Psychological Review, 100*, 254–278.

Medin, D.L., Lynch, E.B., Coley, J.D., & Atran, S. (1997). Categorization and reasoning among tree experts: do all roads lead to Rome? *Cognitive Psychology, 32*, 49–96.

Mervis, C. B. & Rosch, E.H. (1981). Categorization of natural objects. *Annual Review of Psychology, 32*, 89–115.

Messick, D.M., & Mackie, D.M. (1989). Intergroup relations. *Annual Review of Psychology, 40*, 45–81.

Miller, G.A. (1956). The magical number seven plus or minus two: some limits on our capacity for processing information. *Psychological Review, 63*, 81–97.

Miller, N., Urban, L.M., & Vanman, E.J. (1998). A theoretical analysis of crossed social categorization effects. In C. Sedikides, J. Schopler, & C.A. Insko (Eds.), *Intergroup cognition and intergroup behavior* (pp. 393–420). Mahwah, NJ: Erlbaum.

Minsky, M.L. (1986). *The society of mind*. New York: Simon & Schuster.

Moscovici, S. (1976). *Social influence and social change*. London: Academic Press.

Moscovici, S. (1980). Towards a theory of conversion behavior. In L. Berkowitz (Ed.), *Advances in experimental social psychology* (Vol. 13, pp. 209–239). New York: Academic Press.

Moscovici, S. (1984). On social representations. In R. M. Farr & S. Moscovici (Eds.), *Social representations*. Cambridge: Cambridge University Press.

Moscovici, S. (1985). Social influence and conformity. In E. Aronson & G. Lindsay (Eds.), *Handbook of social psychology* (Vol. 2, pp. 347–412). Reading, MA: Addison-Wesley.

Moscovici, S. (1993). The return of the unconscious. *Social Research, 60*, 39–93.

Moskowitz, G.B. (1993). Individual differences in social categorization: the influence of personal need for structure on spontaneous trait inferences. *Journal of Personality and Social Psychology, 65*, 132–142.

Moskowitz, G.B. & Roman, R.J. (1992). Spontaneous trait inferences as self-generated primes: implications for conscious social judgement. *Journal of Personality and Social Psychology, 62*, 728–738.

Mullen, B. (1991). Group composition, salience, and cognitive representations: the phenomenology of being in a group. *Journal of Experimental Social Psychology, 27*, 297–323.

Mullen, B. & Hu, L. (1989). Perceptions of ingroup and outgroup variability: a meta-analytic integration. *Basic and Applied Social Psychology, 10*, 233–252.

Mullen, B. & Johnson, C. (1990) Distinctiveness-based illusory correlations and stereotyping: a meta-analytic integration. *British Journal of Social Psychology, 29*, 11–28.

Mullen, B., Brown, R., & Smith, C. (1992). Ingroup bias as a function of salience, relevance, and status: an integration. *European Journal of Social Psychology, 22*, 103–122.

Mullen, B., Johnson, C. & Anthony, T. (1994). Relative group size and cognitive representations of ingroup and outgroup: the phenomenology of being in a group. *Small Group Research, 25*, 250–266.

Mummendey, A. (1995). Positive distinctiveness and social distinction: an old couple living in divorce. *European Journal of Social Psychology, 25*, 657–670.

Mummendey, A. & Schreiber, H. J. (1983). Better or just different? Positive social identity by discrimination against, or by differentiation from outgroups. *European Journal of Social Psychology, 13*, 389–397.

Mummendey, A. & Simon, B. (1989). Better or different? III. The impact of importance of comparison dimension and relative in-group size upon intergroup discrimination. *British Journal of Social Psychology, 28*, 1–16.

Mummendey, A. & Wenzel, M. (1997). *Social discrimination and tolerance in intergroup relations: reactions to intergroup difference.* Unpublished manuscript, University of Jena.

Murphy, G.L. & Medin, D. L. (1985). The role of theories in conceptual coherence. *Psychological Review, 92*, 289–316.

Neisser, U. (1987). From direct perception to conceptual structure. In U. Neisser (Ed.), *Concepts and conceptual development: ecological and intellectual factors in categorization* (pp. 11–24). Cambridge & New York: Cambridge University Press.

Nesdale, A.R., Dharmalingam, S., & Kerr, G. K. (1987). Effect of subgroup ratio on stereotyping. *European Journal of Social Psychology, 17*, 353–356.

Nisbett, R.E. & Ross, L. (1980). *Human inference: strategies and shortcomings of social judgment.* Englewood-Cliffs, NJ: Prentice-Hall.

Nisbett, R.E. & Wilson, T.D. (1977). Telling more than we can know: verbal reports on mental processes. *Psychological Review, 84*, 231–259.

Norman, D.A., & Bobrow, D.G. (1975). On data-limited and resource-limited processes. *Cognitive Psychology, 7*, 44–64.

Nosofsky, R.M. (1984). Choice, similarity, and the context theory of classification. *Journal of Experimental Psychology: Learning, Memory, and Cognition, 10*, 104–114.

Nosofsky, R.M. (1986). Attention, categorization and the identification-categorization relationship. *Journal of Experimental Psychology: General, 115*, 39–57.

Nosofsky, R.M., Palmeri, T.J., & McKinley, S.C. (1994). Rule-plus-exception model of classification learning. *Psychological Review, 101*, 53–79.

Nye, J.L. & Brower, A.M. (Eds.) (1996). *What's so social about social cognition? Social cognition research in small groups.* Newbury Park, CA: Sage.

Oakes, P.J. (1987). The salience of social categories. In J.C. Turner, M. A. Hogg,

P.J. Oakes, S. D. Reicher, & M. S. Wetherell, *Rediscovering the social group: a self-categorization theory* (pp. 117–141). London: Blackwell.

Oakes, P.J. (1996). The categorization process: cognition and the group in the social psychology of stereotyping. In W.P. Robinson (Ed.), *Social groups and identity: developing the legacy of Henri Tajfel*. Oxford: Butterworth Heineman.

Oakes, P.J. (in press). The root of all evil in intergroup relations? Unearthing the categorization process. In R. Brown & S.L. Gaertner (Eds.), *Blackwell handbook in social psychology (Vol. 4): intergroup processes*. Oxford: Blackwell.

Oakes, P.J. & Reynolds, K J. (1997). Asking the accuracy question: is measurement the answer? In R. Spears, P.J. Oakes, N. Ellemers, & S.A. Haslam (Eds.), *The social psychology of stereotyping and group life* (pp. 51–71). Oxford, UK and Cambridge, MA: Blackwell.

Oakes, P.J. & Turner, J.C. (1986). Distinctiveness and the salience of social category memberships: is there an automatic bias towards novelty? *European Journal of Social Psychology, 16*, 325–344.

Oakes, P.J. & Turner, J.C. (1990). Is limited information processing capacity the cause of social stereotyping? *European Review of Social Psychology, 1*, 111–135.

Oakes, P.J., Turner, J.C., & Haslam, S.A. (1991). Perceiving people as group members: the role of fit in the salience of social categorizations. *British Journal of Social Psychology, 30*, 125–144.

Oakes, P.J., Haslam, S.A., & Turner, J.C. (1994). *Stereotyping and social reality*. Oxford, UK and Cambridge, MA: Blackwell.

Oakes, P.J., Haslam, S.A., Morrison, B.E., & Grace, D.M. (1995). Becoming an ingroup: reexamining the impact of familiarity on perceptions of group homogeneity. *Social Psychology Quarterly, 58*, 52–60.

Olson, J.M., Roese, N.J., & Zanna, M.P. (1996). Expectancies. In E.T. Higgins & A.W. Kruglanski (Eds.), *Social psychology: handbook of basic principles* (pp. 211–328). New York: Guilford.

Osherson, D.N. & Smith, E.E. (1981). On the adequacy of prototype theory as a theory of concepts. *Cognition, 9*, 35–58.

Osherson, D.N., Smith, E.E., Wilkie, O., Lopez, A., & Shafir, E. (1990). Category-based induction. *Psychological Review, 97*, 185–200.

Ostrom, T.M. (1984). The sovereignty of social cognition. In R.S. Wyer, Jr., & T.K. Srull (Eds.), *Handbook of social cognition* (Vol. 1, pp. 1–38). Hillsdale, NJ: Erlbaum.

Ostrom, T.M. & Sedikides, C. (1992). Out-group homogeneity effects in natural and minimal groups. *Psychological Bulletin, 112*, 536–552.

Park, B. & Hastie, R. (1987). Perception of variability in category development: instance-based versus abstraction-based stereotypes. *Journal of Personality and Social Psychology, 53*, 621–635.

Park, B. & Judd, C.M. (1990). Measures and models of perceived group variability. *Journal of Personality and Social Psychology, 59*, 173–191.

Park, B. & Rothbart, M. (1982). Perception of out–group homogeneity and levels of social categorization: memory for the subordinate attributes of in-group and out-group members. *Journal of Personality and Social Psychology, 42*, 1051–1068.

Park, B., Judd, C.M. & Ryan, C.S. (1991). Social categorization and the representation of variability information. *European Review of Social Psychology, 2*, 211–245.

Pendry, L.F. & Macrae, C.N. (1996). What the disinterested perceiver overlooks: goal-directed social categorization. *Personality and Social Psychology Bulletin, 22*, 249–256.

Pettit, P. (1993). *The common mind: an essay on psychology, society, and politics*. New York & Melbourne: Oxford University Press.

Quattrone, G.A. & Jones, E.E. (1980). The perception of variability within ingroups and outgroups: implications for the law of small numbers. *Journal of Personality and Social Psychology, 38*, 141–152.

Rabbie, J.M., Schot, J.C., & Visser, L. (1989). Social identity theory: a conceptual and empirical critique from the perspective of the Behavioural Interaction Model. *European Journal of Social Psychology*, *19*, 171–202.

Read, S.J. & Marcus-Newhall, A. (1993). Explanatory coherence in social explanations: a parallel distributed processing account. *Journal of Personality and Social Psychology*, *65*, 429–447.

Read, S.J. & Miller, L.C. (1993). Rapist or 'regular guy': explanatory coherence in the construction of mental models of others. *Personality and Social Psychology Bulletin*, *19*, 526–541.

Read, S.J., Vanman, E.J., & Miller, L.C. (1997). Connectionism, parallel constraint satisfaction processes, and gestalt principles: (re)introducing cognitive dynamics to social psychology. *Personality and Social Psychology Review*, *1*, 26–53.

Reed, S.K. (1972). Pattern recognition and categorization. *Cognitive Psychology*, *3*, 382–407.

Reicher, S.D., Spears, R., & Postmes, T. (1995). A social identity model of deindividuation phenomena. *European Review of Social Psychology*, *6*, 161–198.

Resnick, L.B., Levine, J.M., & Teasley, S.D. (Eds.) (1991). *Perspectives on socially situated cognition*. Washington, DC: American Psychological Association.

Rey, G. (1983). Concepts and stereotypes. *Cognition*, *15*, 237–262.

Reynolds, K.J. (1996). *Beyond the information given: capacity, context and the categorization process in impression formation*. Unpublished PhD thesis, Australian National University.

Rips, L.J. (1975). Inductive judgements about natural categories. *Journal of Verbal Learning and Verbal Behaviour*, *14*, 665–681.

Rosch, E.H. (1978). Principles of categorization. In E.H. Rosch & B. Lloyd, (Eds.), *Cognition and categorization* (pp. 28–49). Hillsdale, NJ: Erlbaum.

Rosch, E.H., & Mervis, C.B. (1975). Family resemblances: studies in the internal structure of categories. *Cognitive Psychology*, *7*, 573–605.

Rosch, E.H., Mervis, C.B., Gray, W.D., Johnson, D.M., & Boyes-Braem, P. (1976a). Basic objects in natural categories. *Cognitive Psychology*, *8*, 382–439.

Rosch, E.H., Simpson, L., & Miller, R.S. (1976b). Structural bases of typicality. *Journal of Experimental Psychology: Human Perception and Performance*, *2*, 491–507.

Ross, L., Amabile, T.M., & Steinmetz, J.L. (1977). Social roles, social control, and biases in social perception processes. *Journal of Personality and Social Psychology*, *35*, 485–494.

Rothbart, M. (1981). Memory processes and social beliefs. In D.L. Hamilton (Ed.), *Cognitive processes in stereotyping and intergroup behavior* (pp. 145–182). Hillsdale, NJ: Erlbaum.

Rothbart, M. & John, O.P. (1985). Social categorization and behavioural episodes: a cognitive analysis of the effects of intergroup contact. *Journal of Social Issues*, *41*, 81–104.

Rothbart, M. & Lewis, S. (1988). Inferring category attributes from exemplar attributes: geometric shapes and social categories. *Journal of Personality and Social Psychology*, *55*, 861–872.

Rothbart, M. & Taylor, M. (1992). Category labels and social reality: do we view social categories as natural kinds? In G. Semin & K. Fiedler (Eds.), *Language and social cognition* (pp. 11–36). London: Sage.

Rottenstreich, Y. & Tversky, A. (1997). Unpacking, repacking, and anchoring: advances in support theory. *Psychological Review*, *104*, 406–415.

Rumelhart, D.E. & McClelland, J.L. (1986). *Parallel distributed processing: explorations in the microstructure of cognition* (Vol. 1). Cambridge, MA: MIT Press.

Ruscher, J.B. & Fiske, S.T. (1990). Interpersonal competition can cause individuating processes. *Journal of Personality and Social Psychology*, *58*, 832–843.

Ryan, C. S. & Judd, C. M. (1992). False consensus and out-group homogeneity: a methodological note on their relationship. *British Journal of Social Psychology*, *31*, 269–283.

Sankey, H. (1993). Five varieties of cognitive relativism. *Cognito*, *17*, 106–111.

Schaller, M. (1992). Sample size, aggregation, and statistical reasoning in social inference. *Journal of Experimental Social Psychology*, *28*, 65–85.

Schaller, M. (1994). The role of statistical reasoning in the formation, preservation and prevention of group stereotypes. *British Journal of Social Psychology*, *33*, 47–61.

Schaller, M. & Maass, A. (1989). Illusory correlation and social categorization: toward an integration of motivational and cognitive factors in stereotype formation. *Journal of Personality and Social Psychology*, *56*, 709–721.

Schaller, M., Boyd, C., Johannes, J., & O'Brien, M. (1995). The prejudiced personality revisited: personal need for structure and formation of erroneous group stereotypes. *Journal of Personality and Social Psychology*, *68*, 544–555.

Schaller, M., Rosell, M.C., & Asp, C.H. (1998). Parsimony and pluralism in the psychological study of intergroup processes. In C. Sedikides, J. Schopler & C.A. Insko (Eds.), *Intergroup cognition and intergroup behavior* (pp. 3–25). Mahwah, NJ: Erlbaum.

Scheff, T.J. (1993). Toward a social psychological theory of mind and consciousness. *Social Research*, *60*, 171–204.

Schul, Y. & Burnstein, E. (1990). Judging the typicality of an instance: should the category be accessed first? *Journal of Personality and Social Psychology*, *58*, 964–974.

Schwarz, N. & Bless, H. (1992). Constructing reality and its alternatives: an inclusion/exclusion model of assimilation and contrast effects in social judgment. In L.L. Martin & A. Tesser (Eds.), *The construction of social judgments* (pp. 217–245). Hillsdale, NJ: Erlbaum.

Schwarz, N., Strack, F., Hilton, D.L., & Naderer, G. (1991). Base rates, representativeness, and the logic of conversation: the contextual relevance of 'irrelevant' information. *Social Cognition*, *9*, 67–84.

Schyns, P.G. & Rodet, L. (1997). Categorization creates functional features. *Journal of Experimental Psychology: Learning, Memory and Cognition*, *23*, 681–696.

Sedikides, C., Olsen, N., & Reis, H.T. (1992). Relationships as natural categories. *Journal of Personality and Social Psychology*, *64*, 71–82.

Semin, G. (1997). The relevance of language for social psychology. In C. McGarty & S. A. Haslam (Eds.), *The message of social psychology: perspectives on mind in society* (pp. 252–267). Oxford, UK & Cambridge, MA: Blackwell.

Semin, G. & Fiedler, K. (1988). The cognitive functions of linguistic categories in describing persons: social cognition and language. *Journal of Personality and Social Psychology*, *54*, 558–567.

Semin, G. & Fiedler, K. (Eds.) (1992). *Language and social cognition*. London: Sage.

Shanks, D.R. & Gluck, M.A. (1994). Tests of an adaptive network model for the identification and categorization of continuous dimension stimuli. *Connection Science*, *6*, 59–89.

Sherif, C.W., Sherif, M., & Nebergall, R.E. (1965). *Attitude and attitude change: the social judgment–involvement approach*. Philadelphia: Saunders.

Sherif, M. (1936). *The psychology of social norms*. New York: Harper and Row.

Sherif, M. (1967). *Group conflict and cooperation: their social psychology*. London: Routledge and Kegan Paul.

Sherif, M. & Hovland, C.I. (1961). *Social judgment: Assimilation and contrast effects in communication and attitude change*. New Haven, CT: Yale University Press.

Simon, B. (1992). The perception of ingroup and outgroup homogeneity: reintroducing the social context. *European Review of Social Psychology*, *3*, 1–30.

Simon, B. (1993). On the asymmetry in the cognitive construal of ingroup and outgroup: a model of egocentric social categorization. *European Journal of Social*

Psychology, *23*, 131–147.

Simon, B. (1997). Self and group in modern society: ten theses on the individual self and the collective self. In R. Spears, P. J. Oakes, N. Ellemers, & S. A. Haslam (Eds.), *The social psychology of stereotyping and group life* (pp. 318–335). Oxford: Blackwell.

Simon, B. & Brown, R.J. (1987). Perceived homogeneity in minority-majority contexts. *Journal of Personality and Social Psychology*, *53*, 703–711.

Simon, B. & Hamilton, D.L. (1994). Self–stereotyping and social context: the effects of relative in-group size and in-group status. *Journal of Personality and Social Psychology*, *66*, 699–711.

Simon, B., Pantaleo, G., & Mummendey, A. (1995). Unique individual or interchangeable group member? The accentuation of intragroup differences versus similarities as an indicator of the individual self versus the collective self. *Journal of Personality and Social Psychology*, *69*, 106–119.

Simon, B., Hastedt, C., & Aufderheide, B. (1997). When self-categorization makes sense: the role of meaningful categorization in minority and majority members' self-perception. *Journal of Personality and Social Psychology*, *73*, 310–320.

Simon, H.A. (1974). How big is a chunk? *Science*, *183*, 482-488.

Sloman, S.A. (1998). Categorical inference is not a tree: the myth of inheritance hierarchies. *Cognitive Psychology*, *35*, 1–33.

Sloman, S.A. & Rips, L.J. (1998). Similarity as an explanatory construct. *Cognition*, *65*, 87–101.

Smith, D.J., Murray, M.J., Jr., Minda, J.P. (1997). Straight talk about linear separability. *Journal of Experimental Psychology: Learning, Memory, and Cognition*, *23*, 659–680.

Smith, E.E. & Medin, D.L. (1981). *Concepts and categories*. Cambridge, MA: Harvard University Press.

Smith, E.E., Shoben, E.J., & Rips, L.J. (1974). Structure and process in semantic memory: a featural model for semantic decisions. *Psychological Review*, *81*, 214–241.

Smith, E.E., Medin, D.L. & Rips, L.J. (1983). A psychological approach to concepts: comments on Rey's 'Concepts and stereotypes'. *Cognition*, *17*, 265–274.

Smith, E.E., Patalano, A.L., & Jonides, J. (1998). Alternative strategies of categorization. *Cognition*, *65*, 167–196.

Smith, E.R. (1991). Illusory correlation in a simulated exemplar-based memory. *Journal of Experimental Social Psychology*, *27*, 107–123.

Smith, E.R. (1996). What do connectionism and social psychology offer each other? *Journal of Personality and Social Psychology*, *70*, 893–912.

Smith, E.R. & de Coster, J. (1998). Knowledge acquisition, accessibility, and use in person perception and stereotyping: simulation with a recurrent connectionist network. *Journal of Personality and Social Psychology*, *74*, 21–35.

Smith, E.R. & Henry, S. (1996). An in-group becomes part of the self: response time evidence. *Personality and Social Psychology Bulletin*, *22*, 635–642.

Smith, E.R. & Mackie, D.M. (1995). *Social psychology*. New York: Worth.

Smith, E.R. & Mackie, D.M. (1997). Integrating the psychological and the social to understand human behavior. In C. McGarty & S.A. Haslam (Eds.), *The message of social psychology: perspectives on mind in society* (pp. 305–314). Oxford, UK & Cambridge, MA: Blackwell.

Smith, E.R. & Zárate, M.A. (1992). Exemplar-based model of social judgment. *Psychological Review*, *99*, 3–21.

Smith, E.R., Fazio, R.H., & Cejka, M.A. (1996). Accessible attitudes influence categorization of multiple, categorizable objects. *Journal of Personality and Social Psychology*, *71*, 888–898.

Smithson, M.J. (1996). Science, ignorance and human values. *Journal of Human Values*, *2*, 67–81.

Snyder, C.R. & Fromkin, H.L. (1980). *Uniqueness: the human pursuit of difference*.

New York: Plenum.

Spears, R. & Haslam, S.A. (1997). Stereotyping and the burden of cognitive load. In R. Spears, P. J. Oakes, N. Ellemers, & S. A. Haslam (Eds.), *The social psychology of stereotyping and group life* (pp. 171–207). Oxford: Blackwell.

Spears, R. & Manstead, A.S.R. (1990). Consensus estimation in social context. *European Review of Social Psychology, 1*, 81–109.

Spears, R. & van Knippenberg, D. (1997). *Cognitive load and illusory correlation*. Unpublished manuscript, University of Amsterdam/University of Leiden.

Spears, R., van der Pligt, J., & Eiser, J.R. (1985). Illusory correlation in the perception of group attitudes. *Journal of Personality and Social Psychology, 48*, 863–875.

Stangor, C. R. & Duan, C. (1991). Effects of multiple task demands upon memory for information about social groups. *Journal of Experimental Social Psychology, 7*, 357–378.

Stangor, C.R. & Ford, T.E. (1992). Accuracy and expectancy-confirming processing orientations and the development of stereotypes and prejudice. *European Review of Social Psychology, 3*, 57–89.

Stangor, C.R. & Lange, J. (1994). Mental representation of social groups: advances in understanding stereotypes and stereotyping. *Advances in Experimental Social Psychology, 26*, 357–416.

Stangor, C.R. & McMillan, D. (1992). Memory for expectancy-congruent and expectancy-incongruent information: a review of the social and social developmental literatures. *Psychological Bulletin, 111*, 42–61.

Stangor, C.R., Lynch, L., Duan, C., & Glass, B. (1992). Categorization of individuals on the basis of multiple social features. *Journal of Personality and Social Psychology, 62*, 207–218.

Stapel, D.A., Koomen, W., & van der Pligt, J. (1996). The referents of trait inferences: the impact of trait concepts versus actor-trait links on subsequent judgments. *Journal of Personality and Social Psychology, 70*, 437–450.

Stapel, D.A., Koomen, W., & van der Pligt, J. (1997). Categories of category accessibility: the impact of trait concept versus exemplar priming on person judgments. *Journal of Experimental Social Psychology, 33*, 47–76.

Stryker, S. (1997). 'In the beginning there is society': lessons from a sociological social psychology. In C. McGarty & S.A. Haslam (Eds.), *The message of social psychology: perspectives on mind in society* (pp. 315–327). Oxford, UK & Cambridge, MA: Blackwell.

Stryker, S. & Statham, A. (1985). Symbolic interaction and role theory. In G. Lindzey & E. Aronson (Eds.), *Handbook of social psychology* (3rd. ed., Vol. 1, pp. 311–378). New York: Random House.

Tajfel, H. (1969). Cognitive aspects of prejudice. *Journal of Social Issues, 25*, 79–97.

Tajfel, H. (1977). Social psychology and social reality. *New Society, 39*, 65–66.

Tajfel, H. (1981). Social stereotypes and social groups. In J.C. Turner & H. Giles (Eds.), *Intergroup behaviour* (pp. 144–167). Oxford: Blackwell.

Tajfel, H. & Turner, J.C. (1979). An integrative theory of intergroup conflict. In W.G. Austin & S. Worchel (Eds.), *The social psychology of intergroup relations* (pp. 33–47). Monterey: Brooks/Cole.

Tajfel, H. & Turner, J.C. (1986). The social identity theory of intergroup behaviour. In S. Worchel & W.G. Austin (Eds.), *Psychology of intergroup relations* (pp. 7–24). Chicago: Nelson-Hall.

Tajfel, H. & Wilkes, A.L. (1963). Classification and quantitative judgement. *British Journal of Psychology, 54*, 101–114.

Tajfel, H., Flament, C., Billig, M.G., & Bundy, R.F. (1971). Social categorization and intergroup behavior. *European Journal of Social Psychology, 1*, 149–177.

Taylor, S.E. (1981). A categorization approach to stereotyping. In D.L. Hamilton (Ed.), *Cognitive processes in stereotyping and intergroup behaviour* (pp. 83–114). Hillsdale, NJ: Erlbaum.

Taylor, S.E., Fiske, S. T., Etcoff, N.L., & Ruderman, R.L. (1978). Categorical and contextual bases of person memory and stereotyping. *Journal of Personality and Social Psychology, 36,* 778–793.

Terry, D.J. & Hogg, M.A. (1996). Group norms and the attitude-behavior relationship: a role for group identification. *Personality and Social Psychology Bulletin, 22,* 776–793.

Thagard, P. (1989). Explanatory coherence. *Behavioral and Brain Sciences, 12,* 435–467.

Thagard, P. (1992). *Conceptual revolutions.* Princeton: Princeton University Press.

Thurstone, L.L. (1931). The measurement of attitudes. *Journal of Abnormal and Social Psychology, 26,* 249–269.

Trope, Y. (1986). Identification and inferential processes in dispositional attribution. *Psychological Review, 93,* 239–257.

Turner, J.C. (1985). Social categorization and the self-concept: a social cognitive theory of group behaviour. In E.J. Lawler (Ed.), *Advances in Group Processes: Theory and Research* (Vol. 2, pp. 77–122). Greenwich, CT: JAI.

Turner, J.C. (1987). The analysis of social influence. In J.C. Turner, M.A. Hogg, P.J. Oakes, S. D. Reicher, & M. S. Wetherell, *Rediscovering the social group: a self-categorization theory* (pp. 68–88). Oxford: Blackwell.

Turner, J.C. (1991). *Social influence.* Milton Keynes: Open University Press.

Turner, J.C. & Bourhis, R.Y. (1996). Social identity, interdependence and the social group: a reply to Rabbie et al. In W. P. Robinson (Ed.), *Social groups and identity: developing the legacy of Henri Tajfel.* Oxford: Butterworth Heinemann.

Turner, J.C. & Oakes, P.J. (1989). Self-categorization theory and social influence. In P.B. Paulus (Ed.), *Psychology of group influence* (2nd ed., pp. 233–275). Hillsdale, NJ: Erlbaum.

Turner, J.C. & Oakes, P.J. (1997). The socially structured mind. In C. McGarty & S.A. Haslam (Eds.), *The message of social psychology: perspectives on mind in society* (pp. 355–373). Oxford, UK & Cambridge, MA: Blackwell.

Turner, J.C. & Onorato, R.S. (in press). Social identity, personality and the self-concept: a self-categorization perspective. In T.R. Tyler, R. Kramer & O.P. John (Eds.), *The psychology of the social self.* Hillsdale, NJ: Erlbaum.

Turner, J.C., Hogg, M.A., Oakes, P. J., Reicher, S. D., & Wetherell, M. S. (1987). *Rediscovering the social group: a self-categorization theory.* Oxford: Blackwell.

Turner, J.C., Wetherell, M.S., & Hogg, M.A. (1989). Referent informational influence and group polarization. *British Journal of Social Psychology, 28,* 135–147.

Turner, J.C., Oakes, P.J., Haslam, S.A., & McGarty, C. (1994). Self and collective: cognition and social context. *Personality and Social Psychology Bulletin, 20,* 454–463.

Tversky, A. (1977). Features of similarity. *Psychological Review, 84,* 327–352.

Tversky, A. & Gati, I. (1978). Studies of similarity. In E. Rosch and B. Lloyd (Eds.), *Cognition and categorization* (pp. 79–98). Hillsdale, NJ: Erlbaum.

Tversky, A. & Kahneman, D. (1973). Availability: a heuristic for judging frequency and probability. *Cognitive Psychology, 4,* 207–232.

Tversky, A. & Kahneman, D. (1974). Judgement under uncertainty: heuristics and biases. *Science, 185,* 1124–1131.

Tversky, A. & Koehler, D.J. (1994). Support theory: a nonextensional representation of subjective probability. *Psychological Review, 101,* 547–567.

Uleman, J.S., Newman, L.S., & Moskowitz, G.B. (1996). People as flexible interpreters: evidence and issues from spontaneous trait inferences. *Advances in Experimental Social Psychology, 28,* 211–279.

Ullman, S. (1989). Aligning pictorial descriptions: an approach to object recognition. *Cognition, 32,* 193–254.

Upmeyer, A. (1981). Perceptual and judgemental processes in social contexts. *Advances in Experimental Social Psychology, 14,* 257–308.

Upshaw, H.S. (1965). The effect of variable perspective on judgements of opinion statements for Thurstone scales: equal appearing intervals. *Journal of Personality and Social Psychology, 2*, 60–69.

Upshaw, H.S. (1984). Output processes in judgement. In R.S. Wyer, Jr. & T.K. Srull (Eds.), *Handbook of social cognition* (Vol. 3, pp. 237–256). Hillsdale, NJ: Erlbaum.

Upshaw, H.S., & Ostrom, T.M. (1984). Psychological perspective in attitude research. In J.R. Eiser (Ed.), *Attitudinal judgment* (pp. 23–41). New York: Springer.

Urban, L.M. & Miller, N. (1998). A theoretical analysis of crossed categorization effects: a meta-analysis. *Journal of Personality and Social Psychology, 74*, 894–908.

Vanbeselaere, N. (1996). Reducing intergroup discrimination by manipulating ingroup/outgroup homogeneity and by individuating ingroup and outgroup members. *Communication and Cognition, 21*, 191–198.

van Knippenberg, A. & Wilke, H. (1988). Social categorization and attitude change. *European Journal of Social Psychology, 18*, 395–406.

van Knippenberg, A., van Twuyer, M., & Pepels, J. (1994). Factors affecting social categorization processes in memory. *British Journal of Social Psychology, 33,* 419–431.

van Knippenberg, D. & Wilke, H. (1992). Prototypicality of arguments and conformity to ingroup norms. *European Journal of Social Psychology, 22*, 141–155.

van Overwalle, F. (1998). Causal explanation as constraint satisfaction: a critique and a feedforward connectionist alternative. *Journal of Personality and Social Psychology, 74*, 312–328.

van Overwalle, F. & van Rooy, D. (1996). A connectionist approach to causal attribution. In S. J. Read & L. C. Miller (Eds.), *Connectionist and PDP models of social reasoning and social behavior*. Hillsdale, NJ: Erlbaum.

van Twuyer, M. & van Knippenberg, A.F.M. (1995). Social categorization as a function of priming. *European Journal of Social Psychology, 25*, 695–701.

Verplanken, B., Jetten, J., & van Knippenberg, A.F.M. (1996). Effects of stereotypicality and perceived group variability on the use of attitudinal information in impression formation. *Personality and Social Psychology Bulletin, 22*, 960–971.

Wattenmaker, W.D. (1995). Knowledge structures and linear separability: integrating information in object and social categorization. *Cognitive Psychology, 28*, 274–328.

Wattenmaker, W.D., Dewey, G.I., Murphy, T.D., & Medin, D.L. (1986). Linear separability and concept learning: context, relational properties, and concept naturalness. *Cognitive Psychology, 18*, 158–194.

Wegner, D.M. & Erber, R. (1992). The hyperaccessibility of suppressed thoughts. *Journal of Personality and Social Psychology, 63*, 903–912.

Weisz, C. & Jones, E.E. (1993). Expectancy disconfirmation and dispositional inference: latent strength of target-based and category-based expectancies. *Personality and Social Psychology Bulletin, 19*, 563–573.

Whitney, P., Davis, P. A., & Waring, D.A. (1994). Task effects on trait inference: distinguishing categorization from characterization. *Social Cognition, 12*, 19–35.

Whorf, B.L. (1956). *Language, thought and reality: selected writings*. New York: Technology Press/Wiley.

Wierzbicka, A. (1988). *The semantics of grammar*. Amsterdam, PA: Benjamins.

Wilder, D.A. (1978). Perceiving persons as a group: effects on attributions of causality and beliefs. *Social Psychology, 41*, 13–23.

Wilder, D.A. (1981). Perceiving persons as a group: categorization and intergroup relations. In D. Hamilton (Ed.), *Cognitive processes in stereotyping and intergroup behaviour* (pp. 213–257). Hillsdale, NJ: Erlbaum.

Wilder, D.A. (1984). Predictions of belief homogeneity and similarity following social categorization. *British Journal of Social Psychology, 23*, 323–333.

Wilder, D.A. (1986). Social categorization: implications for creation and reduction of intergroup bias. *Advances in Experimental Social Psychology, 19*, 291–355.

Wilder, D.A. (1990). Some determinants of the persuasive power of ingroups and outgroups: organization of information and attribution of independence. *Journal of Personality and Social Psychology, 59*, 1202–1213.

Wilder, D.A. & Thompson, J.E. (1988). Assimilation and contrast effects in the judgements of groups. *Journal of Personality and Social Psychology, 54*, 62–73.

Wisniewski, E.J. & Medin, D.L. (1994). On the interaction of theory and data in concept learning. *Cognitive Science, 18*, 221–281.

Wisniewski, E. J., Imai, M., & Casey, L. (1996). On the equivalence of superordinate categories. *Cognition, 60*, 269–298.

Wittenbrink, B., Gist, P. L., & Hilton, J.L. (1997). Structural properties of stereotypic knowledge and their influences on the construal of social situations. *Journal of Personality and Social Psychology, 72*, 526–543.

Wittenbrink, B., Park, B., & Judd, C.M. (1998). The role of stereotypic knowledge in the construal of person models. In C. Sedikides, J. Schopler, & C.A. Insko (Eds.), *Intergroup cognition and intergroup behavior* (pp. 177–202). Mahwah, NJ: Erlbaum.

Wittgenstein, L. (1974) *Philosophical investigations*. Oxford: Blackwell.

Wyer, R.S. & Srull, T.K. (1986). Human cognition in its social context. *Psychological Review, 93*, 322–359.

Wyer, R.S. & Srull, T.K. (1989). *Memory and cognition in its social context*. Hillsdale, NJ: Erlbaum.

Yaniv, I. & Foster, D.P. (1995). Graininess of judgment under uncertainty: an accuracy-informativeness trade-off. *Journal of Experimental Psychology: General, 124*, 424–432.

Yzerbyt, V.Y., Schadron, G.H., Leyens, J.-P., & Rocher, S. (1994). Social judgeability: the influence of meta-informational cues on the use of stereotypes. *Journal of Personality and Social Psychology, 66*, 48–55.

Yzerbyt, V.Y., Rocher, S., & Schadron, G. (1997). Stereotypes as explanations: a subjective essentialistic view of group perception. In R. Spears, P.J. Oakes, N. Ellemers, & S.A.Haslam. (Eds.), *The social psychology of stereotyping and group life* (pp. 20–50). Blackwell: Oxford.

Yzerbyt, V.Y., Rocher, S., McGarty, C., & Haslam, S.A. (1998a). *Illusory correlation as meaningful differentiation revisited*. Unpublished manuscript, Catholic University of Louvain-la-Neuve.

Yzerbyt, V.Y., Rogier, A., & Fiske, S.T. (1998b). Group entitativity and social attribution: on translating situational constraints into stereotypes. *Personality and Social Psychology Bulletin, 24*, 1090–1104.

Zadeh, L.A. (1965). Fuzzy sets. *Information and Control, 8*, 338–353.

Author Index

Subject Index

Note: Page numbers in **bold** refer to glossary definitions.